Mothers and Children

JEWS, CHRISTIANS, AND MUSLIMS FROM
THE ANCIENT TO THE MODERN WORLD

SERIES EDITORS
R. STEPHEN HUMPHREYS, WILLIAM CHESTER JORDAN, AND PETER SCHÄFER

Imperialism and Jewish Society, 200 B.C.E. to 640 C.E.
by Seth Schwartz

A Shared World: Christians and Muslims in the Early Modern Mediterranean
by Molly Greene

Beautiful Death: Jewish Poetry and Martyrdom in Medieval France
by Susan L. Einbinder

Power in the Portrayal: Representations of Jews and Muslims in Eleventh- and Twelfth-Century Islamic Spain
by Ross Brann

Mirror of His Beauty: Feminine Images of God from the Bible to the Early Kabbalah
by Peter Schäfer

In the Shadow of the Virgin: Inquisitors, Friars, and Conversos *in Guadalupe, Spain*
by Gretchen D. Starr-LeBeau

The Curse of Ham: Race and Slavery in Early Judaism, Christianity, and Islam
by David M. Goldenberg

Resisting History: Historicism and Its Discontents in German-Jewish Thought
by David N. Myers

Mothers and Children: Jewish Family Life in Medieval Europe
by Elisheva Baumgarten

Mothers and Children

JEWISH FAMILY LIFE IN
MEDIEVAL EUROPE

Elisheva Baumgarten

PRINCETON UNIVERSITY PRESS
PRINCETON AND OXFORD

Copyright © 2004 by Princeton University Press
Published by Princeton University Press,
41 William Street, Princeton, New Jersey 08540
In the United Kingdom: Princeton University Press,
3 Market Place, Woodstock, Oxfordshire, OX20 1SY

ALL RIGHTS RESERVED

British Library Cataloging-in-Publication Data is available

Library of Congress Cataloging-in-Publication Data

Baumgarten, Elisheva.
    Mothers and children: Jewish family life in medieval Europe / Elisheva Baumgarten.
      p. cm.—(Jews, Christians, and Muslims from the ancient to the modern world)
    Rev. ed. of author's thesis (Ph.D.—ha-Universitah ha-'Ivrit bi-Yerushalayim, 2000)
    originally titled: Imahot vi-yeladim ba-hevrah ha-Yehudit bi-Yeme ha-Benayim.
    Includes bibliographical references and index.
    ISBN 0-691-09166-8 (cl: alk. paper)
    1. Childbirth—Religious aspects—Judaism. 2. Motherhood—Religious aspects—Judaism. 3. Judaism—Customs and practices. 4. Parent and child—Religious aspects—Judaism. I. Title. II. Series.
BM726.B3813 2004
306.874′3′08992404—dc22   2003066386

This book has been composed in Electra
Printed on acid-free paper ∞
www.pup.princeton.edu
Printed in the United States of America
1 3 5 7 9 10 8 6 4 2

For Yaacov, Yonatan, and Ayelet, with love

CONTENTS

Illustrations	*ix*
Acknowledgments	*xi*
Abbreviations	*xv*
INTRODUCTION	1
CHAPTER ONE. Birth	21
CHAPTER TWO. Circumcision and Baptism	55
CHAPTER THREE. Additional Birth Rituals	92
CHAPTER FOUR. Maternal Nursing and Wet Nurses: Feeding and Caring for Infants	119
CHAPTER FIVE. Parents and Children: Competing Values	154
CONCLUSIONS	184
Notes	*191*
Glossary	*241*
Bibliography	*243*
Index	*269*

ILLUSTRATIONS

FIGURE 1. Circumcision and Baptism, Joshua in Gilgal	60
FIGURE 2. Zipporah As Circumciser	66
FIGURE 3. Isaac's Circumcision (*Regensburg Pentateuch*)	73
FIGURE 4. Isaac's Circumcision (*Verduner Alter* of Nicholas of Verdun)	74
FIGURES 5a and 5b. Hollekreisch	94, 95
FIGURE 6. *"Von der Geburt"*	103
FIGURE 7. *"Ceremonien in Kinds-Nöthen und Kindbett"*	104
FIGURE 8. *"Felicitas cum septem filiis"*	179
FIGURE 9. The Mother and Her Seven Sons	181

ACKNOWLEDGMENTS

My debts, institutional and personal, material and spiritual, are great. Financial support for the project came from a variety of institutions. The Nathan Rotenstreich Fellowship at the Hebrew University, the Memorial Foundation for Jewish Culture, and the American Association of University Women provided support for the first stages of this project and made possible the dissertation from which this book has grown. A postdoctoral grant from the Yad Hanadiv Rothschild Foundation as well as funding from the Braun Chair at Bar Ilan University allowed the revision and completion of this manuscript.

My work would have been impossible without the help of librarians at the National Library, Hebrew University, Jerusalem, in the General Reading Room, the Hebrew Manuscript Institute, and especially in the Judaica Reading Room. I also thank the library at the Center for Advanced Judaic Studies at the University of Pennsylvania, and especially Judith Leifer and Etty Lassman, for all of their help.

My interest in the Jewish family and in medieval Ashkenaz began as a student in the Department of Jewish History at the Hebrew University. I wish to thank my teachers in the department and especially in the medieval section, for their encouragement and support over the years. Professor Robert Bonfil, my dissertation advisor, has been a model of superb scholarship and judicious criticism. His generous support and critique have accompanied all of my work, and words cannot express my debt to him. Other teachers and colleagues in Israel, first and foremost Avraham Grossman and Shulamith Shahar, accompanied this project from its inception, and I wish to express my deep thanks to them for their advice. Special thanks go to Robert Brody who read an early draft of the manuscript and saved me from many mistakes. I also benefited from the critique and suggestions of Gadi Algazi, Yoram Bilu, Harvey Goldberg, Menahem Ben-Sasson, Ora Limor, and Israel Ta-Shma and I thank them for their comments and advice. In addition, I wish to express gratitude to my colleagues at Bar Ilan in the Department of Jewish History and in the Gender Studies Program for their support and encouragement, and for making my transition into full-time teaching so comfortable.

It is a pleasure to acknowledge my tremendous debt to two additional scholars. My thanks to Emanuel Sivan with whom I took my first steps in social history and gender studies and who has accompanied my work throughout the years. It was in his class, as a first-year student, that I first became acquainted with the work of Natalie Davis. I met with Natalie Davis in Jerusalem in the spring of 1998. Her helpful suggestions and assistance at that time and since then are a continual source of encouragement and inspiration. I thank her for her generosity and constant support.

Outside Israel, I have been blessed with supporting teachers and colleagues, and I owe a great deal to them as well. My greatest thanks goes to David Ruderman, who invited me to the University of Pennsylvania and generously provided ideal conditions for research and teaching both at the Center for Advanced Judaic Studies and on campus. His enthusiastic interest in and support of this project helped make its completion possible. The Alice Paul Center for Women and Gender Studies at the University of Pennsylvania provided me with a room of my own during the second year of my stay in Philadelphia, and I thank Dana Barron, Demi Kurz, and Luz Marin for their generous hospitality and friendship during this period. The two years I spent in the United States allowed meetings with colleagues at a variety of institutions. Presentations of part of this book at Dartmouth, Yale, Columbia, Stanford, and the University of Pennsylvania during 2000/2001 allowed me to reexamine my ideas and revise my thinking. Discussions with Caroline Bynum, E. Ann Matter, and Haym Soloveitchik during the time spent in the United States and afterward contributed to this book. A special thanks goes to Ivan Marcus whose advice and criticism have been a tremendous help and from whom I have learned much.

My fellow graduate students in Jerusalem and elsewhere have been critical readers as well as faithful partners for ongoing discussion in and out of the Judaica Reading Room. I thank Adam Shear, Aviad Hacohen, Daniella Talmon-Heller, Dena Ordan, Ephraim Shoham-Steiner, Jennifer Harris, Kimmy Caplan and Richelle Budd Caplan, Nils Roemer, Oren Falk, Rami Reiner, Roni Weinstein, Sharon Koren, Yehuda Galinsky, Yochi Fisher-Yinon, and especially Ze'ev Elkin and Rachel Greenblatt for their help. My students at the Hebrew University, the University of Pennsylvania, and Bar Ilan University have criticized my ideas and argued with me, helping me understand what it was I wanted to say, and I have learned much from them. Nevertheless, all mistakes remain mine alone.

A special thanks to Brigitta van Rheinberg at Princeton University Press for her enthusiasm and support of this project, and to the editors of this series. I also wish to thank Deborah Tegarden and Alison Kalett, the production editors, for their infinite patience and for their continuous help through out the period of our work together. The readers for the Press offered helpful and thought-provoking comments on the manuscript and I thank them for their criticism and suggestions. I also wish to acknowledge Jackie Feldman, a scholar in his own right, who improved the manuscript and helped smooth the transition of my work from Hebrew into English. Chapter 2 of this book appears in a condensed form in the collection: Elizabeth Mark, (ed.). *The Covenant of Circumcision: New Perspectives on an Ancient Jewish Ritual,* 2003. Brandeis University Press; reprinted by permission, University Press of New England.

My parents, Al and Rita Baumgarten, helped in more ways than can be recalled—reading drafts of the manuscript, encouraging me, and providing ongoing support. I hope they will recognize some of what I have learned from them in what follows. My sisters, Shoshana, Margalit, and Naama, all took interest in this project and helped as well. Yaacov Deutsch has read this manuscript more times than he cares to remember, making suggestions, referring me to articles and sources, and discussing many of the issues explored here. He has been my most severe critic and greatest support, and this book would never have been completed without him. Words cannot express my gratitude for his love and companionship over the years. It is to him and to our children, Yonatan and Ayelet, that I dedicate this book.

ABBREVIATIONS

AJS Review	*Association of Jewish Studies Review*
CCCM	*Corpus Christianorum: Continuatio medievalis*
EJ	*Encyclopedia Judaica*
HdA	*Handwörterbuch des deutschen Aberglaubens*, ed. Hans Bächtold-Stäubli. Re-edited by Eduard Hoffmann-Krayer; Forward by Christoph Daxelmüller, 10 vols. (Berlin, 1927–41, repr. Berlin and New York, 1987)
JQR	*Jewish Quarterly Review*
LdM	*Lexikon des Mittelalters*, ed. Robert Auty, 8 vols. (Munich-Zurich, 1977–1993)
Maḥzor Vitry	*Maḥzor Vitry*, ed. Simon haLevi Horowitz, (Nürnberg, 1892)
PL	*Patrologia, Series latina*, ed. J. P. Migne
REJ	*Revue des études juives*
Sefer Or Zaru'a	R. Isaac b. Moses, *Sefer Or Zaru'a*, 4 parts, 2 vols., (Zhitomir, 1862)
Sefer Tosafot haShalem	*Sefer Tosafot haShalem: Commentary on the Bible*, ed. Jacob Gellis, 10 vols. (Jerusalem 1982–95)
Semag	R. Moses b. Jacob of Couçy. *Sefer Miẓvot haGadol*, 2 vols. (Venice, 1547, repr. Jerusalem, 1961).
Semak	R. Isaac b. Joseph of Corbeil. *Sefer 'Amudei Golah haNikra Semak* (reprint Jerusalem, 1979).
SHB	R. Judah b. Samuel Ḥasid, *Sefer Ḥasidim*, ed. Reuven Margaliyot (Jerusalem, 1957)
SHP	*Sefer Ḥasidim* (Das Buch der Frommen), ed. Judah Wistinetzki. (Frankfurt, 1924, 2d edition).
WCJS	*World Congress of Jewish Studies*

Meir b Barukh of Rothenburg's writings

She'elot uTeshuvot (Crimona)	*She'elot uTeshuvot*, Crimona edition (repr. Jerusalem, 1986)
Shut Maharam (Prague)	*Sefer Shut Maharam b. Barukh*, Prague edition, ed. Moses Arye Blakh (Budapest, 1895)
She'elot uTeshuvot (Lvov)	*She'elot uTeshuvot*, ed. R. N. Rabinowitz (Lvov, 1860)

Mothers and Children

Introduction

IN HIS FIRST LETTER to Héloise, Abelard draws a sharp distinction between family life and the life of the philosopher[1]:

> What harmony can there be between pupils and nursemaids, desks and cradles, books or tablets and distaffs, pen or stylus and spindles? Who can concentrate on thoughts of scripture or philosophy and be able to endure babies crying, nurses soothing them with lullabies, and all the noisy coming and going of men and women about the house? Will he put up with the constant muddle and squalor that small children bring into the home?[2]

The focus of this study is the cradles and the nurses and the noisy coming and going of men and women about the house . . . exactly that which Abelard intended to dismiss — the connection between these aspects of medieval life and the more accessible lives of scholars. This study follows the Jewish family in medieval Germany and northern France during the High Middle Ages, from the birth of a child until that child was ready for formal education.[3] An understanding of the family unit, the most basic building block of the medieval Jewish community, is essential in order to broaden our knowledge of Jewish family life in the past and to comprehend the Jewish community. During the period of their lives examined here, children were under the supervision of their mothers and other women. The girls remained under this influence until they got married, whereas the boys left the female sphere sooner and began their formal religious education under the guidance of male tutors and teachers at the age of five, six, or seven. As mothers played a central role in their children's existence during these years, this study has placed special emphasis on their lives. It is, however, a book about both mothers and fathers, about their shared goals and their distinctive roles.

Each aspect of Jewish life studied here is compared with that of the Christian surroundings. Each issue is evaluated not only in the context of Jewish society, but in that of European society as a whole. In some cases, these two separate groups are, in fact, one, for Jews and Christians lived in close proximity and, as neighbors, maintained daily contact with each other. In other cases, the inner structure of each society commands our attention, as the practices studied were conducted on distinctly parallel planes, with no direct contact between the two societies. By examining Jewish families along with Christian ones, we may identify shared social structures and mentalities, as well as differences.

Family History and Gender Studies

Until recently, motherhood and childhood were considered subjects without history.[4] Many scholars of Jewish society, like those studying other societies, took for granted that the lives of mothers and children in the past were similar to those of their modern contemporaries,[5] but in recent decades, social historians have revealed the great variety of cultural and social patterns that have characterized different societies, demonstrating the extent to which this assumption was incorrect. Among the first, prominent studies to examine these topics was research on the lives of medieval families; and to a great extent, interest in the topics of motherhood and childhood began with the examination of medieval European culture.

Central to this investigation of family life in the past was Philippe Ariès's book *L'enfant et la vie familiale sous l'ancien régime*.[6] This book generated a polemic that precipitated a new historical discourse. As Barbara Hanawalt has recently argued in her summary, and assessment of several decades of this debate, despite the refutation of many of Ariès's arguments, his book is still central to all studies of childhood and family life.[7] A central focus of the initial debates following the publication of Ariès's book was his characterization of the emotional attachment of parents and, especially of mothers, to their children. Many of the conclusions attributed to Ariès in this context—such as the lack of parental love toward their children and especially the lack of grief over the death of children (as a consequence of high infant mortality)—became fundamental tenets of a school of research that sought to portray premodern parent-children relationships as characterized by neglect and indifference.[8] While detailed research over the past three decades has persuasively argued that medieval parents were, in fact, emotionally attached to their children and has refuted many of the other claims made by Ariès and his followers, there is no doubt that his study was a central factor motivating much of the subsequent research. Important surveys and detailed studies written by Shulamith Shahar, Barbara Hanawalt, Pierre Riché, Danielle Alexandre-Bidon, Monique Closson, Didier Lett, James Schultz, and most recently Nicholas Orme among many others, have demonstrated the complexity of medieval childhood.[9]

While Ariès focused only on childhood, some of his followers and critics expanded the field of study to include questions dealing with parenting in the past. Different models of parenthood and, especially of motherhood, were studied, giving rise to the awareness that being a mother or father in the past was not the same as parenthood today. While a small portion of this research was motivated by ideological purposes, particularly the work of radical feminists such as Elisabeth Badinter,[10] most of this scholarship drew a new picture of a historical phenomenon that had received little attention in previous research.[11] Book-length studies by historians such as Clarissa Atkinson and, more recently, Mary Dockray-Miller, as well as a number of authors of essays published in edited volumes on medieval motherhood, have examined attitudes toward motherhood and the medieval reality of mothers' lives, while other scholars have studied birthing and infant feeding practices.[12]

This study of motherhood was instigated by an additional set of interests as well. The feminist revolution revived interest in the lives of women in the past. At first, heroines were sought out and the actions of women in the public sphere were emphasized, and little attention was devoted to the lives of unexceptional women. Feminist scholars tended to ignore the private lives of women and their traditional functions — as mothers, wives, and daughters. Many feminist historians, like many other feminists during the 1970s and 1980s, saw a basic conflict between motherhood and feminism. Consequently, motherhood was one of the last topics to be addressed by feminist historians.[13] When private life was studied, the questions investigated were usually limited to marriage and marriage practices.

Fifteen years ago, the first book on motherhood in medieval Christian society was published; since then, more have followed. Along with the study of motherhood and the lives of women, a new awareness has affirmed the necessity of examining the roles and understandings of men as fathers in the past.[14] These studies of fathers are only beginning to be published, almost fifteen years after the first appearance of studies on motherhood. While some of the studies of motherhood, particularly those popular two decades ago, addressed questions of emotional attachment, most recent studies have focused on understanding the historical context and culture of family life in the Middle Ages.

Although much has been published on childhood and on the lives of women in the past, few studies have examined women and children together. The history of childhood has been adopted by social historians, as well as by scholars interested in psychoanalysis. The history of women has been examined by historians interested in the family, who have often studied the role of women as part of their discussion of marriage and of the division of labor in society. These scholars were interested in women as one of the components of the family, but often not as a topic in and of itself. By contrast, feminist research concerning the lives of women in the past adopted other methods of inquiry. In these studies, the interest was in women as a separate group, often portrayed as at odds with male hierarchies, resisting or submitting to them. Research that sought to outline an exclusively women's "History of Their Own," always included a chapter devoted to family life. These chapters were, however, often lopsided, presenting only women's stories, while all but ignoring the men.

Over the past two decades, women's studies has shifted to include both genders, as scholars have realized that one cannot study women and their lives without examining men and their place in society. This shift has led to an inclusion of the lives of men and of society at large in the study of the lives of women. Feminists have demonstrated the extent of men's presence, even when the main subject of their inquiry is women, thus reversing the attempts to isolate a separate female sphere. Such a female sphere was suggested both by more traditional historical writings, which allocated women a place only in the domestic sphere, as well as by feminist historians, who sought a point of entry into women's lives in the past. A prominent example in this context is birth, an area that in premodern times, was supervised by women and took place exclusively in the presence of women. As, however, gender perspectives were introduced to research, this supposedly female sphere, like others, came to be seen as a reflection of the society in its entirety, rather than the world of women alone.

In addition, not only is the constant inclusion of both men and women necessary for historical analysis, but as many of the sources studied, especially in the medieval period, were written by men, new methods had to be developed for examining these sources. Only so could scholars come to understand the perspective from which they were written and how that perspective presented the women mentioned in these sources. As noted over a decade ago by Christaine Klapisch-Zuber, the women presented in the medieval sources are often idealized; their descriptions are not of actual medieval persons. Consequently, we must take care to distinguish the sources referring to actual women and their deeds from sources referring to an ideal of womanhood, whether fair or wicked.[15] In our case, in which the writers were all men, and generally wrote their observations about women for a male audience, these distinctions are of utmost importance.[16]

In summary, the study of motherhood and childhood, and the broader study of family life share many characteristics. In both cases, historians today are studying topics that, a few decades ago, were not considered worthy of historical analysis. Scholars of family life have demonstrated time and again that, although biological functions such as birth and lactation, as well as the basic needs of infants and children, have not changed over time, the ways societies understand and satisfy these needs has. One can no longer explain these needs or functions as simply "natural." They must be understood within their specific cultural and historical contexts.[17]

Jews in Christian Europe

The literature concerning the development of research on gender and family history is one part of the foundation for this study, providing a methodological basis for the research and a model for some of the questions posed in the pages that follow. As mentioned above, many of the scholars who pioneered the study of family life in the past were also historians of medieval Europe. As a result, their work provides not only a methodological basis but a substantive one as well. This substantive foundation has been complemented by a growing number of studies concerning women and families in medieval Europe over the past decades. The Jewish communities examined in this study shared many aspects of this well-documented world. The question of how to view Jewish society in light of this research and within the broader medieval context provides an additional foundation for this study. I will now briefly describe the Jewish communities of medieval Ashkenaz that are at the heart of this book.

This study focuses on the Jewish family in medieval France and Germany during the High Middle Ages. The earliest sources examined are from the ninth century and the latest sources are from the early modern period. The bulk of the source material was, however, written in the High Middle Ages, between the time of the First Crusade and the Black Death. Since changes in the family often evolved over time, the long period of time examined allows for an assessment of the variation in society that took place over the years.

A time framework similar to the one generally employed in studies of medieval northern France and Germany was chosen for two reasons. As is the case in Christian Europe, the Jewish sources from before the eleventh century are relatively sparse. Despite this relative dearth, the ninth and tenth centuries were formative periods both for the Jewish communities and for their Christian neighbors and institutions. The relative wealth of sources from the late eleventh century onward reflects the vitality of the lives of the Jews of Ashkenaz. This situation parallels that of the Christian world, where we find a wealth of sources from the twelfth century on,[18] as many scholars of childhood and family life in the Middle Ages have pointed out.[19] The early materials from the Carolingian period are very valuable, however, as they reflect a period in which changes that shaped the institutions of the High Middle Ages were initiated. This is equally true of the scarce but important documents we have of community agreements and halakhic opinions from the ninth and tenth centuries.[20]

The terminus ad quem of this study, the mid-fourteenth century, also has shared significance for Jewish and Christian society. The Black Death has been shown to be a turning point in many different contexts, an event that provoked extreme changes in both attitudes and practices. While in some cases, these changes reflect processes that began in the twelfth and thirteenth centuries, many became prominent only after the Black Death. Consequently, many studies about family life in medieval Europe end with the Black Death, just as many studies concerned with early modern Europe begin their inquiry at this point.[21] The Black Death was also a moment of change for the Jewish communities in Europe and, as such, serves as a suitable period for the end of our inquiry. The Black Death changed the face of European Jewry. Following the Black Death, the process of expulsion of Jews that had begun in England at the end of the thirteenth century, and continued in France at the beginning of the fourteenth century, spread to some cities in Germany as well.[22] In addition, many Jews in German communities began to move to Poland during this period. As the population moved eastward, the result of these migrations, both forced and voluntary, created a new Jewish geography.[23] My examination of sources from after the Black Death demonstrates some of the effects of those changes and investigates to what extent changes that began earlier were accentuated, continued, or transformed after the mid–fourteenth century.

The communities examined are situated in today's northern France and Germany, and are generally called "Ashkenaz" in Jewish historical writing. Although these areas did not belong to a single geopolitical entity during the Middle Ages, and Jewish sources themselves reflect some differences between the localities, the corpus of sources that provides the basis for this study is, for the most part, shared by the two communities.[24] Jews settled along the banks of the Rhine during the ninth and tenth centuries, in cities that over time became central Jewish establishments. The "Shum" communities—Speyer, Worms, and Mainz—were home to many important rabbinical figures as well as to the financial leaders of the time (the two vocations often went hand in hand).[25] Additional German communities were home to rabbinic authorities and successful traders as well. Over time, Jewish settlement spread eastward, and new centers of business and learning were established.[26]

The Jews of northern France, like their brothers and sisters in Germany, were also a vital part of the urbanization of Europe during the Carolingian era.[27] Jewish families established themselves along the trade routes and in the large urban centers. By the High Middle Ages, larger communities, numbering several hundred families, lived in the big cities in France, while many smaller Jewish communities were established, some numbering only a handful of families. The Jews of these communities in France and Germany maintained close contact with other Jews who shared their customs—Jews living in Bohemia, Austria, and Italy (where many of the Ashkenazic Jews originated).[28] Some sources from these areas will be examined here as well.[29] I have not included the Jews of England in this discussion, since the Hebrew sources from England are of a different nature from those on the continent, and, despite the existing contacts between Jews in England and in Ashkenaz, the communities' traditions are not the same.

My decision to jointly examine the areas that are today part of Germany and northern France, distinguishing between them only when such distinctions arise from the sources, does not ignore the fact that these were separate geographic units with distinctive sociopolitical features. Some sources demonstrate that the medieval Jews themselves were well aware of such distinctions. Historians have differed over the importance of these distinctions. While some have argued for examining the two traditions jointly, others have argued for distinguishing between the Jews of northern France and those of Germany.[30] My approach assumes that the customs and practices in both areas were, for the most part, shared.[31] Scholars who went to study in the yeshivas frequently traveled between France and Germany, as did many of the business people. In the tenth and eleventh centuries, students often traveled from France to Germany, and in the twelfth and thirteenth centuries, German students often traveled to France to study. As we shall see, in the context of family life, both areas shared many features and, in fact, can be defined as a single broad region.

In short, the geographical and chronological frameworks examined here accord with those commonly employed when studying Christian society. As was the case in some of the first studies that examined family life, as well as women's history in medieval Europe, the geographic scope of our project is rather broad. As in those projects, I have focused on northern Europe, to the exclusion of the southern parts of Europe — Spain and Provence.[32] This division suits the study of Jewish society, as Spain and Provence had legal and philosophical traditions different from those of Ashkenazic Jews, while Muslim rule, under which the Jews had lived in previous centuries, gave rise to substantial differences in religious customs as well as legal traditions.

Over the past two decades, Christian family life and gender divisions in medieval society have been studied extensively. In the course of this period, there has been a gradual shift from studies examining longer time frames and larger geographic areas to research with narrower geographic and chronological foci.[33] One can hope and assume that, as more social and cultural research pertaining to the Jews in medieval Ashkenaz is undertaken and published, our ability to distinguish between communities and localities will improve.

Jewish Life in Medieval Europe

As stated at the outset, the premise of this study is that it is impossible to comprehend the history of medieval Jews without an in-depth understanding of the society in which they lived. This premise has been debated and contested since the earliest studies on Ashkenazic Jewry written by *Wissenschaft* scholars in the nineteenth century. Certainly, the Jews formed a distinct social and religious group that saw itself, and was perceived by others, as separate from its surroundings. Moreover, the medieval Jewish communities, as well as their Christian neighbors, strove to create separate and even opposing identities, cultivating their own unique customs, some of which were designed to set Jews apart from Christians. Some of these distinctions, within the family framework, will be examined below.

At the same time, however, within the medieval cities, the Jews in Germany and northern France were in contact with their Christian neighbors on a daily basis and had to deal with many of the same mundane worries and troubles. Clearly, on the most basic level, the everyday needs of a Jewish family were similar to those of their Christian neighbors. The Jews needed to support themselves financially, as did their neighbors, and they too married, gave birth, and died. In the context of family life, giving birth, and raising children, we can assume that Jews and Christians who lived in similar material surroundings and environments shared many of the same concerns. This similarity is aptly illustrated by medieval accounts of medical techniques and beliefs related to child care, as well as other categories of medical care.[34]

Aside from daily concerns, Jews and their neighbors shared a common language — the local vernaculars in which they conducted their everyday business and family life.[35] They also shared many beliefs, values, and principles, in spite of their separate and, at times, conflicting religions. These shared values are expressed through the shaping of their respective rites of passage and their social institutions, as well as through shared outlooks on life.[36] While these similar worldviews sometimes led to intense interfaith polemics, they were also the foundation upon which those polemics were built.[37] As such, it is important to outline the similarities as well as the differences between Jewish and Christian family lives.

These shared approaches and attitudes derived not only from common living conditions and beliefs, but also from daily contact. Medieval sources provide many examples of everyday contact between Jews and Christians, especially between Jewish and Christian women, including trade and daily neighborly life. Through these connections, Jews and Christians became familiar with one another's customs. On the family level, Christian women lived inside Jewish homes as servants and as wet nurses, sharing many aspects of the family's daily routine.[38] This certainly provided opportunities for exchanging opinions and beliefs. Christian women who worked for Jews learned about Jewish customs and taught Jews their own practices. These more intimate contacts between Jews and Christians are central to this study.

One might argue that since these Jewish-Christian contacts took place within a very clear framework in which Jews were masters and mistresses and Christian women at their beck and call, such contacts are of limited value in illustrating shared worlds. These contacts were, however, so commonplace, that they must be taken into account as part of any attempt to understand medieval Jewish life. As we shall see, many Jewish families, including very poor ones, had Christian servants and wet nurses. In addition, in spite of the very clear hierarchy within the Jewish home, the relationships between the Jewish masters and their servants were shadowed by a reverse hierarchy in which Christians had the upper hand over the Jews.

Contact with household servants was only one of the many facets of daily Jewish-Christian relationships. During the medieval period, there were no ghettos, and Jews and Christians were neighbors. Despite the clear preference Jewish community members showed for living in close proximity to one another, they almost always had Christian neighbors as well.[39] These shared neighborhoods created many points of meeting and contact: Jewish and Christian women shared ovens, Jews and Christians met by the local wells and cisterns, borrowed food, and knew each other's daily routines. Medieval *responsa* indicate that Jewish and Christian women borrowed dresses from one another and were familiar with intimate details of one another's customs.[40] To these informal connections, we may add commercial contacts between Jews and Christians.[41] Certainly, a Christian man or woman who came to the home of a Jewish moneylender was witness to various aspects of Jewish life. Likewise, Jews became aware of aspects of Christian life by receiving securities that had specifically religious connotations, or when business or other contacts required them to become familiar with the Christian ritual calendar. As Cohen and Horowitz have suggested, members of coterminous different cultures were probably more familiar with one another's rituals than with their respective ideologies.[42]

Our focus will be on the more intimate and domestic contacts between Jews and Christians, especially those between women. The presence of Christian women in Jewish homes, as well as the shared world of medical practitioners and practice, are both central to understanding medieval Jewish family life. Medical practice is a central component of birth and child care. Jews and Christians exchanged knowledge and techniques and, in some cases, practitioners as well. In addition, medieval medicine had strong religious components — the relics and amulets used, the verses chanted and the explanations given for different practices were often based on religious texts and interpretations.[43]

In spite of the many contacts between Jews and Christians, the Jewish community, as noted at the outset, saw itself and was seen by others as a separate entity. In many of the cases examined here, Jewish and Christian society will be compared, and I will point to parallel practices and developments as well as to central differences between Jewish and Christian practice. Many scholars have debated how ideas were transferred from one society to the other, especially in cases in which we cannot attribute shared outlooks and practices to daily contacts alone. When scholars of the nineteenth century identified parallel customs, they were often most interested in tracing the origin of the practice to either a Jewish or a Christian source, rather than explaining the culture and period in which the two parallel practices existed.[44] As my main interest is in the lives of medieval Jews and Christians in their cultural context, I will not be concerned with tracing practices back to their alleged point of origin in Judaism or Christianity. My assumption is that Jews, as a minority society, were more influenced by their Christian neighbors, than the Christians, as a majority culture, were influenced by the Jews. Jews absorbed and appropriated some of the ideas and values of their social environment, more often than not unconsciously. Ivan Marcus has called this kind of cultural appropriation "inward acculturation," as it did not lead to Jews' joining Christianity and giving up aspects of their Judaism; rather, it involved the absorption of new ideas into Jewish society.[45]

This approach presents a change from that adopted by past historians. It allows a departure from the attempt to portray Jews as living in a world separate from that of their Christian neighbors. This method also emphasizes that Jews belong to European culture. As Robert Bonfil has shown, this approach also raises new questions: If the Jews are indeed part of their surrounding society, then their lives must be studied in light of their environment.

To a certain extent, this method, which has been developed in different ways by a number of scholars recently,[46] was already examined and discussed by historians of medieval Ashkenaz in the nineteenth century. However, an additional dominant emphasis in many of those studies was the history of persecution that was a central component of medieval Jewish life.[47] This emphasis also underlined the difference between the unpleasant contact of Jews with their Christian surroundings, and the religious and creative spirituality enjoyed by leaders of the Ashkenazic communities. As a result, subsequent scholarly approaches usually restricted their gaze to the world of scholarship, positing an unfriendly world beyond the spiritual environment. Family life, according to this approach, was an internal aspect of Jewish life because it was regulated by the Torah and by the leaders of the Ashkenazic communities. With few exceptions, it was presented as a world apart, not connected to the daily contact that existed between Jews and Christians.

The social, rather than the religious or intellectual history of the Jews, was the subject of a number of studies in nineteenth-century Germany and England, but was first brought to the forefront of research through the writings of Salo Baron and Jacob Katz. Baron's approach, which held sway in the twentieth century, especially in North America, concentrated on the social history of the Jews and refused to see the Middle Ages only as a period of persecution. Yet despite the tremendous scope of Baron's research, he did not devote attention to Jewish family life.[48] Another prominent social historian, Jacob Katz, devoted his attention to the family in medieval and early modern times. Katz's analysis, however, was based on a sociological prototype, and he was not interested in understanding the daily life of the family or the place of women and children within the family framework.[49]

Well before Baron and Katz, scholars of the late nineteenth and early twentieth centuries such as Moritz Güdemann, Israel Abrahams, and others were interested in cultural history, and the Jewish family had a prominent place in their work. On the whole, these scholars, many of whom lived in Germany, were interested in situating Jewish history, and specifically medieval European Jewish history, within the context of the dominant Christian culture.[50] They pointed to many parallels and shared features of Jewish and Christian life, while maintaining the position that, even in cases in which practices were shared, an inherent difference existed between the Jews and their neighbors. While aspects of family life were examined within the Christian context, an underlying assumption was that the Jewish family was a special haven from the rough, and at times anti-Jewish and unkind world Jews inhabited.[51]

After World War II, and especially with the establishment of the State of Israel, medieval Jewish life in Europe attracted much interest. In these studies, the self-organization of the medieval Jewish communities became a central topic. The family, however, the basic building block of these communities, received little attention.[52] The lack of attention to family history, as well as to the place of women and children in medieval Jewish society, was not merely a reflection of the interests of historians who studied Jewish culture. It also reflected the foci of historical research generally during these years; family history and gender studies were not yet prominent in medieval studies. Jewish historical research turned to the family and gender studies only several years after this trend was initiated in general studies of the medieval world in the late eighties and early nineties of the twentieth century.[53]

In addition to the interest in medieval Jewish community life, the past decades of medieval research have followed the more traditional study of the history of Jewish thought—the works and lives of the great rabbinical figures, whose writings also provide most of the evidence for this study.[54] Many studies on Jewish-Christian relations were also published.[55] Only recently have scholars attempted to illuminate the social settings in which these intellectual pursuits took place and connect between these two topics, by examining the works and lives of rabbinic scholars in the context of Jewish-Christian relations. These new emphases in research follow many years in which scholars assumed that Jewish intellectuals functioned in a rather rarefied and isolated intellectual environment.[56]

The tendency, prevalent until quite recently, to examine Jewish life in medieval Ashkenaz in isolation from the lives of non-Jewish neighbors contrasts with research on the Jews of medieval Spain, which has emphasized the shared features and joint culture of Jews, Muslims, and Christians.[57] There are a number of reasons for this difference: First and foremost, the focus of most scholars studying medieval Ashkenaz was the halakhic corpus composed by scholars during the Middle Ages. These sources are mainly in Hebrew and were not written in order to describe social conditions or situations; rather, they focus on legal and exegetical topics. Scholars' major interest has been in the authors and their intellectual creativity, in the rabbis, and in the contact between them. Their wives, children, and unlearned neighbors were of little concern. Thus, family life was disregarded. An apt illustration of this point can be found in the information we possess regarding the families of the sages themselves. Only a small number of their wives are known by name, and, even in those cases, little else is known about them.[58]

A second reason for the tendency to examine internal Jewish communal life in relative isolation has to do with the extant sources. Most of the sources examined in the past, as in this study, are traditional Jewish sources written in Hebrew. These sources are religious writings focused on the interpretation of Holy Scripture and other canonical texts. As such, they seem to invite examination from an internal Jewish perspective. The second focus of research—Jewish-Christian relations—also promoted separate examination of religious traditions. The discussion of Jewish-Christian polemics assumed difference, for if there is no difference, there is no argument. Despite recent tendencies to concentrate on the dialogue between Judaism and Christianity, the main focus of scholarship in this area has been on the presentation of the differences between Jews and Christians, rather than on their shared aspects.[59]

With the growing interest in the lives of women in the past, this too has been changing. One of the most important works reflecting this outlook is that of Avraham Grossman, a prominent scholar of sages' lives who has recently turned his attention to the history of medieval Jewish women and, especially, to issues relating to marriage and family.[60] Grossman has emphasized the more ancient elements of Jewish tradition, which are important for any attempt to understand medieval Jewish texts, along with comparing Jewish practices to those of their Christian and Muslim neighbors. However, although Grossman does compare Jewish and Christian society in his work, both societies remain distinctive entities, and his comparisons, unlike those of some scholars of Spanish Jewry, single out parallels, rather than describe shared mentalities and frameworks.

A third possible reason for this attitude toward Ashkenazic Jewry lies in the events that have been emphasized in the history of the Middle Ages: the persecutions and expulsions the Jews experienced in Ashkenaz and beyond. From the eleventh century onward, we find many accounts of these persecutions as well as of the rise of accusations such as host-desecration accusations and blood libels.[61] The tremendous impact of these events, as reflected in research, led to a growing perception of medieval Ashkenazic Jewry as a community living in hostile surroundings. Many of the earlier studies that examined Jewish-Christian relations also emphasized the antagonism that existed between Jews and Christians in medieval society. Recent research, however, has sought to reexamine these relationships, and, while scholars do not deny the existence of this hostility, they have also emphasized the shared facets of Jewish and Christian practice and belief.[62]

This study is based on the premise that, although Jews and Christians belonged to two distinct religious groups, they lived in the same time and place and often shared many aspects of their lives, despite hostilities that existed between them. Furthermore, these features were not only common to both religious groups, but were also part of a shared dialogue. Thus, medieval Jews and Christians must be studied both as part of a larger joint society and as members of independent religious societies. In some cases we will witness shared practices and frameworks, while in others, the separate structures will be salient. As such, the comparison between Jews and Christians in the pages that follow will serve to identify cases in which the similarities between both societies were overwhelming. There, we may speak of a single framework of medieval life. In other instances, where we will be struck by the distinct differences between Jews and Christians, we will inquire as to whether this diversity resulted from religious differences or from some other cause.[63]

This comparison also serves another, albeit secondary purpose. As mentioned, there is a substantial body of research about family life in medieval Christian Europe. In some cases where the Jewish sources were lacking in certain details, but the known features indicated great similarity between Jewish and Christian practices, I have used this knowledge to help fill in the missing details. The dangers of such practice are obvious, since, in such cases, Christian society serves as both a comparison and a parallel. I believe, however, that the benefits of this method, when exercised cautiously, outweigh the dangers. In order to monitor the conclusions of such comparisons, I also make reference to some Jewish practices in other diasporas, beyond Ashkenaz. Although social research is still lacking for the Jews of Muslim lands and for the Jews of Spain, Goitein's monumental *Mediterranean Society* as well as work on Provence, Spain, and Italy have served as controls.[64]

The methods employed here seek to identify parallels, joint practices, and shared beliefs. Due to the nature of the sources, however, this methodology meets with a central difficulty that must be noted at the outset. While we may isolate parallels and shared traditions and actions, it is rarely possible to reconstruct chains of causation and proof or processes of contact, dissemination, and exchange. I would like to emphasize that this is not the purpose of this study, and that, in this respect, it differs from previous research, especially nineteenth-century *Wissenschaft* studies, which focused on the question of who influenced whom and how. Rather, as I suggest explicitly in the book, I believe that Jews and Christians living in medieval Ashkenaz were part of the same cultural surroundings and shared a store of ideas, values, and beliefs. In some cases, these shared values were expressed in similar ways, while in other cases, due to religious and social differences (for example the fact that Jews were part of a minority culture, while Christians were not), they were expressed differently.

The nature of the topics examined in this book might lead some to dismiss many of the resemblances I discuss as arising merely from "common sense." After all, they might argue, children all over the world have the same basic needs, and parents caring for these children experience similar processes and share similar obligations. To use just one example examined here, that of birth, one could argue that throughout history, the biological process of birth has not changed, and that this explains the sharing of medical practices among Jews and Christians in medieval Europe. However, as noted, scholars of gender and of the history of childhood have shown that these biological processes take on diverse cultural significance in different cultures. Moreover, medieval medicine contained many elements that were closely tied to religious ideas and concepts and hence, cannot be treated as a value-neutral category. Also, as I demonstrate in chapter 1, procreation and celibacy have been at the heart of the Jewish-Christian debate since ancient times. Therefore, we cannot simply assume that Christian and Jewish practices surrounding procreation, fertility, and childbirth will "naturally" resemble one another. Rather, it is important to demonstrate the similarities between them as well as the differences. The other chapters of the book support this conclusion. In them I show that ceremonies and educational processes that have been presented in other studies as exclusively Jewish or exclusively Christian are actually based on shared social structures and values.

Parents and Children in Medieval Ashkenaz

Fifteen years ago, Louise Tilly and Miriam Cohen drew attention to the fact that family history and gender studies have rarely been researched jointly.[65] While there has been some change over the years, as gender became a more prominent category of analysis, most studies of both medieval Jewish and Christian society have chosen to focus either on mothers or on children, but not on both. This book examines both parents and children, with special emphasis on mothers and motherhood. In this way, I intend to situate the medieval Jewish family within its wider framework, both in relation to fathers and the broader context of Jewish society, while devoting special attention to medieval Jewish women, who have become subjects of historical inquiry only recently.

The joint examination of motherhood and family life enables us to challenge preconceptions concerning both Jewish society in particular and medieval society in general. By examining parenting practices and attitudes toward infants and children, we become acquainted with material and social aspects of everyday life in the Middle Ages and increase our knowledge of the religious beliefs and values of the period. In medieval society, as in many premodern societies, women were seen as responsible for children's welfare during their early years. This fundamental social situation gave rise to shared needs among Jewish and Christian families. At the same time, religious beliefs and values are other factors that shaped cultural attitudes and practices. In the case of medieval Jewish and Christian society, I explore the extent to which religious difference led to distinct practices, and I attempt to outline the areas in which religion made a difference.

The History of Childhood and Women's and Gender Studies in Medieval Jewish Culture

Just as much of the literature concerning childhood in medieval Christian society was grounded in the Ariès controversy, so too, studies of childhood in medieval Jewish society have taken Ariès as their point of departure. Three studies of medieval Jewish attitudes toward children have been written to date. Simḥa Goldin has examined the history of medieval Jewish childhood, comparing Jewish and Christian society. Israel Ta-Shma examined attitudes to children in *Sefer Ḥasidim* and argued for differences between Jewish and Christian society over many issues.[66] Another scholar who has devoted his attention to attitudes toward children and, especially, to education is Ephraim Kanarfogel.[67] These studies, accepting the theories of Ariès and his followers concerning medieval childhood, assumed that Christian parents did not love their children and were not saddened by their deaths. These scholars suggested that in Jewish society, by contrast, the situation was better.[68] Although they acknowledged that some of Ariès's conclusions *did* apply to the Jewish community—for example, the idea that childhood was a more poorly demarcated period of life and that the lack of distinguishing terms for concepts of childhood attests to this fact.[69] They argued that Jews, unlike Christians, loved and cared for their families. This argument was made without acknowledging the vast body of literature written on precisely this topic over the past three decades.

The idea that Jews were somehow better than their Christian neighbors can be found in the many studies in the nineteenth century that compare Jews and Christians in medieval society. Even those nineteenth-century scholars who pointed to the many similarities between Jewish and Christian practices proclaimed the superiority of Jews over their neighbors. For example, Israel Abrahams noted: "In most of these particulars, I can hardly think that the life of the Jewish child differed from that of his gentile brother. But the Jewish view of domesticity showed itself in the success with which life was made lovable to the child notwithstanding the rigours of the discipline to which he was subjected." Throughout his book, he emphasizes time and again: "The home was the place where the Jew was at his best."[70]

The study of childhood is but one component of the transformation the study of Jewish history has undergone over the past two decades. Social history and, more specifically, gender studies have now become a central area of study. However, this change in methodology and subject matter followed the path of its precedents in non-Jewish Western historical research. Some studies have examined Jewish marriage practices, while others have analyzed men's attitudes toward women or women's history in the public sphere, as teachers and educators of women. Few studies have examined motherhood or have sought to place women within a broader context of family and community.[71] Furthermore, much of the work on Jewish women in the past has emphasized our inability to recover their voices, as well as the misogynic attitudes toward women in ancient sources.[72] These studies, many of them written in the wake of current ideological debates, either sought to demonstrate the oppression of women in Judaism or were written in a more apologetic vein and wished to prove the opposite.

In addition, when comparing Jewish and Christian women's lives, some scholars have emphasized the superiority of one culture over another, just as we found in the discussion of childhood. They often emphasized how much better attitudes were toward women in Jewish society, and the superior rights they enjoyed, or emphasized that negative attitudes toward women in Judaism were the result of non-Jewish influence. It is our contention that this type of analysis is not productive, as it often tends to apologetics rather than historical examination. Any attempt at determining which society was better or worse leads to value judgments based on principles that are anchored in modern life and are of limited value in understanding the past.[73] Although it is easy to slip unconsciously into such comparison,[74] I have tried to circumvent such discussions by avoiding labeling practices when discussing medieval Jewish society.[75]

I have tried to distance myself from both the apologetic and the triumphalist (ethnocentric) positions. I have taken as a given that medieval Jewish society, like all of medieval society, was patriarchal, and that its communities were governed by male hierarchies. My purpose has been to explore the fabric of this society and examine the social ideologies, hierarchies, and practices that characterized it. Where possible, I have also explored our capacity to accurately recover the actual women's voices through the testimonies provided by male writers. These voices are frequently found in descriptions of conflicts or arguments over various practices.

In addition to the aspiration to provide a fuller picture of motherhood, fatherhood, and family life, two other issues are central to this study. The first is the examination of birth rituals and the understanding of ritual frameworks regulating birth for parents and children in medieval Ashkenaz. The second is the examination of the daily contacts between Jews and Christians in the sphere of family life.

The study of ritual has become a central tool for historical analysis over the past years. Jews and Christians in the Middle Ages, as in most societies, celebrated birth, marriage, and death with elaborate ritual. As scholars have shown, examining these rituals offers new insights into the place of individuals in their societies, as well as the social settings and religious ideologies that framed these rituals.[76] Over the past years, ritual theory has been used extensively to understand different aspects of medieval Christianity,[77] and the beginnings of such an approach can be seen in Jewish studies over the past decade.[78] In the medieval context, the rite of passage that marked the beginning of boys' education, as studied by Ivan Marcus, is the most notable example of such research on medieval Ashkenaz.[79] Few studies, however, have studied the social aspects of rituals, and most have focused exclusively on the religious symbolism that was part of the ritual in question.[80] Moreover, only circumcision has been studied extensively, despite the fact that other, less formal rituals existed as well.

The issue of daily contacts between Jews and Christians has been studied in the economic sphere and, most recently, in the context of Hebrew Bible and New Testament exegesis and the connections between Jewish and Christian scholars. Our focus is on the more mundane contacts, especially between women inside and outside the house. Wet nursing and midwifery, as well as advice shared between women about health and child care are all part of these contacts. By demonstrating these close contacts between Jewish and Christian women, and the world shared by both groups, we hope to open up new vistas for research. The evidence pointing to a world shared by Jewish and Christian women encourages historians of both Jewish and Christian society to search for and learn from comparisons between them. In that way, at times by filling in the blanks, we can piece together a fuller picture of the knowledge women shared in medieval society, as well as a sketch of a central channel through which Jews and Christians, both men and women, learned and adopted ideas that became part of Jewish and Christian life alike.

The Sources

The sources that provide the basis for this study are varied and were, for the most part, written in northern France and Germany during the High Middle Ages. They include halakhic responsa (questions and answers addressed to prominent rabbinical authorities), exempla such as those in *Sefer Ḥasidim*, ritual books, comprehensive books of commandments (*sifrei mizvot*), biblical and talmudic commentary as well as commentary on liturgical poetry (*piyutim*), medical tractates, polemical compositions, chronicles, lists of the dead, and gravestones. In addition to sources originating in the Jewish communities, canon law, municipal records, medical texts, commentaries on the Bible (Old and New Testament) and *legenda* provide knowledge about the Jewish communities, their Christian surroundings, and the contacts between Jews and Christians. Some of the Hebrew sources are found in printed editions that have been published extensively since the mid-nineteenth century. Other sources remain in unpublished manuscripts. The majority of these sources were not written with the intention of discussing family life; rather they address a variety of concerns, both legal and theological, and the details about family life emerge from the narrative.

Sefer Ḥasidim provides unique information about parent-children relations and about attitudes toward children and family life. Scholarship about this book has debated the nature of the group that adhered to the instructions of Sefer Ḥasidim and constituted the audience of the book. While some have suggested seeing Ḥasidei Ashkenaz as a unique and separate group, others have suggested that many of the moral lessons recommended in the book pertained to all of Ashkenazic society.[81] While I do not intend to discuss this issue in the book, I propose reading many of the stories concerning women, children, and family life as representative of Ashkenazic society as a whole.[82] Even if Ḥasidei Ashkenaz were as small and sectarian a group as some have suggested, this does not mean their family life was completely different from that of their Jewish neighbors. As a way of checking these conclusions, I have sought to compare between attitudes expressed in Sefer Ḥasidim and those expressed in other contemporary Jewish and Christian sources in order to determine how normative these ideas were.

Working with the sources described above involves a number of difficulties, both technical and more substantive. As I stated above, these texts were all written by and for men. This perspective poses difficulties for the evaluation of the opinions and attitudes of women cited in these writings. Unlike many of the parallel Christian sources, the men writing these texts had families and were not removed from family life. Despite this, one cannot forget that their readers were only men. I have tried to demonstrate how, in some cases, one can discuss women's attitudes and opinions in spite of these limitations. This difficulty is compounded by the fact that most of the sources were not meant to discuss the family. Consequently, the evidence in the sources must be examined both in its context and in a broader perspective. The attempt to combine information from sources belonging to different literary genres requires that we be cognizant of the rules of each genre when piecing the sources together. Most of the sources examined here have been discussed in previous literature by scholars who specialized in medieval Ashkenaz. In the tradition of gender studies, I have examined these sources in new ways, posing different questions.

It is also crucial to note the sources we are lacking. Besides the obvious fact that we have not a single source written by a woman, we also have no sources providing demographic or statistical information,[83] nor do we have maps or city plans to provide us with a layout of the cities in which Jews lived. We also have no Jewish parallel to the medieval hagiographic sources that describe the saints' lives—sources that have been used extensively to study family life in medieval Christendom.[84]

While I have used a variety of sources in comparing Jewish and Christian society, my most basic resource for Christian society has been the extensive research on medieval women, men, and children. In some cases, I have based my comparison on these secondary sources, while in other cases I have returned to the medieval sources themselves. As the main focus of this study is Jewish society, most of the sources are Jewish sources.

Family Life in Medieval Ashkenaz

In the chapters that follow, the narrative begins with pregnancy and ends with boys' entry into formal education, at age six or seven. This narrative was chosen because it enabled a combined analysis and discussion of several kinds of sources. This is necessary, since one type of source may provide a wealth of information on one topic, but none on others. For example, a huge body of legal literature discusses common breast-feeding practices. By contrast, there are almost no legal writings on birth.

While we can find a wealth of information about the process from birth until early childhood, the lack of demographic and statistical information prevents us from outlining other basic information about the family and its characteristics. I have relied on the suggestions made by others on the composition and character of medieval Jewish families as well as their living conditions. The following summary will provide an overview of the research I have utilized for the study.

Living conditions are especially important because young children—boys who had not yet begun school (at the local synagogue or their tutor's home) and young girls—spent most of their time at home. When they went out of their homes, young children were usually accompanied by adults. Since we know that these children's mothers were mobile and could be seen in many public spaces—around the home, at synagogue, as well as in the streets and marketplace — we can assume that they often took their young children with them, even if there is little evidence of such outings. There is substantial evidence, however, of their visits to the synagogue. These visits began long before they were ripe for education and attended the synagogue to study with the local tutor.[85] Both young boys and girls attended the synagogue with their parents. The synagogue was a central communal meeting place for social and spiritual functions. Archeological evidence reflects the tremendous importance the Jewish communities attributed to their communal places of worship — both as an antithesis to the local churches and as a sanctuary.[86]

Over the past years, a wealth of research has been published on the locations of medieval Jews habitations. These studies are, for the most part, the result of research done in Germany, where scholars have been interested in understanding the development and settlement of Jews in Germany during the Middle Ages.[87] Few of these studies have, however, examined the lifestyles and living conditions of individual families within the city. Fifty years ago Alexander Pinthus raised some of these questions in his study *Die Judensiedlungen der Deutsche Städte. Eine stadtbiologische Studie*, and little has been done in this direction since.[88]

In contrast to the lack of sources on Jewish living conditions, we know that the Jews' Christian neighbors lived as nuclear families, and that each couple usually had a room of their own and formed an independent economic unit.[89] These units were often tied to broader family frameworks in their daily life, but they almost always lived independently.[90]

With the exception of studies concerning the age of marriage and especially child brides,[91] little research has been done on Jewish family structures.[92] Kenneth Stow is one of the few scholars who has addressed this topic, and he has argued that the Jews, like their urban Christian neighbors, lived in nuclear families.[93] The medieval Jewish sources, also, point to the complex networks that existed between and within families, especially insofar as economic relationships and partnerships were concerned.[94] Sources that discuss economics and business deals may potentially shed additional light on family structures, since so much of Jewish business took place within the home.

As we shall see in the following chapters, especially regarding rituals, the wider family framework was also central in religious and social life. Family background was an essential component in matchmaking agreements and was a central factor in determining social status.[95] Few sources, however, discuss the involvement of grandparents in the upbringing and education of their grandchildren. Consequently, we cannot outline the nuclear family's relationship with broader family networks in the context of early childhood. While we can assume that grandparents and siblings were involved in the upbringing of children, especially in cases in which a young bride gave birth, there are few details on these relationships.[96] These issues all require further research, research that was not undertaken in the context of this study.

The first chapter traces family life from marriage and the period before conception, to birth and practices surrounding birth, including attitudes toward procreation and the preference for boys over girls. The social organization around birth, the work of midwives, the connections between Jewish and Christian women, as well as the gendered conceptions of birth are all addressed in this chapter. The second and third chapters discuss birth rituals — the more institutionalized rite of circumcision, as well as the less formal rites for girls, boys, and women after birth. This discussion outlines the understandings of the rites in both individual and more communal terms. The place of women in these rites, and the changes in the rituals over time are central to the discussion. From the ritual framework, I turn to examine daily practices and attitudes toward children and child care. Chapter 4 discusses breast-feeding and wet-nursing practices and exposes a complex world of interactions between Jews and Christians. Chapter 5, the final chapter, discusses attitudes toward children and child care, from the division of labor to the place of child care in religious and ethical thought. All the chapters compare Jewish and Christian sources and practices.

In the conclusion, I summarize the insights that arise from this examination of Jewish society within the wider Christian context. I argue that the only way to understand Jewish family life in the past is by studying Jewish families within their cultural context. Medieval Jewish attitudes and beliefs must be understood in the context of earlier Jewish traditions as well as in those of the contemporary environment. Practices and ideas were shared by Jews and Christians, at times in spite of substantive differences in religious belief, and notwithstanding the dissimilar explanations provided for similar customs. By examining the changes that took place in the lives of families in medieval society — mothers, fathers, and children — we may further our understanding of the ways in which Jews in medieval Europe developed and preserved their separate identities, while being full partners in medieval society. Our quest to see and understand women's lives and history, from a gender perspective, constitutes a first step toward a more inclusive Jewish history — a history in which medieval Jewish women can find their place in a narrative alongside the rabbis and students whose works are so well known and so often studied. If we rephrase Abelard's statement in Jewish terms, we are seeking to examine the connections between pupils and nursemaids, thoughts of scripture and babies being soothed by lullabies, and above all the noisy coming and going of men and women about the house.

Chapter One

BIRTH

> For the first three months the embryo dwells in the lower compartment; the next three months in the middle compartment; and the final three months in the upper compartment. For the first three days, one should pray to God that the infant won't decompose; from three to forty days he should pray that it will be a male; from forty days to three months, he should pray that it not be a sandal;[1] and from three months to six months, he should pray that it not be stillborn; and from six to nine months he should pray that the baby will be born safely. And can a man bring the baby out safely? No, rather the Holy One, blessed be He creates for the infant doors and hinges and brings him out safely.
> — Midrash Yeẓirat haValad

THE MIDRASH'S DESCRIPTION of the creation of the fetus was a popular one in the Middle Ages. It outlines the stages of pregnancy and birth and provides explanations of the process. But the story of parents and children begins long before men and women become fathers and mothers. This chapter will focus on the conceptual and practical aspects of birth in the medieval Jewish communities of Ashkenaz. Most research on birth has concentrated on the history of ideas on procreation, with little attention devoted to the more practical and day-to-day aspects of birth.[2] The most common issues concerning birth, as discussed in previous research, are outlined in the Midrash that opens this chapter. The Midrash designates three persons: God, who is responsible for the creation of the embryo; the father, who prays for the baby throughout the pregnancy; and the baby itself. A fourth figure in this Midrash, though never mentioned by name, is the mother, who carries the baby in her womb and gives birth to him. While this chapter will discuss all four persons, I will devote most of my attention to the mother, who has received the least consideration to date.

The chapter will be divided into three interrelated parts. The first deals with medieval Jewish understandings of the biological experience of birth, as well as religious understandings and beliefs concerning birth. I will then discuss how these beliefs and understandings were expressed in the context of fertility and infertility. Finally, I will examine the extant evidence on birth practices in medieval society. The distinctions between these three sets of issues are somewhat artificial, and, insofar as they are interrelated, I will identify the connections. These artificial distinctions do, however, facilitate a more balanced gender analysis of birth. Most intellectual history approaches to procreation have been circumscribed by the textual material, which reflects the thoughts of the men who wrote them, whereas analyses of the social functions of birth have devoted far more attention to women.[3] In the context of medieval Ashkenazic Jewry, neither of these analyses has been undertaken in previous research, and as such, this chapter will provide analyses of attitudes toward procreation and of the social history of birth.

We should note at the outset that the study of birth, as scholars, and especially feminist scholars have shown, is complex. While it is relatively easy to ascertain what medieval people thought about God's role or the role of men in procreation, revealing the roles of women, beyond the bare fact that they bore children, is a difficult task. Although birth was women's business and only women attended births, it is very difficult for scholars to gain access to the birthing chamber and other arenas in which women may be found. Furthermore, the male expectations and social orders, ever present outside the birthing chamber, undoubtedly filtered into that female space as well. Thus, the study of birth is actually the study of "the intercourse of birth with patriarchy."[4]

Procreation and Its Significances

Medieval Understandings of the "Nature" of Women

Feminist scholarship, since its beginnings, has devoted extensive energy in the attempt to define and identify female spheres and characteristics. While feminist categories have been enthusiastically adopted by some scholars, others have avoided them as overly essentialist. All agree, however, on the significance of women's ability to give birth. As the anthropologist Helen Callaway remarked, birth is "the most essentially female function of all." Gender methodologies have attempted to shift the weight from the biological function of giving birth to the role of culture in defining the birth process. This is the course we will follow.[5]

Medieval society assumed that giving birth and being a mother was an inherent feature of female identity. Exactly how this inherency was understood, is, however a matter of great interest. Women in medieval Jewish society, as in all premodern patriarchal societies, bore secondary status. They were expected to serve their husbands in many ways; giving birth to children, especially male children, was just one of them. In addition, in medieval times women were educated to be mothers. In medieval Jewish society, as in its Christian counterpart, motherhood was one of the central aims of female education.[6] Although the expectations fostered by such education became relevant when the girls reached sexual maturity, the education of girls as future mothers began from a very young age.

Jewish sources speak of the centrality of birth and motherhood for a woman's identity in several contexts. Although they never systematically discussed women's ability to give birth or the expectations of women, we do find pertinent information in discussions of sterility and barrenness. Descriptions of barren women emphasize their profound sorrow and grief and put forth the belief that the happy woman, the woman who has realized her true potential, is the woman with children. This idea is clearly expressed in commentaries on piyutim (liturgical poems) and on the Bible, especially with respect to Sarah, Rebecca, and Rachel, who are all described as suffering from barrenness prior to the births of their sons. In a thirteenth-century commentary on the piyut *Ta'alat zu kehafez* for the New Year (Rosh haShana), Rebecca is described as an *asura*, a prisoner, until she finally gives birth. The commentator explains that barren women are like prisoners in their homes; only once God grants them the long-awaited and coveted sons may they walk around proudly. The text continues, discussing the stress on marital relations posed by barrenness in the case of Rebecca and Isaac. It claims that Isaac was also an *asur* (prisoner) because of Rebecca's barrenness. Quoting the verse from Gen. 25:21, "Isaac pleaded with the Lord on behalf of his wife because she was barren," the commentator remarks: "'And Isaac pleaded with the Lord on behalf of his wife': they argued with each other and Isaac said to her 'you are barren' and she replied to him, 'you are barren.'"[7] In the discussion that follows, although both Isaac and Rebecca are described as suffering as a result of their childlessness, Rebecca is seen as the more miserable of the two.

Many later sources repeat the anguished plea of another biblical matriarch, Rachel, concerning her barrenness. Her cry: "Give me children or I shall die" (Gen. 30:1) becomes the staple plea of barren women. A medieval commentary on the Kalir's piyut for Rosh haShanah *"Even hug mazok neshiya"* explains the line: *"Ke'akeret bayit batehal nukra"* (As a housewife at the beginning she was alienated), explaining:

> At the beginning she was alienated from giving birth, from being a housewife; "Rachel was barren" — she was alienated. But in the end, as in the days of the ripening of her first fruits, like a fig at its beginning, "she gave birth to Joseph" — which is the purpose (*takhlit*) of all mothers.[8]

A number of issues are expressed here. The commentator is playing with the multiple etymologies of the verb *akar*: *akara* (barren) and *akeret bayit* (housewife), and the word *ikar* (the center or main part). Rachel was barren so she could not be an akeret bayit. When she gave birth to Joseph, she was fulfilling the purpose (ikar) of her womanhood by becoming a mother.

Another compelling example can be found in R. Judah the Pious's (1150–1217) commentary on Genesis. He explains the phrase "Sarah's lifetimes" (Gen. 23:1)[9] as meaning that Sarah had two lifetimes — one before she gave birth and one afterward. He explains that her real life began only after she had offspring, since a woman without children is like a dead person.[10] While sources provide some expressions of the sorrow of men without offspring, as when it is said that a man without children is like a dead person,[11] it is more common and more categorical in discussions on women. In the Biblical examples above and frequently used in medieval literature, while the husbands of the barren women are surely not pleased with their situations, their wives are distraught.

The idea that the fertile wife is the happy and good wife appears not only in theoretical discussions of happiness or barrenness but also in practical advice on how to choose a wife. *Sefer Hasidim* contains a few directives on the topic. Aside from the religious attributes one should seek in searching for a spouse, the author says that it is important to make sure that the chosen woman will be able to give birth. He suggests: "And one should check the woman because most daughters take after their mothers. If their mother miscarries so will her daughter. Therefore one should pray that God grant him a woman of *middot* [good qualities]."[12] Note that here, the good quality mentioned is not a spiritual attribute, but rather the woman's physical ability to bear children. Once again, this demonstrates that, at least when dealing with women, the distinctions between what we today would consider biological or physical, as opposed to cultural attributes, were blurred.

This idea is repeated in an additional comment in *Sefer Hasidim*. There, the author explains that men should love and show affection to their wives because of their wives' ability to bear children, even in cases in which much love does not exist between the couple.[13] He bases his explanation on Jacob's relationship with Leah and explains that Leah justifiably expected Jacob to love her after she gave birth to his children (Gen. 29:32), and as a result, all men, even those who do not love their wives *ahava shebalev* (with their hearts), should show affection to their wives because of the children they bear. In short, according to the men whose writings have reached us, women were expected to have children, and this was their purpose and goal. As will be seen throughout this book, women's cultural role included not only giving birth, but all the tasks linked to having and caring for young children.

Jews and Christians: Attitudes toward Reproduction

These cultural understandings of male and female reproductive "nature" become more complex when different religious beliefs emphasize different aspects of them. Such is the case with Jewish and Christian attitudes toward reproduction. The disparity between Jewish and Christian attitudes is well known and has been the root of many debates over the centuries. While Jews saw the commandment to procreate — *"pru urvu"* (be fertile and increase) (Gen. 1:28) — as an important foundation of Jewish belief, Christians did not. Many scholars have referred to this distinction as limiting the possibilities for comparison between Jewish and Christian family life, and as justification for studying each society separately.[14] Even scholars who have examined Jewish and Christian family institutions in tandem have emphasized the theological gap that exists in this context.[15]

The Christian preference for celibacy was central from its beginnings.[16] Indeed, most of the extant medieval records dealing with attitudes toward procreation were written by the same small and select group that chose celibacy as its way of life. Men who lived in monastic frameworks understood their choice as an expression of their ability to refrain from worldly pleasures and remain pure. Women who chose to be nuns viewed their celibacy, especially if they were virgins, as a ticket to the male spiritual environment and an escape from their fate as women.[17] Yet despite the many references to these men and women in medieval literature, we must remember that this was not the majority choice. Most Christians throughout the ages were married, not celibate.

Because they esteemed the ideal of celibacy, Christian society treated married life as the less ideal choice. Nevertheless, in their discussions of noncelibate married women, the medieval authors resembled their Jewish peers. The cultural significance of women as childbearers is also evident in these authors' descriptions of women who forewent motherhood to become brides of Christ. As a number of scholars, especially Caroline Bynum, have shown, images of birth and of maternity are prominent in descriptions of all women, including those who do not actually give birth.[18]

Jews, as is well known, did not share this attitude toward celibacy. While only few Christians actually chose the monastic way of life, all saw this as an ideal, albeit one that posed too big a challenge for most. In contrast, all Jews saw procreation as an obligatory and positive commandment. Jewish and Christian attitudes toward the biblical commandment of procreation from antiquity through the Middle Ages have been examined in a recent study by Jeremy Cohen. Cohen examined Jewish and Christian attitudes toward the biblical command. His study altered the prevailing tendency to present Jewish and Christian attitudes as completely distinct. Cohen emphasized that in spite of their fundamental difference, there were also areas of similarity. For example, Cohen maintained that despite the ideal of celibacy, some Christian scholars included procreation as part of the *ius naturalis* (natural order). In other words, procreation was not simply a commandment to be interpreted allegorically, but one that had practical implications. Thus, Cohen demonstrates that among the eastern Church Fathers, procreation within a family framework was understood as a positive commandment.[19]

Procreation was often reassessed and discussed in Western Christian thought throughout the Middle Ages. While some claimed that procreation was a biblical commandment no longer relevant to Christian lives, other interpreters began to attribute more importance to the commandment to procreate within the marital framework. For example, in some cases, the biblical commandment was recited at the wedding ceremony.[20] Thus, it became an important part of the blessing for a newlywed couple. This change in the ceremony was part of a major shift in Christian understandings of marriage that, in the twelfth century, made marriage one of the sacraments.[21] At the same time, fertility became a far more important part of the church's understandings of marriage.

This change brought Jewish and Christian understandings of procreation somewhat closer. Studies concentrating on Christian society have emphasized the growing importance of marriage and family in medieval Christian theology and explained the changing significance accorded the family as a consequence. In reality, we cannot determine which came first. Most certainly, thought and practice developed simultaneously and influenced each other. Marian devotion, as well as devotion to the other members of Jesus' family, especially his grandmother Anna, were also part of the growing importance of family in medieval thought.[22] These developments led to a more positive assessment of procreation in Christian thought.[23]

The increasing convergence of Christian theology and Jewish rabbinic legislation is not limited to attitudes toward procreation. Cohen and others have pointed to shared attitudes toward other aspects of sexual relations besides the question of whether the commandment pru urvu should be seen as practical or allegorical. For example, Cohen has shown that Jews and Christians shared similar understandings of the conjugal relationship. Based on the composition *Ba'alei haNefesh*, written by R. Abraham b. David of Posquières (Ra'abad) in the twelfth century, Cohen shows how the Ra'abad's explanations and justifications for sexual relations between a man and his wife are similar to those provided by theologians such as Ivo of Chartres (1040–1115), Gratian (d. 1160), and Thomas Aquinas (1224–1274).[24] All these commentators, both Jewish and Christian, attributed great importance to the intent of the men engaging in sexual relations. Cohen argues that the Ra'abad linked the obligation of *onah* (conjugal obligations toward one's wife) to the duty of procreation in a manner different than that of his predecessors, but resembling the approach of his Christian contemporaries. Ra'abad argued that if the intent behind the relations was pure, the deeds were too. And conversely, if the intent was not pure, the deeds were not either.

Dalia Hoshen, who focused on the ideal relationships between men and women in the writings of Maimonides and the Ra'abad, promoted this idea more forcefully. She proposed that medieval Jewish sages saw celibacy in a more favorable manner than their predecessors and, consequently, restricted the conditions in which sexual relations were to be advocated.[25] Putting these findings together, we see that while the importance of procreation within the marital framework grew in medieval Christian thought, Jewish authorities took an increasingly negative view of marital sexual relations performed with improper intent.

Hoshen and Cohen concentrate on the philosophy of Maimonides and of the Ra'abad, both of whom lived south of the areas of this study and far away from the locales of the theologians they cite — Paris, Bologna, and Köln. If we turn to northern France and especially Germany, we find that, although Ashkenazic Jews living in those countries attached great importance to procreation, some of the writings of Jews of those countries display a more positive approach to abstinence. For example, the author of *Sefer Hasidim* writes of a hasid who did not want to have sexual relations with his wife after the death of a Zaddik (righteous man).[26] This source, combined with the well-documented attitude of Hasidei Ashkenaz that encouraged avoiding women as much as possible,[27] seems to indicate a shared approach of Hasidei Ashkenaz and their Christian neighbors, an issue that Talya Fishman has recently raised in other contexts.[28]

These allusions to shared approaches are far from inconsequential. They point to shared beliefs and a common mentality. In spite of these points of contact, however, procreation was viewed as a central point of contention between Jews and Christians in the medieval world. For example, in polemical debates, it was often one of the issues discussed. In *Sefer Nizahon Vetus*, the Jews accost the monks and needle them on their stupidity and their concealed lustfulness. One of the issues the Jewish disputants mention is their doubt as to the possibility that anyone can live a truly celibate life. Thus in *Sefer Nizahon Vetus*, the Jews argue:

> Ask them: If the Christian priest is supposed to take the place of the biblical priest, why doesn't he get married and have children like Aaron the High Priest? Moreover, the first commandment given to Adam dealt with being fruitful and multiplying, yet you refrain from this and instead pursue fornication and wine, which capture your fancy.[29]

The book discussed this matter again in another passage, where the Christian priests are compared to eunuchs who practice castration. They are accused of wallowing in licentiousness in secret. The author ends that part of the argument by stating:

> Furthermore it is written "Your wife shall be as a fruitful vine" (Ps. 128:3), and before that it is written, "Blessed is everyone that fears the Lord" (Ps. 128:1). Thus we see that having children is a mark of the God-fearing man.[30]

In this debate, the Jew argues over the spiritual character of celibate men, and the whole passage focuses on their decision not to marry and its consequences. Were they to debate with married Christian neighbors, however, this argument would not have been as powerful. Although these married Christian men might have admitted that there was yet another, higher level of devotion that they did not practice, nevertheless, they would have seen their bearing of children as a way of fulfilling the word of God, much as their Jewish contemporaries did.

The Jewish and Christian attitudes toward procreation as described above, raise new possibilities for comparative study of Jews and Christians in medieval Europe. The suggested similarity between the needs and beliefs of Jewish and Christian families with regard to procreation is central to this book's argument. I wish to compare Jewish families to Christian families, rather than to the minority that chose to live celibate lives. As is clear from studies of birth in medieval Europe, Christian couples were interested in bearing offspring, and, when children were not born soon after marriage, they sought solutions to the problem.[31] This argument for a shared attitude toward procreation within family frameworks will be the basis of the discussion that follows, where we will discuss and compare Jewish and Christian attitudes toward fertility and sterility.

Men and Women

Before we discuss medieval approaches to fertility and infertility, let us briefly examine the system that emerges from the biological and theological elements outlined above from a gender perspective. Although I will restrict my discussion to the topic of procreation, these concepts can also teach us much about the construction of women's religious identity in general. One of the ideas suggested by the author of *Sefer Niẓaḥon Vetus* is that having children is a characteristic of the God-fearing man. Thus, although both men and women were involved in procreation, it was considered a gendered task and was incumbent only upon men. Jewish women were not obligated to perform the commandment of procreation. This religious understanding was based on the biological understandings, which serve as both reason and justification for the exclusion of women. Although Amoraic sources do debate women's obligation to procreate, medieval sources are emphatic on this point. The medieval commentators, first and foremost Rashi, repeat the Talmudic interpretation of the verse "Be fruitful and multiply and fill the earth and conquer it" (Gen. 1:28) and explain: "It is man's nature to conquer, it is not woman's nature."[32] This explanation assumes that women are not naturally inclined to certain types of activity. This "biological" explanation is not limited to women's inability to perform procreative commandments. In cases of other commandments from which women are exempted, we find similar explanations.[33]

This view accords with the medieval medical understanding of women as receptacles of the fetus, whose bodies were designed to protect the baby during pregnancy.[34] Thus, in Christian religious thought, the Virgin Mary served as the *mediatrix* between God and humanity by protecting Jesus in her womb throughout her pregnancy; as such, her example became a paradigm to be imitated by medieval women.[35] Jewish texts also present this view of women's bodies—as containers for the fetus on its way to this world.[36] The Jewish texts adopt Galen's two-seed theory.[37] According to this theory, both mother and father contribute to the creation of the embryo, each with his or her own seed. In the Talmud, the implications of this theory are outlined in terms very similar to theories found in contemporary Latin sources: The mother is said to contribute to the more tangible and earthly features of the fetus — the skin, blood, and hair, whereas the father contributes bones, nails, and the brain.[38] Most discussions of these topics in both Jewish and non-Jewish sources emphasize the father's role and minimize the mother's role, turning her into the means of bringing the infant into the world rather than a central active figure, and her status in the context of birth is unmistakably subordinate.

In Jewish sources, procreation is linked with a second legal issue — the number of children needed to fulfill the religious obligation of procreation. This topic, discussed already in Tractate *Yevamot*, does not seem to have been a topic of much debate in medieval Jewish society. The accepted opinion was that of *Beit Hillel* — one daughter and one son. By contrast, *Beit Shammai* believed that the Law required two sons. This obligation is discussed in *Sefer Hasidim* in a story about a man who had only one child and was worried about his ability to fulfill the commandment of procreation while his wife was nursing their infant, as the nursing would prevent the conception of another child.[39] The precise obligations of this commandment were also important in cases in which a man lost his wife prior to his fulfillment of the commandment and wanted to remarry. In cases in which a man had not yet fulfilled the commandment, he was allowed to remarry earlier,[40] thus demonstrating a clear difference regarding remarriage of widows and widowers with small children, a topic that will be taken up in chapters 4 and 5.

A final point concerns the importance that medieval people, Jews and Christians alike, attached to the birth of male offspring. The approach of Beit Shammai who argued in the Mishna that one must have two sons in order to fulfill the obligation of procreation is a good illustration of this attitude. Medieval Jewish and Christian societies are not unique in this respect, since most premodern societies agree on this point. Jewish sources attest to the great disappointment that accompanied the birth of daughters. Fathers explicitly prayed for the birth of male offspring, and from the moment of conception, special prayers were recited to help women bear sons.[41] Beginning with the Mishna, and throughout medieval literature, men are warned not to pray once the sex of the baby has been determined. This does not mean, however, that the birth of a daughter was not greeted with some sorrow.[42] As a thirteenth-century commentator on Genesis commented, girls were not important; boys were the ikar. Consequently, he writes that in the passages on the naming of Jacob's children, while a reason is given for each of the boy's names, no explanation is provided for why Dinah was named as she was.[43] While the Jewish expressions of this partiality are unique to Jewish sources, this preference was well known among Christians as well.[44]

CHAPTER ONE

INFERTILITY

The issue of fertility and infertility serves as a window enabling us to examine the interaction of the ideological and biological views discussed above with the pressures exerted on these processes in real life. In medieval Europe, fertility was central to the success of a match. Since children were often betrothed and at times even married before reaching sexual maturity, the birth of children was seen as evidence that the match made by parents, often for financial reasons, was indeed a fruitful one.[45] As comparative anthropological studies have shown, the birth of a first child in situations like this often reaffirms and solidifies marriage ties.[46] I would even suggest that, in the case of arranged child marriages, this stage in the life of a couple was more important than the marriage ceremony itself.[47]

By examining medieval attitudes toward fertility, we may view both sides of the same coin. On the one hand, people suffering from infertility are an important topic of discussion. But our inquiry may also teach us much about the treatment of the birth of children in a "normal" fertile situation. If each marriage union, Jewish and Christian alike, was expected to produce offspring, then the treatment of infertile couples provides a useful locus for the examination of shared and differing attitudes of Jews and Christians toward procreation. A central question will be whether or not the differing attitudes toward procreation have any influence over the ways in which Jewish and Christian society treated infertility.

The practical methods of dealing with infertility in medieval Jewish and Christian society were not all that different. The ideas expressed in the sources of the two societies, in the case of couples who did not succeed in conceiving, concurred in their aim to determine who was responsible for the problem. Infertility was believed to be hereditary or the result of a physical fault or bewitchment. Women were usually blamed for infertility, and only in rare cases was the cause of infertility attributed to men. In addition, there was a grave difference between the reasons given to explain female and male infertility. While female infertility was usually ascribed to physical problems, and only rarely associated with witchcraft, male fertility was most often explained as the result of a spell, usually cast by women.

This understanding can be seen as somewhat ironic: Men were given most of the credit for the creation of a healthy fetus, but women were held responsible for problems in conception.[48] This difference also emphasizes the responsibility allocated women over birth. In addition, in a society in which male pride rested in part on having many children, a man who was sterile faced great embarrassment.[49]

An issue that surfaces frequently in the context of infertility is the status of a marriage in which one of the spouses was unable to have children. The solutions to these problems were varied in both Judaism and in Christianity and were linked to theoretical understandings of the duty of procreation and of the marriage bond as well as to social issues. These understandings shaped the ways in which infertility was identified and diagnosed, and especially the implications of infertility.

Infertility was identified in a number of different ways. The most common method, in both Jewish and Christian society, was a physical examination.[50] It seems that women were examined routinely, since midwives regularly examined women who wished to conceive. For example, in Jewish communities, midwives accompanied women on their monthly visits to the ritual bath and were expected to help promote fertility.[51] If a woman seemed to have some kind of physical problem, a midwife might have commented on it. In addition, many cures and potions to promote fertility were available. It seems that the prevailing attitude was not to let nature take its course, but rather to promote and encourage fertility.[52]

These examinations do not seem to have been common for men. The fact that these examinations were routine for women and rare for men only emphasizes the implied responsibility of women concerning birth. Part of the reason for this discrepancy was that, for men, such procedures incurred shame. While it was easy to note, without a physical exam, that a man's voice was not deep or that he had no facial hair, a true physical exam required a more intimate inspection. In Christian society, where men were also examined only infrequently, such examinations were usually performed by midwives.[53] We have little evidence on this point in the Jewish sources. In one of the few references to such an examination, R. Eliezer b. Joel haLevi (Ra'aviah, ca. 1140–ca. 1212) discusses a case in which a woman claims her husband is impotent. He mentions the possibility of verifying this accusation by having this man examined, but he says that such a procedure would involve an extreme embarrassment.[54] Christian sources also discuss midwives' examinations of men charged with impotency and note the shame involved in such a procedure. Perhaps the disgrace that was associated with such an examination and the accusation of a man was behind the common opinion that male infertility was the result of women bewitching men.[55] Many cures and charms for releasing men from bewitchment can be found in the sources.[56]

Medieval people were also aware of the fact that sometimes women and men seemed to be fine physically and still had infertility problems. Therefore a number of other solutions existed that were supposed to enable a diagnosis of problems that had no visible manifestations.[57] For example, a thirteenth-century manuscript of the *Midrash Lekah Tov* discusses a test for determining who was sterile and who was fertile. R. Tuviah b. Eliezer (ninth century) recommended placing a man's semen in a cup of cold water. If the semen takes the shape of a man, then he is fertile and if not, he is sterile. For a woman, R. Tuviah recommended taking the leaf of a pumpkin and having the woman urinate on this leaf. If the leaf dries up, the woman is sterile, and if not, she is fertile.[58] This experiment is suggested in the medieval Latin medical treatises known as the *Trotula* as well.[59] Most of the techniques proposed in the Jewish sources for testing sterility involve examining women. They include inserting garlic into the womb of the barren woman as well as a number of magical cures, such as using the placenta of a woman who had given birth in order to aid conception.[60] Christian medical writings also include similar cures and it seems that the fertility tests and cures were common to Jews and Christians.[61]

These examples illustrate medieval society's concern with solving infertility problems. In some cases, however, these problems could not be solved. Were there differences between the ways Jews and Christians dealt with couples diagnosed as infertile? Given the differing attitudes toward divorce and procreation, we would expect Jewish and Christian legal authorities to propose different solutions in difficult cases.

Infertility As Grounds for Divorce

In medieval Christian society, if one spouse was diagnosed as barren, sterility could serve as grounds for divorce. This issue, however, was highly controversial. During the first centuries of Christianity, sterility was seen as grounds for divorce whether the husband or the wife was held responsible for the problem. This was also the prevailing attitude in the early Middle Ages and was, to some extent, strengthened by Germanic attitudes toward fertility. However, in the eighth and ninth centuries, the question of fertility as grounds for divorce was reappraised, and new distinctions were introduced.[62] Theologians suggested distinguishing between situations in which sterility was a problem from the onset of a relationship and situations in which sterility ensued at some point after marriage. From the ninth century onward, it became much more difficult to invoke infertility as grounds for divorce, especially if the couple was not sterile at the start of their conjugal relationship. A woman who complained that her husband was incapable of fathering a child could still obtain an annulment in some cases, but, as part of the attempt to limit the number of legally separated couples, this became increasingly difficult. Accusations concerning infertility were investigated very thoroughly. Although impotence was generally accepted as grounds for divorce, the proofs of impotence were highly disputed. Often, professionals such as midwives were employed in order to verify such charges. If a man charged his wife with impotence, they would check the woman and, in some cases, the man as well.[63]

It is illuminating to compare the developments of Jewish attitudes toward divorce in Ashkenaz, specifically in cases of infertility, to Christian developments in the Middle Ages. There is, of course, a fundamental difference between Jewish and Christian attitudes: In Jewish society, divorce was viewed more positively and was regularly contracted. Hence, in our study of attitudes toward divorce in cases of infertility, we will need to compare and contrast Jewish and

Christian positions. First, however, a few words concerning divorce and change are in order.

One of the most famous developments regarding Jewish family law in the Middle Ages in Ashkenaz concerns divorce and occurred during the tenth or eleventh century, the same period in which Christian scholars were reassessing and severely limiting divorce in Christian society. According to Jewish law, the divorce writ (*get*) is given by a man to his wife. Consequently, if a woman instigated a divorce claim, a refusal on the part of her husband, to give her a writ of divorce, was a major obstacle. The famous *Takkanot* (Statutes) attributed to R. Gershom (ca. 960–ca. 1028), *Me'or haGolah* (Light of the Exile), decreed that a man cannot marry two women and, more important, that a man cannot divorce his wife against her will. Although different interpretations of this decree have been suggested, and the exact date at which his mandates became law is debatable, there is no doubt that these issues were central during the formative years preceding the Crusades, and that R. Gershom's rulings were the standard from the twelfth century onward.[64]

The problem of infertility was just one issue linked to the ban of bigamy and that of divorce without the wife's consent. However, infertility is an important instance, since it was a condition to which R. Gershom's prohibition against divorcing a woman against her will did not apply. In cases in which the woman was found to be infertile, the situation was governed by the gendered obligation of procreation. According to Tractate Yevamot, a woman is considered barren if she has not borne a child during a ten-year period. I such cases, her husband was expected to divorce her and marry another woman, so that he might fulfill the religious obligation of procreation. During the Middle Ages in Ashkenaz, men were expected to wait ten years before initiating such a divorce process. Once ten years had passed, men were supposed to divorce their wives and move on. According to the tradition passed down by different legal authorities, and despite R. Gershom's ruling prohibiting divorcing a woman against her will, in this case, the religious obligation demanded that the man divorce his wife. Yet the influence of R. Gershom's ban complicated matters. If prior to his ruling, a man could have married a second woman in order to demonstrate his virility, he now had to divorce his first wife in order to do so. In cases in which both husband and wife claimed that the other was to blame for infertility, the ban limited opportunities for justifying the man's claim.[65]

Attitudes toward the issue of female infertility changed during the course of the Middle Ages as well. Elimelekh Westreich has argued that during the tenth and eleventh centuries, in the case of couples who tried to conceive for ten years without interruption and failed to do so, female infertility was cited as legitimate cause for divorce. In these cases, R. Gershom's ban notwithstanding, the man was supposed to be forced to divorce his wife and marry another woman. In the twelfth century, this approach underwent substantial change. Subsequent to the ruling of the Ra'aban (R. Eliezer b. Nathan, (ca. 1090–ca.

1170), less importance was attributed to procreation. Men were no longer forced to divorce their infertile wives and were certainly not allowed to marry a second woman in order to fulfill the commandment of procreation.[66]

The attitudes of the German and French sages to infertility varied according to the problem at hand. A woman demanding a divorce writ on grounds of her husbands' impotence suffered consequences far different than those undergone by a man claiming that his wife was barren. Since women were not commanded to procreate, they could not claim, as the men did, that they were kept from fulfilling a religious obligation. There were, however, other arguments they could enlist in order to facilitate a divorce. A woman could argue that without offspring, she would remain lonely at the end of her days and become a burden on society. The Aramaic expression "I wish to have a staff in my hand and a spade for my burial" (*ḥutra ledah umara lek'vurah*)[67] is used to exemplify the idea that these women want children so that they will have someone to provide for them in old age. This idea expresses the belief in the inherent need of women to be mothers. It also is a telling comment on women's position in the ideological framework. As they have no religious obligation to procreate, they cannot make claims based on religious grounds to justify their demand for divorce. Women could, however, make claims based on what were perceived to be their natural qualities, or perhaps, what was seen by the society as their natural weakness. A woman whose nature is "not to conquer" is "naturally" expected to need and desire children so as not to be lonely and bitter in her old age.

The main point that comes up again and again is, however, the legislators' reluctance to intervene in issues that involved trusting women about male infertility. The legislators voiced the fear that women might lie in order to be released from an undesirable marriage. They also expressed hesitation in accepting women's testimony on their husband's impotence, since according to Jewish law, women's testimony is not valid. However, the Mishna and the Talmud already stated that in cases dealing with infertility, women are to be believed.[68] The issue was also one of great discomfort, since accusing a man of infertility was an embarrassing ordeal.

By law, releasing women from marriage in impotence cases often involved not only a writ of divorce, but also the return of a sum of money from the *ketubbah* (marriage agreement) to the divorcee. This money was often the locus of argument between spouses during the Middle Ages. The enforcement of the ruling accepting a wife's testimony and the returning of the ketubbah money underwent change in the course of the Middle Ages. In the eleventh century, Rashi commented on the divorce of a woman whose husband was impotent, stating that she is to be divorced and given her ketubbah monies. At the same time, he makes a comment that implies that this divorce was less automatic than might be assumed. He says: "One should ask him to give her a writ of divorce, but one does not force him."[69] These instructions differ from the ruling in previous cases in which men are forced to divorce their barren wives. Rashi's grandson, Rabbenu Tam (1100–1171) restates the position that men whose wives claim they are impotent must divorce their wives, yet once again it is not clear to what extent this ruling was actually enforced.[70]

While the legal authorities agree that in certain situations men should be forcefully persuaded to divorce their wives, we can also discern changes over time with respect to attitudes toward women who complained of their husband's impotence. As mentioned above, already in the Mishna we find a certain opinion voicing suspicions of women who might fabricate infertility claims. This opinion, which stood in opposition to the decision to accept women's testimony regarding the infertility of their spouses, seems to have been widely accepted by the Ge'onim in Babylon. In the Middle Ages, if the husband denied his impotence, the woman was not immediately believed. Those supporting the ruling accepting a woman's testimony, on the other hand, claimed that no woman would lie about an issue such as this one. The reservations that are mentioned in this context are telling if we consider that there are no discussions in the Mishna[71] or at a later date, concerning men who unjustly accuse their wives of infertility. Only women are accused of making false accusations.

From the twelfth century on, the legal authorities accepted women's testimony but demanded that they pay a certain price for the right to divorce. In the twelfth century, R. Isaac b. Avraham (Rizba) supported the acceptance of women's evidence. His response, however, reveals how equivocal his approach was. He discusses a case in which a woman has been living with a man for three years and found him impotent. He tried to convince the couple to wait an additional year and explains that he himself had difficulties when he was first married and advises the couple to give themselves a little more time. It is important to note that in this case the husband himself admitted that he had difficulties. Rizba, however, poses the woman a new challenge. As opposed to earlier opinions, such as that of Rashi mentioned above, he says that the wife may demand a divorce but that she must forfeit her ketubbah. This financial measure was certainly a major obstacle for any woman suing for divorce, but the Rizba justified this requirement by explaining that only if she sued without demanding money could she be believed.[72]

A different responsum from the twelfth century, addressed to Ra'aviah, relating a case that seems to have lasted for many years, broadens our understanding of the way male impotence was addressed. In this case, the couple had been married for sixteen years and the husband was accused of being impotent. In addition to the wife's testimony, this man also bore the outward signs of a *saris* (eunuch). He had no facial hair and a high voice. His wife had been complaining for quite some time and had even gone so far as to lock the doors of the synagogue during prayers, refusing to allow her community to leave the synagogue until her plea was heard. This was a standard procedure in medieval communities when a person bore an unresolved claim against someone else in the community.[73] It seems that in this case, rabbinic authorities went to great lengths to convince her not to press charges and to attempt a conjugal union. Finally, they submitted a decision to grant her a divorce and give her her ketubbah. It is clear, however, that this case dragged on for quite some time and that this woman had to insist in order to retain her financial rights.[74]

In these examples from the twelfth century, the wife's complaint is eventually accepted and a divorce is procured for her. Yet it is important to note that in both cases, the wife's testimony is not the only evidence. In the case brought before the Riẓba, the husband admitted that he had a problem. In the second case, the husband displayed the outward signs of a eunuch. The many years one of the women in fact spent with her husband — sixteen — and the Riẓba's ruling that she give up her financial rights as a condition for divorce are evidence of the growing struggle women faced when demanding divorce and of the rabbinic attempts to limit their ability. The two twelfth-century sages examined here had different opinions regarding monetary arrangements. Riẓba thought that a woman who claimed her husband was impotent should forfeit her rights to her ketubbah in order to be believed, whereas Ra'aviah said that if her claim can be proved, she is to receive her ketubbah. During the thirteenth century, this issue is discussed further. Grossman has suggested that the increase in the number of impotence claims might have resulted from the regulations instituted limiting women's abilities to procure divorce writs. Consequently, one of the only claims available to women was an accusation of impotence.[75]

Although Riẓba's approach became the standard one, and women who claimed that their husbands were impotent were expected to give up their ketubbah, some authorities did not accept even this ruling. R. Meir of Rothenburg (d. 1293), who wished to limit the phenomenon of divorce, and especially divorce instigated by women, suggested that in his day too many women were attempting to procure divorces on grounds of impotency.[76] He thus argues that impotence should not be automatic grounds for divorce. His opinion, however, was not accepted and the Riẓba's ruling continued to prevail.[77] In short, women could obtain divorces if they argued that their husbands were impotent, but they did have to give up some money in the process, and this money was especially precious to a divorcée who probably wished to remarry. Furthermore, this accusation was viewed with increasing suspicion. In many cases, women came under pressure from various quarters and had to be both daring and insistent in order to present their cases. If we try to map out a general trend, it becomes clear that women's ability to procure a divorce on the grounds of infertility became more restrictive over time.[78]

The grounds for women's entitlement to a divorce writ were not religious per se; rather, they were based on understandings of women's nature and of her role in childbirth and procreation. Women's rights were restricted by a basic tendency to mistrust women and not accept their word against that of a man who claimed he was not impotent. On the other hand, we can see how, as a result of legislation such as R. Gershom's bans against divorcing women against their will and a relative devaluation in the centrality of the commandment of procreation, it became more difficult for a man to divorce his wife. We see here how "natural" understandings of women became religious factors. This is a good example of the difficulty in distinguishing between culture and nature when examining attitudes toward women.[79]

What is most striking in the comparative context is how in both Christian and Jewish society in northern Europe and, more specifically in Germany, the ability of couples to get divorced was revised and rediscussed throughout the Middle Ages. While Jews and Christians differed on fundamental issues concerning divorce as a regular social phenomenon, both societies shared the desire to restrict divorces within the frameworks that allowed them. Some of the influential Jewish and Christian figures mentioned here lived in close geographical and chronological proximity. Reginus of Prum (840–915) was born near Speyer and died in Trier, and lived in Prum not far from the younger churchman Burchard of Worms (965–1025), whose writings on divorce were highly influential. Both of them sought to minimize or prevent divorce as much as possible, and their writings were highly influential in the eleventh and twelfth centuries.[80] Both these figures lived in the Rhine area, close to important Jewish centers, and R. Gershom Me'or haGolah was, in fact, a contemporary of Burchard's.

It is clear from the medieval Jewish responsa literature that the Jews were acutely aware of the customs of their neighbors concerning divorce. We learn of this familiarity in a question that does not refer to infertility, but to other grounds for divorce. Rashi refers to Christian customs when discussing a case in which a man wishes to divorce his wife because she has developed a physical deformity that repulses him. He says that this man should remain married to his wife, as do the gentile neighbors, and he comments that this behavior is worthy of imitation.[81] This attitude seems to be the product of the specific geo-cultural milieu in which Burchard, R. Gershom, and Rashi lived, as such discussions of divorce and bigamy were not common in other Jewish diasporas, where the divorce process in cases of infertility seems to have been much more expeditious.[82]

Despite this similarity, we should note that this comparison is very limited, as it pertains mainly to infertility, rather than to other practices related to divorce. Infertility was only one reason for divorce in Jewish society whereas the majority of divorces were most likely the result of other marital difficulties. In Christian society, on the other hand, infertility was one of the only grounds for divorce. Recent research has indicated that the rate of divorce was quite high in Jewish society, but it is impossible to assess how many of these divorces were related to infertility. This basic distinction notwithstanding, this comparison certainly demonstrates shared attitudes. While we have no hard evidence of dialogue between Jewish and Christian authorities or communities, it is possible to outline a general trend during the Middle Ages, of authorities who sought to limit the cases of divorce. This development becomes all the more important in the Christian medieval context outlined above, in which marriage became an important sacrament and procreation an important part of this sacrament.

Fertility

Infertility is the exception that teaches us about the norm. Although it is not as easy to provide details about the lives of couples who were fertile, as they are not mentioned as frequently in the sources, documenting the norm is no less important. A basic assumption in medieval society was that fertility was the norm. A couple was expected to have children as quickly as possible after marriage. As R. Meir of Rothenburg stated in one of his responsa: "Most women conceive and give birth."[83] Although pregnancy and birth certainly concerned both men and women in medieval society, the sources we have, written only by men, provide a very partial glimpse of this reality. Not only were pregnancy and birth experienced by women, but in those times, these women were cared for by other women. This is not to say that birth was a private affair; the opposite is true. As recent research has emphasized, birth was very much a social affair, as the parturients were attended by a number of women in their communities. But birth took place in a gendered space, without the physical presence of men. As such, the extant sources provide only very partial access to the women's space of birth. The information we do possess on the birthing space, entirely written by men, can serve as a commentary on how men and patriarchy saw birth.[84]

The gap between the information we have about birth in medieval Europe and the knowledge that birth was the privileged domain of women has sparked substantial scholarly interest in the topic over the past two decades. Although previous scholars dismissed medieval birth practice as a topic too difficult to examine due to the lack of sources, recently, some scholars, especially feminist scholars, have been eager to investigate this world.[85] Approaches toward this topic, however, have changed substantially over time. While early work regarding birth treated the birthing process as a female space to which men had no access and in which common power hierarchies were reversed and women were "on top," recent research has suggested that birth must be viewed as an integral part of patriarchal society.[86] The existence of this female space was not autonomous and cannot be understood independently of the space of the society at large.

While birth in medieval Christian society has been the subject of intense scrutiny, the study of birth in medieval Jewish society is still in its infancy. Recently, Ron Barkai has published a book on medieval gynecological texts, in which he discusses obstetric treatises from medieval Spain, but no work has been done to date on Jewish society in Ashkenaz.[87] In the pages that follow I will discuss evidence for the birthing process in Jewish sources. Information about pregnancy and birth is discussed in passing in commentaries on the Bible, the Talmud, and in various piyutim. Some of the commentaries are allegorical and use pregnancy and birth as metaphors, while others sometimes refer to their own day and age in their remarks on biblical events. For example, in explanations of the story of Judah and Tamar (Gen. 38) or that of the midwives in Egypt (Exod. 2), we receive information on the methods of birth in the past and in the contemporary medieval period. Other commentaries explain the laws related to birth such as the laws of the parturient or of circumcision. Additional information can be found in halakhic codes, where mundane instructions on how to treat the parturient at birth can be found, and especially in medical treatises that document common methods of treatment. The information that can be gleaned from all these different sources illuminates the way in which medieval society regarded birth.

I will begin with the allegorical interpretations. From these, we can learn much about birth as a symbol in medieval Jewish society. Birth was understood as the end of a long process, one that was accompanied by pain, fear, and great danger. The parturient was considered in great peril during birth, and every birth was accompanied by the threat of death. The hours during which a woman sat on the *mashber*, (the birthing stool) were both treacherous and perilous.[88] As such, the hour of birth was, in a sense, a Day of Judgment.[89] This idea is expressed clearly in a commentary on the piyut for New Year's Day (Rosh haShana) "*HaYom Harat Olam.*" The author writes:

> "HaYom Harat Olam" [Today is the conception of the world] — for all of man's nourishment is meted out on Rosh haShana. Like a pregnant woman who conceives now and gives birth after time. For this is based on the verse "Like a woman with child, approaching childbirth, writhing and screaming in her pangs" (Isa. 26:17), so we are before you. For the world is impregnated with the deeds of people, good and bad, and on Rosh haShana all the deeds are accounted for and are judged and on that very day it is decreed whether to good or to bad. On that day the world is in peril until it is judged; just as a woman is in danger when she suffers in labor, so we cry out on that day. . . . And that is why we say, after the shofar is blown, [the prayer] "haYom harat olam." Because through the blowing of the shofar, God's mercy on the world is aroused, as if the world were just created. For in *Tishrei* [the month in which Rosh haShana falls] man was created; therefore we say "haYom harat olam." And in the poem "*Elohai gadalta me'od,*" there are 271 verses [*tevot*] corresponding to the number of days of pregnancy [*herayon* (pregnancy) = 271 in *gematriya*] for a pregnant woman . . . and on Rosh haShana the world is like a woman sitting on the birthing stool [mashber], and because a woman is pregnant for nine months, there are nine blessings on Rosh haShana.[90]

The understanding of birth as a time of great danger stemmed first and foremost from reality; death during labor and birth was not uncommon.[91] Traditionally, pain and death during childbirth were attributed to the sin of Eve. The Bible already states that the pain of childbirth is a punishment for that sin: "In pain you shall bear children" (Gen. 3:16). Later, the Mishna explains that death at childbirth is the result of laxity in performing three specific commandments—the separation of the *challah*,[92] the lighting of the Sabbath candles, and the observance of menstrual purity. These were known, in short, as *Miẓvot HaNaH* (*CHallah*, *Niddah*, and *Hadlakat haNer*).[93] A connection between these two explanations was implied. According to some commentators, the reason women were held responsible for these three commandments is related to Eve's sin. As *Midrash Tanḥuma* explains:

> For which transgressions do women die at the time of their childbirth? Thus have our masters taught (Sabbath 2:6): Women die at the time of their childbirth for three transgressions: Because they have not been careful in regard to menstruation, in regard to challah and in regard to the lighting of the Sabbath lamp. These three commandments are also from the Torah. . . . And why are women charged with these commandments? Our sages said: During the creation of the world, Adam was first. Then came Eve and she shed his blood in that he heeded her. . . . The Holy One said: Let her be given the commandment of menstrual blood so that she may have atonement for that blood which she shed. . . . Because Adam was the challah of the world, when she came and defiled him, the Holy One said: Let her be given the commandment of challah so that she may have atonement for the challah of the world, which she defiled. . . . And the commandment of the (Sabbath) lamp exists because Adam was the lamp of the Holy One. . . . But Eve came and extinguished it. The Holy One said: Let her be given the commandment of the lamp in order that she may have atonement for the lamp that she extinguished.[94]

Although the Mishna attributes a woman's death at childbirth to her failure to perform the three commandments that were her domain, and this understanding was accepted throughout the centuries, few medieval sources emphasize this specific cause of guilt. Rather, the consensus seems to be that at the hour of birth, all a woman's deeds are judged and not just her performance of these three female commandments. The author of *Sefer Ḥasidim* warns people not to gossip or discuss any bad deeds the woman may have done, since any reminder of her sins might tip the scales against her.[95] Instead, the parturient was to be prayed for. In fact, the first known mention of blessings for the sick connected to the reading of the Torah are blessings for the parturient.[96] These understandings again highlight the complex web of connections between religious understandings and biological and social realities. Many women died in childbirth, and, as in the case of many other deaths in the Middle Ages, the justification offered was religious.

The belief that women died during childbirth because of their sins is, of course, not uniquely Jewish. It might even have been of greater importance in Christian sources. In Christianity, the origin of pain and death during childbirth was also assigned to Eve.[97] Christians, like Jews, believed that women who gave birth without pain were not in Eve's lot. In Christian tradition, the Virgin Mary was regularly characterized as not having suffered at birth, while in Jewish tradition, only the midwives in Egypt were ascribed this quality.[98] In fact, as Ulrike Rublack has recently shown, women who did not suffer during childbirth were viewed with tremendous suspicion.[99] Pain during childbirth was the lot of women and they were expected to bear this pain with perseverance.[100]

Birth was also a symbol of the mundane world and its trials and tribulations. A central source in this connection was *Midrash Yezirat haValad* (The Midrash of the Creation of the Newborn), which was well known in medieval Ashkenaz.[101] The Midrash is based on Tractate *Niddah* (BT Niddah 30b–31a) and appears in *Midrash Tanhuma* as well as in medieval works such as *Likutei ha-Pardes*, attributed to Rashi, and other medieval manuscripts. The Midrash has two versions; one describes the fetus's encounter with the world before leaving the womb and after being born, whereas the other explains the creation of a fetus in great detail. According to the Midrash, the creation of the embryo is the product of cooperation between God, man, and woman, and is assisted by an angel called Layil (Night) "When a man comes to have intercourse [*leshamesh mitato*] with his wife, God calls the angel responsible for pregnancy and says: "Know that tonight this man is sowing the creation of a man." The Midrash also explains how the fetus is created:

> R. Eliezer says the man sows white and the woman sows red and they mix with each other and from them the fetus is created according to the will of God. . . . The white that the man sows, from it the bones and tendons and brain and nails are formed, as well as the white in the eyes. The red that the woman sows, from it the skin and flesh and blood are created, as well as the black in the eyes. Spirit and soul and image and wisdom . . . and courage — they are given by God.[102]

The Midrash describes the time spent by the fetus inside his[103] mother's womb and divides this period into three parts. It also explains that the sex of the baby is determined within the first forty days. These understandings are medical explanations that can be traced back to Aristotle's medical treatises on obstetrics.[104] For example, it was believed that the male's soul is formed forty days after conception, and the female soul eighty days after conception. These numbers also explain the duration of ritual impurity after birth, as mentioned in the Bible: forty days for males and eighty for females.[105] Consequently, medieval Jewish sources instruct expectant fathers to pray for the birth of a son during the first forty days of a pregnancy.[106] After these first forty days, they believed that the gender of the child had been determined; thus, they prohibited praying for a specific gender.[107]

Although medieval writings discuss the centrality of the father in the formation of the fetus and the development of the different parts of his body, the determination of the gender of the fetus was attributed to his or her mother. The extent of the mother's enjoyment of the act of procreation determined the gender of the child. This belief was shared by Jews and Christians alike.[108]

Medieval Jewish texts provide many other details on pregnancy and birth. Although it was commonly accepted that pregnancy lasted nine months, medieval medical sources understood that the term of pregnancy was somewhere between seven and nine months. Children born after an eight-month term were doomed to death, but those born after a seven- or nine-month term were healthy children. Some halakhic discussions, as well as exegetic texts, distinguish between these two possibilities. For example, most medieval biblical commentators understood the births of the ten tribes as following short pregnancies, whereas Jacob and Esau underwent a full-term birth, as it is written, "when her time to give birth was at hand" (Gen. 25:24).

These ideas on pregnancy had practical implications as well. For example, Hasidei Ashkenaz were very concerned about women giving birth on the Sabbath. Although helping a woman in travail was permitted and overrode the laws of the Sabbath,[109] Hasidei Ashkenaz preferred to avoid such an instance. They determined that the duration of pregnancy as between 271 and 273 days. Consequently, they believed they could calculate the day of the baby's birth. Thus, the readers of *Sefer Hasidim* were instructed to refrain from sexual intercourse on Sundays, Mondays, and Tuesdays, days that might lead to a Sabbath birth.[110]

These many references to birth and its processes in halakhic writings testify to men's intimate knowledge of this world of women. Although men were excluded from the birth chamber, they were well aware of the many activities within. We may even situate the physical location of the father during birth. One commentator derives the names given to Judah's sons from his involvement in their respective births. Judah's first son was called Er (literally, awake); the commentator explains that Judah was awake all night and listened to his wife's screams during labor. The second son was called Onan (lament), for Judah cried and lamented his wife's pain during birth. His third son was called Shelah, (literally, hers), since "the sorrow was hers alone, as he was at *Kziv* at the time of her birth." (Gen. 38:5) In the account of the birth of twins related later in that chapter, commentators remark on the birth of twins in medieval culture and the methods of examining and determining multiple births.[111]

The male authors display familiarity with the female anatomy of birth as well. For example, Rashi explains what the placenta is and says: "It is a kind of clothing that the baby lies in and is called '*vashtidor*' in French."[112] It is interesting to note that, in many of these discussions, including most cases of Rashi, commentators almost always provides a parallel vernacular term when discussing issues related to childbirth.[113] Clearly, the women who provided accounts of birth used these terms, whereas the Hebrew names were not well known.

In summary, our sources document both the religious and personal significance attributed to birth. For women, birth was the fulfillment of a social goal as well as a moment of great danger. For men, the birth of a child fulfilled personal and religious obligations, and family was a symbol of prestige and status.

Medical Care and Practice

When a medieval woman got married she immediately began to hope for the birth of her first child, preferably a son. In Jewish society, midwives accompanied young women to the *mikve* (ritual bath), and newlywed Christian women also consulted with midwives. Once a woman suspected she was pregnant, her pregnancy was confirmed based on a midwife's examination of her stomach and breasts.[114] During pregnancy, women were supposed to guard themselves from harm. Pregnancy was considered a period of great vulnerability, and amulets and charms, as well as incantations, were offered by midwives and others to protect the expectant woman.

Many took part in guarding and protecting the expectant mother. Men often prayed for their wives, as did other family members and friends as well as midwives and other helpers at the scene of birth.[115] Medieval sources often focus on male activities around birth, but the figures most involved in the practical aspects of birth were the expectant mother and the midwife. Both these female figures were supervised and accompanied by men — the father of the baby and others. For example, the midwife's employment was often contracted and always paid for by the father.[116] From this perspective, although men were generally excluded from the birthing chamber, their presence and opinions were strongly felt.

Let us turn to the figure of the midwife, who was central not only for the welfare of the mother throughout her pregnancy and birth, but also for that of the infant after he was born. In Hebrew sources, the midwives are called by a number of different names — *meyaledet* (midwife), *isha ḥakhama* (wise woman), or *ḥakhama*. The second name, *isha ḥakhama* is very much like the term used for midwives in contemporary medieval German and French sources — *Weise Frauen* or *sâges femmes*.[117] As noted above, the midwives were central to the birth process and they accompanied the women throughout the period. Midwives or wise women took care of women not only at times of birth; they also examined women throughout their lives and served, in essence, as their doctors.

In legal cases that required professional assessment of women's health, midwives instructed authorities on medical circumstances.[118] For example, R. Ḥayim b. Isaac Or Zaru'a (late thirteenth century) reports the case of a woman who was ill "in the place of urine." He explains that in order to determine the exact nature of her problem, she must consult with the wise women who know how to distinguish between the different parts of her body.[119] Another instance in which a consultation with a wise woman is mentioned is in the responsa of the Rosh, R. Asher b. Yeḥiel (1250–1327). He discusses a case in which a man accuses his wife of not being "like all other women" — in other words, that she bore physical abnormalities that resulted in female fertility problems. The wise woman is called to verify this accusation.[120]

The term *isha ḥakhama* served as a general name for female medical figures who served in different capacities, primarily providing care for other women, but also as general medical practitioners. For example, a thirteenth-century manuscript refers to a certain Marat Yiska who is called *"Isha ḥakhama leha'ir me'or einayim"* — a wise woman who kindles the light of the eyes (i.e., an eye doctor). The same composition refers to another wise woman who treated an ailing baby.[121] In many cases, the midwife is referred to as an *Isha ḥakhama meyaledet* (wise woman midwife).

As midwifery among Jews, like midwifery in medieval Christian society, was not officially regulated by the community, few records remain. Hence, the identity of these midwives and the course of their training are largely unknown. Nor can we determine how many midwives regularly serviced a given community. If, however, we examine references on gravestones and in lists of Jews killed in attacks throughout the Middle Ages, and include the midwives mentioned in fourteenth-century tax lists, a rough sketch of these female professionals emerges. Midwifery was one of the most highly regarded female occupations. Consequently, it earns special mention in several different sources.[122] It is one of only two female occupations noted on gravestones, along with women who served as prayer leaders (*Mitpallelot haNashim*).[123] Their professional status seems to have become part of the midwife's identity — it also appears in listings of women's gifts to charity. For example, in the list of gifts donated in Nürnberg, one woman, Marat Rikhẓena the Midwife (meyaledet) is listed as having donated money to both the cemetery and the synagogue.[124]

All the midwives referred to in the sources have a few common attributes. They are all described as being widows and grandmothers.[125] For example: A tax list from 1338 mentions two midwives: Schönfraw, die Hebamme; and Seklin, die Hebamme — both are described as widows.[126] We cannot determine, however, if they were the sole midwives of the community.[127] Although we know nothing more about any of these women, they were clearly not young mothers. Many other midwives are referred to as mothers of adult children, grandmothers, and even great-grandmothers. Although women who were grandmothers might certainly have been young enough to bear additional children of their own, they were clearly at a later stage in life. They already had grown children of their own and were no longer tied down by obligations to their own small children.[128]

The grandmotherly age of these Jewish midwives as well as their professional status corresponds with what we know about Christian midwives. As in medieval Jewish sources, our information on Christian midwives is rather sparse, since extant legislation concerning midwifery dates only from the fourteenth century. While the thirteenth century was a time of rapid change and increased legislation in the medical profession, midwifery was one of the last areas to undergo such change. A look at more plentiful early modern sources can confirm some of our medieval findings. For example, early modern records from both England and Germany attest that most midwives were older women who no longer had young children under foot. Most midwives were of the middle class and some only worked in periods when their families needed additional income. Many widows who were midwives began to practice shortly after their husband's deaths, as they were then in need of a steady means of support.[129]

All midwives, both Jewish and Christian, appear to have been mothers themselves. This seems to have been a requirement. They learned their profession by accompanying other more senior midwives and by attending many births. Until the end of the fourteenth century, there was no formal period of apprenticeship. However, only those women recognized as professionals were called midwives. At the end of the fourteenth century, some German cities established licensing requirements for professional midwives, but no such rules seem to have existed within the Jewish communities.[130]

Our knowledge about midwives is hampered by the dearth of records on their practice. The secrets of the trade were passed down from generation to generation. Since the practitioners were all women, few could read Hebrew or Latin and the extent of their literacy is questionable.[131] The extant literature was written by men. Consequently, scholars have questioned the relation between these writings and the actual practices of the midwives. Many of the medical sources that have reached us from Christian Europe are Latin translations of Greek and Arabic treatises. Only one group of these texts, those attributed to the Trotula of Salerno, is said to have been written by women or based on the directions given by women.[132] A number of Hebrew translations of Greek, Latin, and Arabic treatises from Spain and Provence from the late twelfth century onward have survived. Among them is a Hebrew version of Salernus's gynecological treatise *Genicias*, as well as a Hebrew translation of one of the Trotula texts. These treatises, however, as well as others, such as Joel Ibn Falquera's *Zori Haguf* were not known in Ashkenaz before the fifteenth century.[133]

There is only one central extant medical source that we can be sure was well known in Ashkenaz during the High Middle Ages: the physician Assaf's book known as *Sefer Assaf haRofe*.[134] This book originated in the Gaonic period and contains cures copied from Latin, Greek, and Arabic sources. The German manuscript of this book contains some German medical terms as well as references to physicians in Germany.[135] There are several gynecological and obstetrical cures in this book, mostly translations of Galenus's medical treatise.[136] The information in Sefer Assaf is too sporadic to enable detailed understanding of the methods they employed. The same can be said for the references to midwives' practices in the halakhic materials discussed earlier. In addition, in the case of Sefer Assaf, it is questionable to what extent the cures he suggests were really used, as some of them seem very exotic. Moreover, due to their limited literacy, it is not clear if midwives could have used the book.

While references to midwives' practices may be found sporadically in a number of manuscripts, especially from the fourteenth century onward, only one text provides a glimpse into midwives' actual practices.[137] This text is the third chapter of the well-known circumciser's manual *K'lalei haMilah* written in the early thirteenth century by R. Jacob and his son R. Gershom haGozrim, the circumcisers (literally, the cutters).[138] The third chapter contains explicit references to its writer, R. Gershom, and therefore can be dated to the first third of the thirteenth century.[139] R. Gershom recorded the practices of the midwives in his vicinity and thus provides precious evidence of their actions.

R. Gershom's manual is of great importance for understanding birth in medieval society. First of all, it gives us a glimpse of cures used by Jews during birth, which included cooking herbs, smoking substances under the birthing chair, as well as the recitation of a variety of chants and incantations. The cures listed in the manual are similar to those listed in some of the medical treatises of the time, such as Hildegard of Bingen's *Physica* and *Curae et Causae*. More important, the inclusion of the birthing instructions in a circumcisers' manual enables us to better understand birth and its place in medieval Jewish society.[140]

Why was a circumciser interested in birth? If the practice of birthing was the job of women, performed in a female space to which no man was privy, including, by his own account, R. Gershom himself, why is he recording the cures? These questions bring us back to some of the questions raised concerning the involvement of men in the birthing process. The appearance of this circumciser in a central locus, passing on information he learned from midwives to other midwives by way of other circumcisers who read his manual, illustrates the intricacy of the politics of childbirth. Here we find a man placing himself in a position of authority regarding care of women in labor. If most midwives did not know how to read, then any circumciser who could pass on this information gained a new authority over childbirth. It would seem that this is further evidence of the deep involvement of patriarchy in the affairs of birth.

While R. Gershom's treatise can be seen as a sign of male interest and, to a certain extent, intervention in the world of the midwives, it also provides valuable affirmation of the midwives' knowledge and authority. The "wise midwives" (*meyaldot ḥakhamot*) are the ultimate authorities. They know how to expel the placenta and to identify and prevent miscarriages. They also know how to ward off evil spirits and deal with other problems that come up during birth. This stamp of approval of the midwives' authority is of great significance if we compare it with the situation in the sixteenth and seventeenth centuries, when midwives were often accused of witchcraft. As scholars have suggested, this accusation was specifically early modern and is not common in medieval Christian sources.[141] The same can be said of the Jewish sources. Although there are some references to older women bewitching women in childbirth, they seem to be the exception to the rule.

The references to these "bewitching" women and midwives reveal further details about birth and the identity of those involved in the process. For example the author of *Sefer Ḥasidim* relates:

> In one place where there were many women only few of them were pregnant, whereas in another place almost all are pregnant. They asked a wise-man and the wise-man said: "Know that I have investigated [and found] that in the place where they are pregnant it is because the midwives go with the women to the mikve [literally, in the text, 'the house of immersion'] and are happy that the women conceive; but in a place where few women conceive it is because those who go with the women to the mikve are not midwives and they bewitch the women so that they do not become pregnant. [And that way] they [the women] will often be menstrually impure and they will often [need to] immerse [themselves] and give them [the midwives] a salary. Therefore, one must carefully choose an honest [kosher] and trustworthy woman, so that she may be trusted when she testifies to proper immersion, and [she should be] a righteous woman who will not bewitch others so that they will [not] become pregnant, for it is easy to cast a spell.[142]

This source traces the very thin line between bewitchment and medicine and also illustrates one of the ways in which midwives were paid for their services. This source also reveals that midwives were commonly believed to possess powers to affect fertility.

Another example of a woman who bewitches others, in this case a woman in labor, can be found in Rashi's commentary on the Talmudic story concerning Yoḥani bat Retavi that appears in the Tractate *Sotah*. Yoḥani bat Retavi is mentioned as an example of a "gadabout widow" (*Almana shovavit* — BT Sotah 22a) who brings destruction upon the world. The Talmud mentions Yoḥani bat Retavi without explaining what she does. Rashi explains:

> She was a widow witch, and when the time came for a woman to give birth she would close her womb with magic and after she [the woman in childbirth] would suffer much, she [Yoḥani] would say "I will go and beg mercy. Perhaps my prayer will be heard," and she would go and reverse her magic, and the baby would come out. Once she had a day laborer in her home when she went to the home of the woman giving birth and her hired help heard the noise of magic rattling in a dish like an infant making noise in its mother's womb, and he came and removed the covers of the dishes and the magic escaped and the infant was born. Henceforth, everyone knew that she [Yoḥani] was a witch.[143]

Yoḥani's magic is also mentioned by R. Judah the Pious who was also familiar with the tradition referred to by Rashi. He states: "She was a woman who bewitched women so that they did not give birth, since the soul [of the infant] was in the bowls until she opened [them]."[144] It is important to note that

Yoḥani is not called a midwife in any source. Rather she is referred to as a witch (*makhshefah*). She does not help the women physically or prescribe herbs; rather, she prays for them.

I would suggest that this source does not indicate an ambiguous category of midwife. Rather, Yoḥani is one of a number of attendants at birth. As mentioned at the outset of this chapter, every birth was attended by a number of women. The midwife clearly bore professional authority. Also present was a woman who prayed for the parturient. This Jewish woman, perhaps a widow who was known to be righteous, would pray for the Jewish women, just as nuns often attended the births of Christian woman and prayed for them.[145] R. Gershom's text supports this suggestion. He distinguishes between different attendants and explains that the wise women encourage the parturient and give her directions how to "bear her fate" (in other words, endure labor), while other women, described as nursing the woman in labor, hold her down.[146] A similar division of labor among the attendants of birth can be found in the Spanish *Sefer haToladot*. The text describes a midwife who massages the laboring woman's body while other attendants explain to her how to react to her contractions.[147] Besides these attendants, a praying woman might also have been present. In the medieval texts, the midwife or the other attendants are not suspected of witchcraft.

As mentioned before, the midwives were responsible for the welfare of their clients, but many other measures were taken to safeguard women during pregnancy and childbirth. They were fed healthy and wholesome foods, and all their wishes were to be indulged.[148] Pregnant women were not allowed to leave the house on their own and were instructed to wear special amulets and belts. These amulets are mentioned in the halakhic literature concerning the wearing of amulets on the Sabbath. They are generally called by their Talmudic term "*avnei tekuma*." These were stones, some of them red rubies or garnets, which were believed to protect women from miscarrying.[149] A different stone mentioned in the sources is the *aetites*, which cannot be clearly identified.[150] Other women hung a gold coin or parts of an animal's body around their necks. A popular amulet was a rabbit's heart. Another custom of women was to wear their husband's belts. These belts were often embroidered with protective formulas.[151]

These beliefs are found in many cultures and were also part of the surrounding contemporary Christian culture. Beliefs concerning foods that were good for the pregnant woman, stones that protected her and her fetus, as well as belts, were all standard care for pregnant women. There were, however, clear religious differences between the Jewish and Christian practices. While we know that the Christian amulets and belts were inscribed with praises to the Virgin Mary and other patron saints of birth, such as St. Margaret, Jews did not use these same formulas. Hildegard of Bingen tells of a stone, sardonyx, that Christian women used during pregnancy to alleviate pain, and during birth to help expedite labor. They put this stone on their stomachs and prayed to Jesus for protection.[152] While Jews used similar stones during labor, they did not pray to Jesus. This is merely one of many examples of a shared culture with clear religious distinctions.

Not only were pregnant women protected during pregnancy, the rooms they gave birth in were also prepared to safeguard them from harm. One of the main threats from which the Jews believed women during labor and after birth must be protected was the figure of Lilith. Amulets were hung around the lying-in room and the parturient concealed an iron knife under her pillow. This knife was supposed to protect her, by summoning the Matriarchs — Bilhah, Rachel, Zilpah, and Leah (*BaRZeL* = iron in Hebrew). Large bowls used for magic were positioned at the entrance to the room. In addition, the midwives knew and whispered biblical verses as well as mystical formulas such as the verse from Isa. 51:14 "Quickly the crouching one is freed," which was supposed to expedite delivery. Notwithstanding the internal Jewish explanations given for them, none of these protective measures was unique to medieval Jewish society in Ashkenaz. Some of them may be found among Christians, whereas others may be found in other Jewish communities.

The affinity between the Jewish and Christian customs related to birth is evident in one additional issue related to midwives. As it seems that many medical techniques were shared by Jewish and Christian midwives, we might inquire into the relations between Jewish and Christian midwives and between Jewish parturients and Christian midwives. The issue of Christian practitioners attending Jewish women at birth is already raised in the Tractate *Avodah Zara*. The Mishna states that a gentile woman may assist a Jewish woman during childbirth, and the Talmud concurs, adding the further stipulation that the gentile midwife not be left alone with the parturient. The same law states that a Jewish midwife may not assist a gentile woman.[153] The reason given for this prohibition is that in doing so, they would help in giving life to a child of idol worshipers. Jewish women were not permitted to be alone with Christian women because of the fear that the Christian midwife might kill the baby.

These laws and the reasoning behind them seem to indicate a deep suspicion toward non-Jewish midwives. Some of the previous discussion in this chapter can explain this suspicion. While the techniques the midwives (Jewish and Christian) used were similar, the medical practice was accompanied by many other actions with a distinct religious flavor. Calling out to the Virgin Mary during birth was certainly encouraged by Christian midwives, just as the prayers uttered by Jewish women were distinctly Jewish. Religious beliefs were often part of the standard medical practice. This might have posed difficulties for Jews and Christians in particular situations.

In fact, Jews did employ Christian midwives, as the ecclesiastical rulings of the period demonstrate. The laws prohibiting the employment of Christian midwives by Jews were reiterated several times. An examination of ecclesiastical legislation reveals, however, that unlike the prohibition against employing Christian wet nurses, which was reissued regularly, the ban on employing

Christian midwives was less frequently repeated. While the prohibition against employing Christian wet nurses is repeated more than fifteen times during the period from the last third of the twelfth century until the mid–thirteenth century, the employment of Christian midwives is mentioned in only three documents.[154] Even more significant is the fact that we find no prohibition against the employment of Christian midwives in the documents of the Third Lateran Council, whereas the employment of Christian wet nurses by Jews is forcefully condemned.[155] The only time the employment of Christian midwives is mentioned in Jewish sources is in restating the legal decision that they may not attend a woman alone. By contrast, Christian wet nurses are mentioned many times.[156]

The reason for this difference in attitudes toward the employment of Christian midwives, as opposed to Christian wet nurses, is not stated in the texts and one can only surmise its rationale. One possibility is that the smaller number of references to Christian midwives is a reflection of reality. Whereas every child whose family hired a wet nurse needed his or her own wet nurse, the same midwife could help a number of Jewish women give birth. Therefore, even if the community had only one Jewish midwife, she could help perform many deliveries, obviating the need to turn to a Christian woman for help.

A completely different argument for the relative paucity of references to Jews employing Christian midwives in Christian and, especially, in Jewish sources is related to the medical profession in general. It is clear from studies of the period that Jews regularly employed Christian medical professionals. Two Ashkenazic sources from the thirteenth century provide good examples of how widespread this practice was. On the one hand, R. Elḥanan (d. 1184), the son of R. Isaac the Elder (known as R'i haZaken) states that a baby should not be left in the home of a Christian doctor or healer for a lengthy period of time. He says: "As for a baby [male or female] who needs a cure from a non-Jew, it seems from [this ruling] that they should not be left in the home of the non-Jew on their own without any Jew present for a month or two."[157] Although R. Elḥanan's ruling aimed at limiting the time spent by a child in a Christian home, the details of this ruling reveal much. Children may stay at a healer's home for more than a month if they have an adult Jew with them, and they may also stay for a shorter time by themselves. This, in and of itself, is evidence of regular contact between Jewish and Christian medical practitioners.

Rabbi Isaac b. Moses gives his permission for contact between Jews and Christian medical professionals and states: "And it seems in my eyes, to me the author, that all this [the restrictions concerning the use of Christian medical professionals] is restricted to cases when the service is for free; but if it is paid for, it is allowed."[158]

There are many examples of the employment of Christian doctors by Jews in Ashkenaz. The Ashkenazic manuscript of Sefer Assaf mentions by name a number of Christian doctors who live along the Rhine valley. A story in *Sefer*

Ḥasidim mentions a Jew who held a Christian medical textbook in security for a loan.[159] R. Gershom's manual, mentioned before, recounts an event in which it was necessary to turn to a Christian doctor when the Jewish midwife was not successful in curing a baby injured during his circumcision ceremony. The baby was finally cured when the *mohel* (circumciser) went to a non-Jewish doctor and bought a bandage from him.[160]

The case brought by R. Gershom suggests that one turned to Christians for help only when other attempts failed. In his case, he tells of a Jewish midwife who also tried to help before the Christian doctor was contacted. Other sources, however, tell of contacting Christian practitioners immediately. For example, Rabbi Judah b. Asher (Rosh) tells of an eye disease he had as a child, which a Jewish wise woman healed after a Christian woman had failed to cure him.[161] These few examples display some of the many contacts that existed between Jews and non-Jewish medical professionals. Although we find some preference for using a Jewish practitioner, it does not seem to have been the general rule.

I would suggest one of two possibilities with regard to the employment of Christian midwives. The first option is that Jews preferred to employ Jewish midwives whenever possible. If so, the relative indifference of Christian law to the employment of Christian midwives by Jews reflects the application of this principle in practice. Another option would be that Jews employed Christian midwives routinely, as they did Christian doctors. But as medical professionals, unlike wet nurses or servants, did not have to live in the home, church authorities did not see this relation as problematic, and few comments were made on the practice. I would suggest that the two options are not in contradiction; Jews regularly employed Christian midwives, although they may have preferred Jewish professionals. Perhaps in smaller Jewish communities, where there were no Jewish midwives, it became necessary to call upon the services of Christian neighbors.

Research done on midwifery in early modern Europe in recent years supports many of these suggestions. For example, studies on midwifery among minority religious groups, such as the Quakers in seventeenth-century England, reveal that they preferred to employ a midwife of their own religious group. Protestant women also preferred Protestant midwives over Catholics. At times, however, women of other religious groups were employed due to the lack of "in-house" professionals or as a result of the expertise others were believed to possess. In such cases, the groups made sure to have the woman in labor attended by one of their own number at all times.[162]

The fear of religious conversion of the mother during birth was real, as birth was a time of great pain and fear. Jews, like members of other religious groups, feared that a midwife of a different religious persuasion might convince a panicked woman to convert. While Jewish sources do not mention this fear, they often cite the words of the Talmud that warn of the possibility that the midwife might kill the baby. However, a number of Latin sources tell of conversion "miracles" at time of birth. For example, Vincent de Beauvais (d. 1064), as well as others, relates cases in which the Virgin Mary appeared to a Jewish woman in labor and convinced her to convert.[163] Early modern sources claim that some Jewish women called on Mary during birth, praying for her help, even when they did not intend to convert.[164]

The great fear that seized women at the time of birth and which made birth seem like a Judgment Day had other consequences besides conversion. Among Christians, many women confessed as they went into labor, so that if they died during childbirth they would be absolved of their sins. Many women revealed secrets, including the conception of children out of wedlock. In fact, midwives were considered prime witnesses in paternity suits in medieval Christian society.[165] *Sefer Ḥasidim* also relates a case in which a woman revealed the true paternity of her child while in labor.[166] It is possible that women preferred to reveal these secrets to midwives of their own religious persuasion.

There was an additional element of the Christian midwife's practice that might have deterred Jews from employing them. Midwives were responsible not only for the mothers, but also for the infants after birth. Not only did they clean and check the babies after they were born, but they also performed a religious function. Christian society displayed a growing concern with the need to baptize babies as quickly as possible so that they would be admitted to heaven if they died. From the early thirteenth century on, it became customary for midwives to baptize babies in the vernacular. If the baby survived, this action was confirmed by a member of the clergy.[167] Perhaps some Jews feared that a Christian midwife might baptize their babies.

Although they bore mutual suspicions and Jews preferred Jewish midwives, Jewish and Christian women remained in daily contact. It is likely that, just as Jewish and Christian doctors were in constant contact, so too were the midwives. We also know that Jewish and Christian women exchanged remedies.[168] Although we have no hard evidence of contact between Jewish and Christian midwives in medieval Ashkenaz, I would suggest that such contact was likely.

A Child Is Born

After birth, the midwife and the attendants devoted their attention to the infant and its postpartum mother. Usually, they prepared food intended to strengthen the parturient; a chicken was often slaughtered for her. In order to guard her and her child from any lurking evil spirits, she was never left alone. Immediately following birth, the baby was washed, sprinkled with salt, and swaddled. Salting, a widespread custom among Jews and Christians, as well as in other societies, was understood as a protective measure. The practice of swaddling was also widespread. Babies were wrapped in large cloth diapers in a way that was believed to help shape their bodies.[169]

The newborns remained with their mother and her attendants during the weeks following birth. If the newborn was a boy, he was separated from this group of women for the first time on the day of his circumcision. On this occasion, his father first formally recognized him as his son. After the circumcision ceremony, the infant was returned to the sphere and care of the women. Female infants remained with their mothers. There is no definitive evidence concerning their naming, a topic that will be taken up later in the book. The parturient rested in bed (known as the *Kindbett*) during the period following birth. Sources from the fifteenth century mention a lying-in period of five to six weeks, but we have no evidence from the twelfth and thirteenth centuries. In any case, it is clear that the first weeks after birth were spent with women who took care of the new mother and supervised the infant's welfare.

This brings us back to some of the issues raised at the beginning of the chapter. The process of birth did, in fact, take place in a female environment. Women were actively involved in all stages of birth. We do not know where the men were and what roles they played. On the other hand, when we turn to sources describing the ideological and religious understandings of birth, only men are present, while women are conspicuously absent. These two glimpses into medieval life seem somewhat disconnected. However, as this chapter has demonstrated, although men were not present at birth, they were part of birth and their interest in what went on within the birthing chamber was intense.[170] Although their involvement was of a very different nature, they too played a part in the dramas of pregnancy and birth. Men prayed for their wives throughout pregnancy. First they prayed that their wives would conceive, then for the conception of a boy and for a healthy pregnancy, and finally, for a safe delivery. The wish for male offspring was also central in men's involvement.

Sources also point to several male authorities who provided advice concerning pregnancy and birth. We read of R. Judah the Pious instructing women on which women should accompany them to the mikve. It is possible that some men had a say in their wives' choices of attendants. Rashi tells us that it was accepted practice for the husband to pay the midwife's fee.[171] Men were charged with summoning the midwife when the moment of birth arrived, and some of the chants and formulas used to protect women during birth were taught to the midwives by men.[172] In addition, patriarchal society expected women to give birth to male offspring. We have no idea how women felt about this, although it is likely that, given the educational ideals of their period and society, they too wished for male offspring.[173]

We can conclude that although the father remained outside the birthing chamber, his presence was felt within. The midwife was a mediator between the waiting men and the mother, both during and after labor. She took care of the expectant woman and conducted business with the father. She supervised the birth and related its proceedings to the men waiting outside the door, bearing the good news when the right time came. If the baby was born dead or died at birth, or if the mother herself died during childbirth, it was she who informed the waiting father. Although the midwife was often the one who informed the father of the sex of the newborn, some sources accept her testimony as to the hour of birth, but do not allow her testimony on the sex of the baby.[174] Perhaps they feared that a midwife might declare that the newborn was a boy in order to pacify a waiting father, and this might cause troubles afterward. In any case, this division of midwives' responsibilities accords with the other issues examined. She was to be trusted on practical matters (such as the time of birth), but not with the determination of the sex of a child. When a son was born, she mediated between the female and male space in an additional way. According to R. Gershom the Circumciser's book, it was the midwife who prepared babies for the circumcision ceremony.[175]

The circumciser is a second mediating figure. As will be discussed in detail in the next chapter, he turned a male infant into part of the male community. He entered into the female space both before and after the circumcision to check his patient. This relationship is supported by the text discussed above, in which the circumciser's manual includes a chapter devoted to midwifery techniques. This may be an attempt to supervise this area in which women were the practitioners.

Research on Christian society has illustrated symbols of male involvement in the seemingly female birth process. For example, Gail McMurray Gibson has argued that pictures on trays used for serving the parturient emphasize the male supervision that underscored the events of birth. Along these lines (although perhaps in a more forceful way), I would suggest that the connections between the midwives and the circumcisers, specifically, as well as the wider engagement of men both on the ideological level and from behind the doors of the birthing chamber, reflect male involvement in the birth process.

Birth was the moment of entrance into society. Girls were born into the milieu they would belong to for much of their lives — they too would be mothers in time. Boys had to start the process of joining male society. Both girls and boys had to become part of their communities. The ways in which these initiations were conducted will be taken up in the next chapters.

Chapter Two

CIRCUMCISION AND BAPTISM

> The baptism of Jews includes a peculiar custom: they perform it by cutting.
> —Wolfram von Eschenbach, *Willelham*

IN MEDIEVAL JEWISH SOCIETY, as in all societies, the days after birth were days of great concern for the newborn and his or her mother. Many ceremonies were performed to help the society and the family cope with this concern and to welcome the newborn into their midst. These ceremonies marked the acceptance of the baby into the community and were designed to protect it from evil spirits.[1] Jewish boys were welcomed into both their families and their community by way of the circumcision ritual that took place eight days after birth. This ritual will be the focus of this chapter. We will discuss the meager information we possess on the welcoming of girls into medieval society, along with additional birth ceremonies in chapter 3.

The circumcision ritual was a central religious obligation and a significant community event in medieval Europe. We find details concerning the time of the rite as well as the identity and actions of the participants in a wide range of texts. Because of its centrality, circumcision provides us with a window into the organization, hermeneutics, and practices of medieval Jews.[2] As a male ritual, circumcision reflects, in a condensed form, traditional gender divisions and understandings within medieval Jewish society. Since circumcision was also central in medieval Jewish-Christian discussions and polemics between Jews and Christians, it provides a useful case study for these relations and their social implications. We may better understand the specific social and cultural significances attributed to circumcision in the Jewish-Christian context by comparing it with baptism.

Over the past years, circumcision has been the topic of much research and discussion. Two books have been written on the topic, and a number of essays and collections of essays have been published. Nissan Rubin[3] described the practice of birth ceremonies during the period of the Mishna and the Talmud; Lawrence Hoffman discussed the development of the circumcision rite in Gaonic times, devoting special attention to its gendered implications.[4] The two authors utilize different anthropological approaches to circumcision and discuss their applicability to Jewish sources.

Both discuss three central approaches to circumcision in anthropological studies. The first approach, the psychoanalytic one, has attempted to integrate Freudian theory and interpret circumcision as an expression of the fear of castration. A second approach analyzes circumcision as a male rite de passage from childhood to sexual maturity and adulthood.[5] A third approach, adopted by both Hoffman and Rubin, explains circumcision as the Jewish rite of child initiation, the initial male experience the newborn undergoes. This approach, like the other approaches, does not analyze circumcision as a birth ritual, but as a male ritual. Although these two categories are not mutually exclusive, the emphasis on the male aspects of the ritual often comes at the expense of analysis of its life-cycle context.

Rubin collected the sources on circumcision from the Mishna and the Talmud and discussed the rite's historical development during that time period. He followed Eilberg-Schwartz, who suggested interpreting the circumcision ceremony as one through which boys are initiated into the "Jewish male cosmic order."[6] Hoffman treats two central aspects of the circumcision ceremony. He discusses the symbolic significance of circumcision, especially of the blood of circumcision, comparing circumcision to early Christian understandings of baptism, as well as the understandings of men and women in rabbinical thought, especially those of the Gaonic Period (eighth to ninth century), when the canon of the ceremony was fixed. Hoffman's study outlines the development of the liturgy and the interpretations of circumcision, but ignores the historical context of those rituals.[7] He extends his study to the medieval period and discusses the participation of women in the ceremony, a topic that will be central in this chapter as well.

Hoffman's and Rubin's studies will serve mainly as background for developments that preceded the Middle Ages. The medieval Ashkenazic circumcision rite will be our focus here, and, in contrast to previous research, I will not focus on the religious significance of the ceremony, but rather examine how we may gain insight into the values and social practices of medieval society through examining this rite.

Over the past decades, the study of ritual has given rise to a number of different approaches. While some have seen rituals as an expressive discourse on society, others have argued that rituals expose power structures within a given society, by affirming its hierarchy or, alternatively, by undermining the accepted social order.[8] As the circumcision ritual is the performance of an obligatory act and a Jewish institutional rite, it cannot be read as an attempt to undermine hierarchy or authority as a whole. The ritual does allow us, however, to examine the way this hierarchy is expressed, while also exposing tensions within medieval Jewish society.

The first parts of this chapter will discuss the circumcision ceremony as it took place in Ashkenaz in the High Middle Ages and will emphasize the changes in the performance of the ritual and in the identities of the participants. A comparison with Christian baptism will accompany this discussion.

The last part of the chapter will suggest a social interpretation of the ceremony and present Jewish society in light of this ritual.

Circumcision and Baptism: Historical Developments

The obligation of circumcision appears in the Bible (Gen. 17) and refers specifically to the circumcision of infant males. In later writings, such as the Mishna, the commandment of circumcision is included among the many obligations incumbent upon fathers educating their sons.[9] Scholars who have studied the ritual have pointed to several phases in its development. Although it is clear that circumcision was practiced well before the early centuries of the common era, we have no information on how the ritual was conducted prior to the Mishna.[10] The Mishna cites the blessings said at the ceremony but provides few other details.[11] The earliest sources providing a full description of the practice of the rite are from the Gaonic Period, in the Siddur of R. Sa'adiah Gaon and Seder R. Amram Gaon. During this period, two elements were added to the ceremony that do not appear in earlier sources—a prayer in Aramaic for the newborn and his mother, and a blessing on the wine, which became an integral part of the ceremony.[12] The custom of preparing a chair for the prophet Elijah was also developed at this time.[13]

The obvious parallel to circumcision is baptism. From the beginning of Christianity it was meant to replace the Jewish rite of circumcision.[14] During the first centuries of Christianity, the differences between circumcision and baptism were very pronounced, as circumcision remained an infant ritual, whereas baptism was a ritual for adults who chose to convert to Christianity.[15] The tradition of baptizing infants became prominent from the fourth century onward. Consequently, the parallels between the two ceremonies, circumcision and baptism, grew. A basic difference between the two rites remained, however—while only boys are circumcised, both girls and boys are baptized. Despite this central gender difference between the two rituals, a difference that also has implications for the understanding of broader differences between Judaism and Christianity, I will not address this issue, as its analysis transcends the bounds of the historical period in question.[16]

Due to the importance of baptism, the ritual was often discussed during the Middle Ages. During the early Middle Ages, the ceremony had a number of variations, depending on the locality in which it was conducted. The ceremony underwent reform during the Carolingian period, as part of an extensive attempt to uproot the remnants of pagan customs remaining within Christian religious activities and to unify practice. Some scholars have argued that the importance of baptism as a sacrament, in comparison to that of the Eucharist, gradually diminished during the Middle Ages. Nevertheless, even if baptism did lose some of its centrality, it remained an essential part of Christian practice.[17] The ritual underwent a number of changes during the Middle Ages. After the Synod of Canterbury (1214), it became increasingly accepted for infants to be baptized immediately after birth. In life-threatening situations, the midwife or father of the baby could perform an emergency baptism.[18] This act did not take the place of the formal baptism ceremony. Babies who were baptized immediately after birth, were not named right away, but in a church ceremony performed later.[19]

More central to our discussion is the reorganization of the institution of co-parenthood during the Carolingian period. The co-parents (often known in modern discourse as godparents) were adults not related to the infant who participated in the baptism ceremony alongside the biological father of the baby. They helped prepare the newborn for baptism and held him/her during the ceremony.[20] This role spread throughout the Byzantine Empire in the fourth century, and gradually became accepted in the western part of the empire as well, particularly under Charlemagne's rule, during the Carolingian period. Prior to this period, babies were prepared for baptism and escorted to the baptism font by their parents and other relatives. No co-parents were chosen to perform this function.[21]

The co-parents had relationships with both the infant they sponsored, for whom they were considered spiritually responsible, and the biological parents. Research has shown that the relationship between the co-parents and natural parents was considered the most binding. The most important role the co-parent had was carrying the infant to the baptismal font and back and holding him/her during baptism. This action, *suscipere* or *excipere* in Latin, was understood as a symbolic rebirth, meant to remove the sin of carnal birth from the child and turn him/her into a Christian. The co-parents answered the questions posed by the bishop or priest who officiated over the ceremony. In addition, they dressed and bathed the infant before baptism and often bought the newborn clothes for the ceremony — a white gown and a small white cap. At times, they also prepared a meal in honor of the baptism and gave the child additional gifts. During the early Middle Ages, it was customary for the co-parent to be of the same gender as the infant. Over time, more co-parents were added. In the fourteenth century, for example, one can often find three co-parents attending a baptism. The number of co-parents chosen varied by locality. In Italy for example, there were often three or more co-parents, whereas in Germany, from the tenth century onward, there seems to have been a concentrated effort to restrict the number of co-parents.[22] Relatives were not allowed to act as co-parents, and marriage between the co-parent and the baptized child was prohibited and considered a form of incest.

A number of studies have examined co-parenting practices in medieval Europe. For example, Christiane Klapisch-Zuber noted that the men chosen as co-fathers were usually of higher social status than the family who chose them. Parents often chose patrons or potential benefactors in order to cement the connection between the two families.[23] Women, on the other hand, chose their co-mothers from among their close friends. This gendered difference is certainly a statement on the roles of men and women in medieval society. When parents had to choose co-parents for their children, they considered the social benefits these connections would create and strengthen. While they did not expect the co-parent to take charge of the newborn's religious education (although this was officially one of their duties), they did hope for an economic agreement with their co-parents or at least for the promise of future prospects. Alliances like co-parenting should be viewed as a strategy for building partnerships and associations between different strata of medieval society.[24]

These findings have been reinforced by the research of two anthropologists — Sidney Mintz and Eric Wolf — who studied co-parenting practices (*compadrazgo*) in Puerto Rico. Wolf studied people in rural, lower-class society and discovered that they preferred to honor close friends and family members, feeling that they could turn to each other for help and support. Mintz studied people in urban, middle-class society and found that they, like medieval Christian urbanites, preferred to honor people one step above them in social rank. I will return to their findings at the end of the chapter.[25]

Before we compare medieval Jewish and Christian ceremonies, one more word about the relative functions of baptism and circumcision is in order. Baptism and circumcision were viewed as analogous in the medieval context. This idea resonates in passages found in *Sefer Niẓaḥon Vetus*, where baptism and its validity are discussed. The author argues that if Christian baptism is based on Jesus' baptism, then

> they should have imitated that baptism in all its particulars. In fact, however, Jesus and John were baptized in the Jordan, which consists of fresh water, while they are baptized in drawn water to this day. Furthermore, just as they derive the requirements of baptism from Jesus' behavior, i.e., from the fact that he was baptized himself, in the same manner they should derive the requirement of circumcision, for Jesus and John were both circumcised.[26]

The link between the two ceremonies is mentioned in Christian sources as well. Wolfram von Eschenbach (1170–1217), the author of the thirteenth-century novel *Willelhalm*, has one of his heroes say: "The baptism of Jews includes a peculiar custom: they perform it by cutting."[27] As both ceremonies are birth rituals, the speaker presents them as essentially the same ceremony, in spite of the different customs attached to them. The connection between both rituals is also portrayed in medieval art. For example a drawing in a thirteenth-century *Bible moralisée* from France (figure 1) depicts the circumcision of the Jews by Joshua in Gilgal, after the crossing of the Jordan (Josh. 5), as a kind of adult baptism.[28]

In medieval Christian Europe, the comparison between the two rites had immediate implications. The two rituals identified and signified Jews and

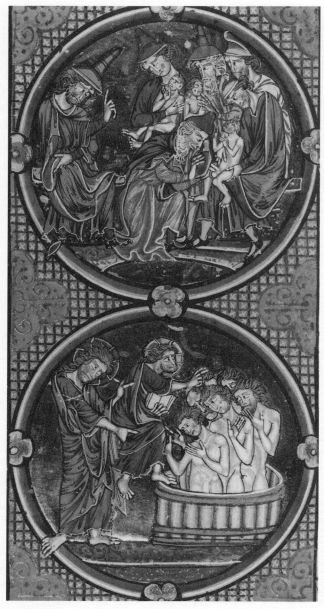

Figure 1. Circumcision and Baptism, Joshua in Gilgal. *Bible moralisée*, France 1220–1229, Vienna Österreichische Nationalbibliothek cod. 1179, fol. 63c. Photo courtesy of Vienna Österreichische Nationalbibliothek, Austria.

Christians, Judaism and Christianity. As the paradigm of the unique features of Jews and Christians, they served to mark the distinction between the two sister religions. Circumcision served the Jewish community as confirmation of loyalty and religious devotion. Baptism, within the Jewish community, was the ultimate symbol of betrayal and conversion during a period in which pressure to convert was ever present.

Circumcision in Medieval Ashkenaz

The liturgy of the circumcision ceremony remained almost unaltered throughout the medieval period with one exception — the omission of the Aramaic prayer for the child and his mother.[29] Yet despite this uninterrupted tradition, the medieval Ashkenazic ceremony introduced a number of nonliturgical customs. The ritual is described at length in many prayer and custom books of the time as well as in responsa and in a manual for circumcisers. While many of the questions raised pertain to circumcisions that take place on exceptional days such as Sabbath, the Day of Atonement, and the Ninth of Av, others describe the normal practice of the ritual.[30] These sources enable us to better understand how this ritual was performed and who participated in it.

The first unique feature of the medieval Ashkenazic circumcision ceremony is that it consistently took place in the synagogue. Evidence from the Second Temple period as well as the period of the compilation of the Mishna and Talmud indicates that the ceremony often took place in private homes.[31] We do not know when the ritual was first performed in the synagogue. Gaonic sources report that the ceremony could take place either at home or in the synagogue.[32] Early modern European sources also indicate a shift back to home ceremonies.[33] During the High Middle Ages, however, Ashkenazic sources consistently indicate that the ceremony always took place in the synagogue, usually immediately after the completion of the morning prayers.

The circumcision of a newborn was a major event in Ashkenazic communities, second only to marriage.[34] The relocation of the ceremony from the private sphere, the home, to the public sphere, the synagogue, demonstrates the importance of the ritual in the eyes of its performers and participants. The community at large participated in the ceremony, responding to verses recited by the circumciser or the person leading the ritual. Although these responses had become part of the liturgy earlier, I would suggest that the significance of having the whole community participate cannot be underestimated. We might note that one of the changes in the baptism ceremony during the Carolingian period was the relocation of the ceremony to the church, where it was well attended by the members of the parents' community.[35]

The sociologist Pierre Bourdieu, who discussed the way rituals, and especially institutional rituals, are performed, has defined rites like circumcision as rites of institution in which communities express their hierarchies and social orders. While these rites symbolize the way the community wishes to present itself, they may also express tensions existing within the social structure.[36] He notes that a useful way of understanding these rituals is by focusing on the participants in the ritual. As we saw before when discussing baptism, recent research has underlined the importance of the roles of the participants, and especially the co-parents. In light of this research and Bourdieu's suggestion, I now turn to examine the ritual of circumcision.

The Participants

Because of the unequal detail in the various extant descriptions of the ceremony, identifying the participants in the ceremony is no simple task. Later sources from the fourteenth and fifteenth centuries often provide more details than earlier sources. It is impossible to know if the additional details in the later sources are evidence of new customs, or simply details that were not previously noted. The analysis that follows is based on the combined information, drawn from all the sources. The examination of the circumcision ritual over time also provides a better picture of both the changing and the fixed details of the ceremony.[37]

The earliest detailed description we have of the circumcision ritual in Ashkenaz appears in *Mahzor Vitry*, a late eleventh- through early twelfth-century compilation of customs written by a number of Rashi's students:[38]

> On the eighth day of circumcision they rise early to the synagogue to pray . . . and they light the candle . . . and they set up two chairs and they spread a mantle [probably a Torah mantle], or some thing of beauty to adorn it. One [chair] is for Elijah who comes and sits there and sees the commandment being performed . . . and one chair is for the *ba'al brit* who sits in it with the child on his knees. And cloths are brought there for the circumciser to clean his hands with them . . . and they wash the child in warm water. And they dress him in fine clothes. A cloth gown and an overgarment and a beautiful hat for his head, as if he were a groom. And they carry him with pomp to the synagogue after the prayers. And the [people in the] congregation rise to their feet for him when the child enters. And they say: "Blessed is he who comes," and the bearer says: "In the name of God." And the father of the boy takes him and blesses [him] "to enter him into the covenant of Abraham," . . . and those standing there say, "As he has entered the covenant, so shall he enter Torah and the wedding canopy (*Huppah*) and good deeds.[39] . . . And the father gives him [the infant] to the ba'al brit. And he [the ba'al brit] sits on a chair and takes him in his hands. And the circumciser recites: "Blessed art thou who has commanded us to circumcise," and he circumcises.[40]

The description of this ritual, as discussed in *Mahzor Vitry*, demonstrates the importance attributed to circumcision and the extensive preparation involved in it, as early as the late eleventh century. This description emphasizes the beautiful cloths and clothes that adorned the newborn and the chairs on which the ceremony took place. Other sources mention that many of the participants wore holiday clothes and that the circumciser, as well as the father of the newborn and the ba'al brit, immersed themselves in the mikve before the ritual.[41] The text also contains many references to other participants—some mentioned by name and others who took part in the preparations, but are not mentioned in any source.

THE NEWBORN

The first and most important participant was, of course, the newborn. As he had no recollection of the ceremony, however, it is difficult to speak of him as a subject. He was prepared with great festivity and splendor. The ritual turned him into a full-fledged member of the Jewish community, from an uncircumcised infant to a Jew who could now theoretically eat from the Paschal sacrifice.[42] This change in the infant's status is apparent in the comments made by R. Jacob the Circumciser in his thirteenth-century circumciser's manual. R. Jacob says:

> Why did they instruct us to call the boy by a name immediately after circumcision? Because until the moment of circumcision, a name of impurity and shame was his, an uncircumcised name. And now that he is circumcised and the commandment of circumcision has been performed, his name must be changed to praise him, a pure and holy name like the names of his fathers Abraham, Isaac, and Jacob.[43]

The circumcision ceremony represented more than just the ushering of a new Jewish member into society. It was also the first formal recognition of the baby by his father, the moment at which he was officially named as the son of his father. Rashi comments that at the circumcision ceremony, the baby leaves his mother's realm for the first time and is acknowledged by his father. He explains the circumcision benediction "*Kol shiv'a*" (seven days) as follows: "Since until then, his father does not yet acknowledge him [during these days], because he has not left his mother's hands and entered into the covenant. Henceforth his father is obligated to recognize him."[44] This idea is also mentioned in the fifteenth-century book of customs written by R. Jacob Mulin (often called Mohar, Segal, or Maharil) (d. 1427). He discusses a case in which an unmarried woman gave birth:

> An unmarried woman gave birth to a son and she gave him to someone [*ploni*] and said that he was his father. And he said "this is not my son." And they wanted to call him the son of ploni, to say ploni b. ploni. And R. Jacob [Mahar"i Segal] warned them not to embarrass him with this, as he would not admit [his paternity].[45]

The act of recognition of the baby on the part of the father at the circumcision ceremony corresponded to a similar process at baptism. Baptism was not only a christening, but also a rite of acceptance into the immediate family and the community at large. Babies born out of wedlock or whose paternity was uncertain were also reminded of their status at the baptism ceremony. The absence of the infant's mother from the baptism ceremony centered attention on the paternal act of public recognition of the baby.[46] The shared social aspects of both rites of passage have frequently been overlooked because of the focus on the male aspects of the circumcision ritual, which have no parallel in baptism. I would suggest that in spite of the undeniably male aspects of circumcision, it is, first and foremost, an initiation rite into a social and religious group. Both circumcision and baptism can and should be studied as rites of passage.

One central difference does exist, however, in the transformation undergone by the infant in the two rites. Whereas Christian children were not considered members of the Christian religion before they were baptized, Jewish children were considered Jewish, though uncircumcised. In other words, the difference between being a Jew before and after circumcision was smaller than that between being unbaptized and Christian. Despite this apparent difference, however, uncircumcised Jews could not participate fully in Jewish rituals, and as such, circumcision did change their religious status. Furthermore, Jewish boys who died prior to being circumcised were circumcised before burial, albeit in a manner different from their living brothers. It was believed that this would expedite their entrance into the Garden of Eden, much as baptism was supposed to pave the way to heaven.[47]

THE FATHER AND THE CIRCUMCISER

The two other main participants in the ritual were the baby's father and the *mohel* (circumciser). Although legally, the father was obliged to circumcise his son, this task was almost always assigned to the circumciser, who was understood to act as the father's emissary.[48] It was considered a great occasion for a father to circumcise his own son, as it rarely took place.

The father's role in medieval Ashkenaz does not seem much different from what we know of earlier periods. The main difference is that while in other diasporas the father held the baby on his lap during the circumcision ceremony and was known, in some cases, as the *av brit*,[49] in Ashkenaz the ba'al brit held the baby during the ritual. The description of the ritual, as presented in *Maḥzor Vitry*, above, has the father taking his son from the ba'al brit, reciting the required blessings and then passing the infant back to the ba'al brit. The father usually hosted a large feast after the ritual and sometimes sent gifts to all his acquaintances present at the celebration.[50]

The circumciser's role did not change much over time either. A central prerequisite for any circumciser was that he be well trained. One of the contexts in which circumcisers are mentioned in the halakhic literature is in discussing how to choose a circumciser. The sources emphasize that expertise, rather than social obligation, was paramount.[51] They also discuss whether it was permissible for a circumciser in mourning to participate in the ritual.[52]

Recent research has indicated an interesting development concerning the circumciser's gender in medieval Ashkenaz. Sources from Antiquity that discuss circumcision often refer to women as *mohalot* (female circumcisers). The Mishna and Talmud discuss the case of a woman who circumcised her sons, who then died one after the other following the circumcision ceremony. The law states that if she has lost her first sons after circumcision, she need not circumcise her third or fourth sons (depending on the opinion accepted).[53] Two passages in First and Second Maccabbees also refer to women who circumcised their sons,[54] while the history of medicine provides ample evidence of the very active role played by women in all the medical professions in antiquity.[55] Furthermore, the Talmud discusses the permissibility of women acting as circumcisers (as opposed to non-Jews who are not allowed to perform the act) and rules that women may act as circumcisers, basing this ruling on the biblical precedent of Zipporah (figure 2).[56]

During the Gaonic period, we find little mention of women serving as circumcisers, although the Talmudic ruling is upheld in different contexts. Yaacov S. Spiegel has shown that the attitude toward women's ability to serve as circumcisers changed in Ashkenaz, especially during the thirteenth century. Spiegel described three different approaches to the issue of women acting as circumcisers prior to this change. One opinion, prevalent among the rabbis in Germany and northern France, permitted women to circumcise, without reservation; a second opinion, which prevailed among some of the rabbis in Spain and Provence and a small number of Ashkenazic rabbis, was that women could circumcise only when no man could do the job; a third opinion, which can be found in sources from the thirteenth century onward, stated that women could not perform the act of circumcision.[57] The latter two opinions became more common during the thirteenth century, and, as Spiegel has demonstrated, by the end of the thirteenth century, the third opinion prevailed.[58] It is possible that this change in legal opinion was of little consequence, as women were rarely called upon to circumcise babies.[59] However, as I will argue later in this chapter, this change is a significant indicator of a wider trend.

BA'ALEI HABRIT

Ba'al haBrit. In the description from *Mahzor Vitry* cited earlier in this chapter, a figure called the ba'al brit appears.[60] The description assigns him a number of different functions. He passes the baby to the father and holds him during circumcision. According to another manuscript of *Mahzor Vitry*, the ba'al brit also carried the infant from his home to the synagogue and brought him into the sanctuary. The *Mahzor* reports an additional custom:

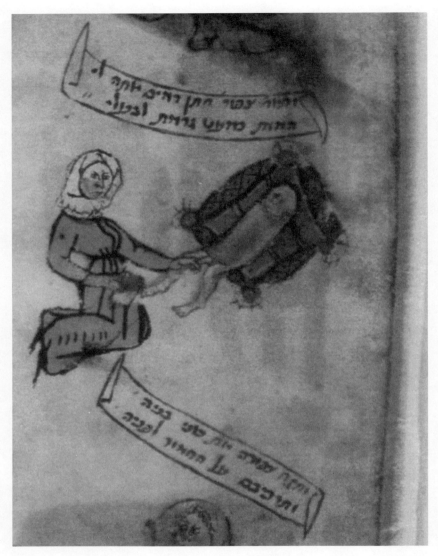

Figure 2. Zipporah As Circumciser. *Second Nürnberg Haggada*, South Germany 1450–1500, MS. 24087 fol. 13b, detail. Photo courtesy of Mr. Nathan Rome, Schocken Institute, Jerusalem.

The tradition of our fathers is Torah and a righteous man should adhere to it. On the eve of the eighth [day] the ba'al brit makes a feast in honor of the commandment. And after the circumcision, the father of the son rejoices with great drinking, eating, and celebration.[61]

In this short description, the tasks assigned to the ba'al brit and the father are nearly identical. Both host meals in honor of the circumcision, both hold the baby at different points in the ceremony, and, according to additional sources, both immersed themselves in the mikve before dressing in their finest clothing in honor of the occasion.[62]

The ba'al brit appears in many Ashkenazic medieval sources. In some cases, the sources discuss whether someone in mourning may serve as a ba'al brit. The halakhic answer reveals the importance attributed to this role. The rabbis ruled that people in mourning could serve as ba'alei brit, because of the importance of the task. The great significance assigned to the role becomes evident from the discussion in the fifteenth-century book of customs of the Maharil (R. Jacob Mulin):

When R. Mahari Segal became a ba'al brit, that which is called *sandek* in the language of the sages, he would wash himself and immerse himself so that the baby should enter the covenant in holiness. And he said: "The task of the ba'al brit is more important than that of the mohel, because his feet are like an altar and it is as if he [the ba'al brit] is sacrificing incense before the circumciser."[63]

This statement, that the ba'al brit is more important than the circumciser is somewhat surprising. After all, without the circumciser, the ceremony could not take place. On the other hand, without the ba'al brit the ceremony could take place without any difficulty and the lack of a ba'al brit was no impediment to the ritual.

The value assigned the role of the ba'al brit is prominent in an additional group of sources. The responsa literature discusses parents who promised friends and relatives that they would be honored as ba'alei brit.[64] These promises, made before birth and before the sex of the child was known, seem to have been standard practice. Halakhic issues arose when more than one person was promised the role of ba'al brit. The rabbis who responded to these cases acknowledged the fact that this promise concerned an honor that might never be performed — after all, many infants died at birth and there was at least a 50 percent chance that the infant would be a girl! However, they explain, that as these promises are routinely made, it is an issue they must discuss.

For example, a responsum from the school of R. Meir of Rothenburg relates a case in which the father promised someone the honor of ba'al brit. As the baby was ill, the circumcision ceremony was postponed, and, in the meantime, the father promised the honor to someone else. The query includes a plea for help, and states: "Please reply for these deeds happen daily and send us your ruling in haste."⁶⁵ The halakhic ruling in such cases was that the first person to whom the honor was promised should receive it.

Another issue that surfaced in these discussions concerns a case in which the mother of the newborn promised someone the honor of ba'al brit. The sources emphatically state that the task of choosing the ba'al brit is not hers. Even in cases in which the father is absent, some sources suggest that the mother should not make this choice. Rather, she should allow the people appointed in the father's stead to decide.⁶⁶ This issue, however, is raised only in sources from the fourteenth century, and I would suggest that the objection to women's choosing of the ba'al brit was not prevalent during the Middle Ages, and probably became more pronounced in the second half of the thirteenth century. I will return to this point later.

The Origins of the Role. One of the biggest questions concerning the role of the ba'al brit is when this role was first established and when it became important. While Ashkenazic sources from the twelfth century onward mention the role, there is little reference to the ba'al brit in earlier literature. In tracing the roots of the role, we must also take note of its additional name—*sandek*. This name, which derives from the Greek (σύντεκνος), is found in earlier sources from the tenth and eleventh centuries.⁶⁷ Although it was not used as often as the term *ba'al brit* during the High Middle Ages, it became the accepted term in late medieval and early modern writings, and has remained so in modern Judaism. The earliest source in which the term appears is the Midrash Shoher Tov on the Book of Psalms. The author of the Midrash explains chapter 35 of Psalms in which David exclaims, "All my bones shall say: Lord who is like you" (35:10). The author enumerates all of the different parts of David's body, which give praise to God, and when he speaks of the knees he states: "With my knees, kneeling at prayer; with my knees I am a *sandikenos* for children who are circumcised on my knees."⁶⁸

This Midrash is difficult to date, since it is compiled of sections belonging to a variety of periods.⁶⁹ It has been suggested that the Midrash can be dated to the tenth century in Italy. The passage that mentions the sandek, however, appears only in a thirteenth-century manuscript from Ashkenaz. In addition, as Buber remarked, the author itemizes all the parts of the body that thank the Lord and brings one example for each body part. Only in our case does he mention two reasons for praising this specific part of the body, the knees. Buber suggested that this is evidence that this passage concerning the sandek was a later addition.⁷⁰

The earliest source mentioning the sandek that we can date with certainty is *Sefer haArukh* by R. Nathan b. Yehiel of Rome (1035–1110). He explains the term by way of the example from Midrash Shoher Tov.⁷¹ The term *sandek* appears in Midrash Shoher Tov and in R. Nathan b. Yehiel's book, while we find it in Ashkenaz along with the term *ba'al brit*, I would suggest that this practice can be traced back to the Byzantine tradition.[72] This would explain why the custom can be found in both Ashkenaz and Italy.[73] For example, in the thirteenth-century Italian book *Sefer haTanya*, the circumcision ritual description includes two ba'alei brit, the "big" and the "little" one.[74] This seems to be a variation on the Ashkenazic custom of having one ba'al brit. In conclusion, although we cannot pinpoint the exact time when this custom originated, it was clearly part of the Ashkenazic tradition. I would also suggest that the frequent mention of ba'alei brit in twelfth- and thirteenth-century sources points to a new and heightened importance of its role.

Although the terms *sandek* and *ba'al brit* do not appear in earlier sources, we should perhaps look for people who might have filled the same role, even if they were called by other names. Obviously, someone had to hold the baby on his lap at the circumcision ceremony. Most sources from before the medieval period, however, mention only the father in this capacity and do not assign much importance to the holding of the baby. See, for example, a Gaonic source attributed to R. Nissim Gaon:

> The elders of the generation told me that on the day that [my] father, our teacher, Abba Aluf, brought me into the covenant, when he came to the synagogue with me on his arm, he sat for one moment on the prepared chair and then he stood up and placed me on the other chair of circumcision. And after he went out, they asked him what the reason for this was, for [they said that] they had never seen anyone doing this. And he said, I have learned from the elders that this prepared chair is for Elijah and he is the angel of circumcision and I sat on it with the child so that perhaps he would bless the child for me, that he find wisdom in his blessing.[75]

This story describes a different custom that does not include the ba'al brit. The father brings the baby to synagogue and holds him. No additional figure, such as the ba'al brit, is mentioned.

The thirteenth-century author R. Isaac b. Moses mentions the holding of the baby by someone other than the father and attributes this custom to R. Sherira Gaon (ca. 906–1006). He says: "Like R. Sherira Gaon said: It is a custom in Israel to prepare a chair covered with a mantle next to the ba'al brit out of respect for Elijah of blessed memory who is called the angel of circumcision."[76] R. Isaac's quotation from R. Sherira is meant to explain the custom of Elijah's chair and not the role of ba'al brit. This custom with the chair is indeed one that can be dated back to *Pirkei deRabbi Eliezer* (eighth century), where no mention of a ba'al brit is made.[77] It is unclear from this source whether this role is performed by someone other than the father and if in fact the ba'al brit is part of the same set of practices we are familiar with for Ashkenaz. Since this reference to the ba'al brit appears only once, in an Ashkenazic source of the thirteenth century, the claim that that this was a widespread Gaonic custom seems far-fetched.

In conclusion, the custom of ba'al brit was of great importance in medieval Ashkenaz. It was often promised to friends and relatives before children were born, and those who were promised the honor, but did not receive it, were offended. The medieval sources reveal a complex set of tasks that the ba'al brit was responsible for — carrying the newborn to the synagogue, passing him back and forth to the father, and holding him during the ritual. The role seems to have originated in the Byzantine tradition and gained growing importance in medieval Italy, Germany, and northern France.

Ba'alat haBrit. Until this point in the discussion, we have focused on the ba'al brit, as he appears in a number of texts. In one manuscript of *Mahzor Vitry*, dated to the first years of the thirteenth century, one extra line appears that tells of another participant, the ba'alat brit, a female ba'al brit. The line reads as follows:

> They brought the baby into the synagogue. The father of the son takes him from the ba'al brit and gives him to the ba'alat brit, and the people standing there say, "Blessed is he who comes," and the ba'al brit says, "In the name of God," and goes and sits in one of the chairs and takes the baby on his knees and they circumcise him.[78]

This source reveals the existence of a female figure and locates her as part of a synagogue ritual, in which the baby was passed from one person to another.

Additional sources provide further information about the ba'alat brit. One group of sources mentions her washing the baby before the circumcision ceremony. These sources discuss restrictions applying to circumcision ceremonies held on the Sabbath, particularly concerning the heating of water to wash the baby before the ritual. Ordinarily, a woman washed the baby. On the Sabbath, the task was sometimes performed by a Christian servant, supervised by a Jewish woman. In *Sefer Ḥasidim* a story is told about a woman who is called a ba'alat brit:

> It happened that there was a woman who washed her two sons and one drowned the other and their mother vowed never to wash during the day. Once she was a ba'alat brit and she washed during the day and died.[79]

The details of this story are unclear. Who did the woman vow to not wash during the day — herself? Her children? Any baby? Is she the mother of the baby being circumcised? The source does not make a connection between the woman and the infant. Additional sources indicate, however, that the ba'alat brit, like the ba'al brit, was not the mother of the baby. In a response from a fourteenth-century manuscript the following story is told:

> Once there was a man who had a son born to him, and his mother commanded him to make her the ba'al brit and his mother-in-law said, "I should merit it." It

seems that as it is the father who is commanded to circumcise him, he must fulfill his mother's bidding.[80]

This source does not provide details on the role of the woman acting as the ba'al brit, but it does speak of the honor connected to the task as well as what might have been a common practice, the bestowal of the honor upon one of the baby's grandmothers. No mention is made in the source of the baby's mother, her role in the ritual or her opinion in this argument. In addition, no men are mentioned in connection with either of the grandmothers.

R. Jacob the Circumciser's book *Klalei haMilah*,[81] as well as a number of other later fourteenth- and fifteenth-century sources, also mention the ba'alat brit. In these writings, however, she is the wife of the ba'al brit. Her role consists of bringing the baby to the synagogue:

> And the wife of the ba'al brit carries him with splendor to the synagogue. As soon as the congregation has finished their prayers, her husband comes out of the synagogue to meet her. He receives the infant from her and brings him into the synagogue to be circumcised, and the congregation stands for him [when he enters] and says, "Blessed is he who comes."[82]

R. Jacob's description differs from that which we saw in *Mahzor Vitry*. Here, the ba'alat brit brings the infant only as far as the synagogue door, whence the ba'al brit takes him in his arms.

Three names for the woman participating in the circumcision ceremony emerge from these sources: ba'alat brit; the wife of the ba'al brit (a term that defines her relationship to the other participants in the ritual), and ba'al brit (in the discussion of the two grandmothers who wanted to serve at their grandson's circumcision ceremony). Although these three terms are almost identical, they are not exactly the same. One explanation for the variety of names might be the fragmentary nature of our sources. One source (*Mahzor Vitry*) only mentions the presence of the ba'alat brit, but does not explain her role. Another source discusses her washing of the infant; a third source talks about bringing the infant to the synagogue, while a fourth only tells of the argument between the grandmothers.

In my opinion, the paucity of information and the variety of details in each source stem from the evolution of the role of the ba'alat brit. Before I trace the development of this role, I must consider one group of sources that can be dated with precision and that describe the diminution of her role. As these sources describe both her actual role and the intended changes, they are of great importance. A central source appears in the book *Sefer Tashbez*, written by R. Samson b. Zadok, a student of R. Meir b. Barukh of Rothenburg (d. 1293), who reports his teacher's opinion:

> The custom that is practiced in most places does not seem to me permissible: A woman sits in the synagogue with the men and they circumcise the baby in her

lap. And even if her husband is the *mohel* [circumciser] or her father or her son, it is not the way [of the world] that such an honored woman should enter among men and in the presence of the Shekhinah . . . especially since she is not commanded to circumcise, not even her own son, as it says "which God commanded him" (Gen. 17:23);[83] "him" and not "her." And if this is the case, why should they circumcise in her lap? Thus, they [the women] snatch this commandment from the men. And whoever can object should object, and whoever acts stringently in this case may he be blessed. Meir son of Barukh . . . About this that my teacher has written. And though I have cried out for many days, no one pays any attention. For it seems very ugly.[84] And even though they are occupied [with the commandment], their thoughts wander. . . . Is it for no reason that the women's section was separated off? Hence, this seems to be a commandment performed in sin . . . and every man who fears the Lord should leave the synagogue, lest it look like he is an accomplice to sinners. Shalom. Meir son of Barukh.[85]

While R. Meir does not use the term ba'alat brit, it is clear that the woman he refers to is performing the ba'al brit's task as she holds the baby on her lap. This source also explains the honor the grandmothers were fighting over. The ba'alat brit was not necessarily the wife of a male participant; she was an independent figure. The source points to possible relationships of the ba'alat brit with the circumciser, who might be her father, husband, or son, but no male figure is mentioned as assisting her. Some manuscripts change the wording of the decision and suggest that perhaps her husband, father, or son was in the audience. Yet, even so, the presence of the woman's husband in the congregation, does not tie the ba'alat brit to a male participant in the ritual.

R. Samson's words reflect the period prior to the end of the thirteenth century. *Sefer Ḥasidim*, R. Jacob the Circumciser's manual, and the manuscript of *Maḥzor Vitry* are all from the thirteenth century. The question concerning the two grandmothers is in a fourteenth-century manuscript, but probably represents an earlier period, as other sources from the fourteenth century follow R. Meir of Rothenburg's lead.[86] In these sources, the ba'alat brit appears only as the ba'al brit's wife. Later sources from the fifteenth century emphasize that R. Meir b. Barukh's ruling won the day and that, despite a struggle against those rulings, his instructions became standard procedure. The Maharil, R. Jacob Mulin, for example, stresses the importance of his ruling.

A picture in the early fourteenth-century Regensburg Pentateuch, representing Isaac's circumcision (Gen. 18:4), illustrates the changed procedure (figure 3). The first part of the picture shows women bringing the infant to the synagogue but stopping at the door of the men's section. The women, dressed in their finest clothing and jewelry, pass the baby into the male realm. The second part of the illustration shows the circumcision ceremony and the infant being circumcised by a male circumciser. This illustration attests to a custom similar to the one R. Meir was advocating. In contrast, an earlier illustration of

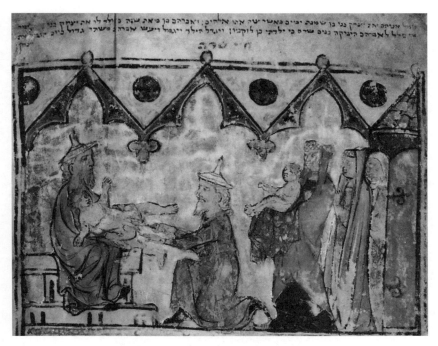

Figure 3. Isaac's Circumcision. *Regensburg Pentateuch*, Israel Museum, Jerusalem, cod. 180/52, fol. 18b, detail, around 1300 Germany. Photo courtesy of Israel Museum, Jerusalem.

Isaac's circumcision ceremony, designed by the famous twelfth-century artist Nicholas of Verdun, portrays Isaac being held by a woman during the circumcision ceremony. Although it is hard to reach firm historical conclusions based on this picture, it depicts the reality that emerges from the sources (figure 4).[87]

This survey of the sources suggests that before R. Meir of Rothenburg's time, women served as ba'alot brit, filling a number of different roles. Sometimes they held the baby while he was being circumcised, sometimes they carried him to the synagogue and/or bathed him. At times, the ba'alat brit had a male partner (who may have been related to her), and in other cases she alone served as ba'al brit. During the second half of the thirteenth century, objections to women serving as independent ba'alot brit were voiced, especially to their holding of the baby on their laps during the ceremony. The wording of the response, however, seems to indicate that this change was not effected easily. Samson ben Zadok states: "Though I have cried out for many days, no one pays any attention." He also suggests that the women are performing an uncivilized act and hints at the illicit sexual connotation of their deed by using the word

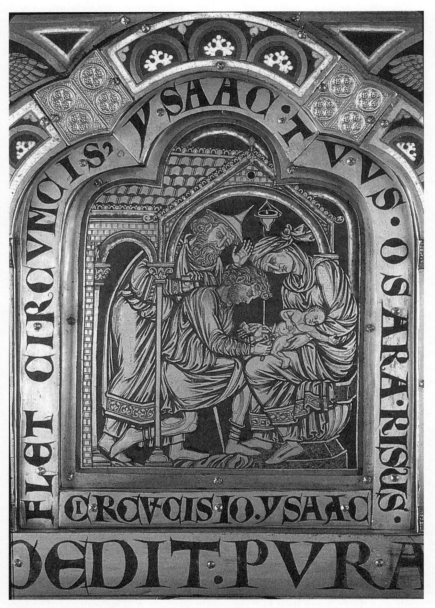

Figure 4. Isaac's Circumcision. Nicolas of Verdun, *Verduner Altar*, Stift Klosterneuburg, Klosterneuburg, Austria. Photo courtesy of Stift Klosterneuburg.

mekho'ar (ugly). His language is especially sharp, in that he advises anyone who fears the Lord to leave the sanctuary. These statements suggest that the change was not readily accepted, perhaps especially by women. After all, birth was an exceptional arena dominated by women; perhaps some of them saw circumcision as an extension of their responsibilities toward the child.

In light of these sources and our discussion of the role of the male ba'al brit, I would suggest that the role of the ba'alei brit became widespread in Ashkenaz during the tenth and eleventh centuries. The task was allotted to men or women and was called by the general term *ba'al brit*, regardless of the gender of the person who held the baby. Sometimes the ba'al brit was a man and sometimes a woman, but both options were common. The task comprised many roles and might be shared by several persons—washing and dressing the infant, taking him to the synagogue and holding him during the ceremony. The distinction between the ba'al brit and the ba'alat brit became more pronounced as objections to women's holding of infants in the synagogue grew. Although it is impossible to pinpoint the first objections, as there might have been an underlying dissatisfaction or discomfort with this custom throughout the Middle Ages, these protests became more audible during the thirteenth century, with the objections of R. Meir and others.

The changes in female involvement in the ritual may account for the wide variety of roles linked with the ba'alei brit in the fragments that have reached us. R. Jacob the Circumciser's account of the ritual, in which the ba'alat brit is the wife of the ba'al brit, marks the beginning of a period in which this became her accepted role in the ceremony, once she was no longer allowed into the male part of the sanctuary. In addition, the fourteenth-century sources' insistence that the prerogative of bestowing the honor of ba'al brit was that of the men, testifies both to women's desire to be part of the ritual process and the struggle around the appointing of a ba'al brit.

This desire is hardly surprising if we remember that during this period of the baby's life he was in the sole care of women. Women took care of him from birth to the circumcision ceremony and they resumed caring for him immediately after the circumcision ritual. R. Meir of Rothenburg and others wanted participants to be male, perhaps in order to emphasize the male character of the ritual. In a comment made by R. Jacob Mulin, the separation of the male circumcision space from the female birth space is conveyed very clearly:

> Our teacher R. Jacob Segel said: Maharam [R. Meir of Rothenburg] declared that the woman who is a ba'alat brit, and takes the infant from the parturient to carry him to the synagogue to be circumcised, should bring him to the entrance of the synagogue but should not enter to be a sandek and have the child circumcised on her lap. For it is an act of immodesty for a woman to walk among men. And he said that certain people who were chosen as sandikin, but whose wives were not with them, go themselves to bring the child from the parturient. But he [Maharil]

was careful. When he was once a sandek and his wife was not with him, he commanded that the child should be brought to him at the synagogue. For it is the way of women to catch onto the cloth of the one entering the birthing chamber to bring the child and escort him to the commandment [of circumcision]. And he [Maharil] said: If Maharam was careful that a woman not enter the men's section, among the men, he [Maharam] also was [careful] that a man not enter among the women, as the more one distances himself from women, the better it is.[88]

It is clear from this passage that the Maharam's ruling forbidding women to serve as ba'alot brit in the synagogue had become commonly accepted by the late fourteenth century, although we might read the repetition of the prohibition as a sign of continuing tension around this issue.[89] This source identifies gendered spaces filled with tensions. The space of birth, the birthing chamber, was women's space. Maharil suggests (and attributes his suggestion to Maharam's [R. Meir's] instructions) that men should avoid entering this space; he also reports the difficulties encountered by men who do enter this women's space. The synagogue, or at least the men's section in the synagogue, is clearly men's space, and women were not to be admitted. This idea of two gendered spaces, the *Kindbetterin*'s room and the synagogue, and the tensions linked with them in the context of the circumcision ceremony, is evident in a passage from *Sefer Leket Yosher*, the fifteenth-century book by R. Joseph b. Moses (1423–1490). He reports one incident in which these tensions became unbearable:

> Once there was a circumcision and the women were delayed in coming to the synagogue and a prominent [rich] man was the ba'al brit . . . and he said to the rich man: "Sit at my house." And when the women arrived at the synagogue with the infant he sent the *shammes* to the women [and said]: "Stand there and wait for us for as long as we have been waiting for you." And the women stood reproached until everyone knew of their foul deed, and the whole community thanked him with the exception of one scholar who said that it was an insult to the child, and that they [the women] should have been punished differently.[90]

In conclusion, while many scholars have pointed to R. Meir's restriction of women's role in the circumcision ceremony, few have attempted to specify what this role actually was and to follow the arguments conducted around it. The study of the role of the ba'alat brit, utilizing the variety of sources that refer to it, rather than merely the prohibition as it appears in *Sefer Tashbez*, brings to light a complex social setting and the tensions it contained. When examining the ba'alat brit in the context of the circumcision ritual as a whole, and not just as an aspect of female religious activity, this change takes on a new meaning. The role of the ba'alei brit was of great importance in the medieval circumcision ritual, as was that of co-parents in the baptism ritual. This change in women's roles evokes a context much wider than that of circumcision.[91] We will now turn to examine one last figure, the mother of the infant, before addressing this more general context.

THE MOTHER

One figure is remarkable in her absence from all the sources examined to this point—the mother of the newborn. Aside from a comment in a fourteenth-century source regarding her ineligibility in deciding who would be the ba'al brit,[92] she has not been mentioned.[93] We must ask where she was and what part she took in the circumcision ceremony. The source that describes the mother's presence most explicitly is also one of the latest sources included in our discussion. R. Jacob Mulin reports that the mother remained at home. He discusses the ba'al/at brit, who "takes the infant from the parturient to bring him to the synagogue."[94] The fact that the mother remained at home is also noted in other fifteenth- and sixteenth-century sources, some of which will be discussed in the next chapter.[95]

One must ask, however, whether the parturient stayed at home throughout the Middle Ages or whether this was a late medieval change. The descriptions of the circumcision ceremony that appear in the Gaonic sources as well as in *Mahzor Vitry* mention that it was customary to let the mother drink from the wine that was blessed during the ceremony. This custom was often accompanied by another custom—the sprinkling of wine on the infant. In Gaonic times, these actions were preceded by two blessings in Aramaic for the health of mother and child.[96] The Ashkenazic sources report sprinkling the child with wine, and some sources report letting the mother drink from the wine, but these Aramaic prayers were no longer recited.[97] Additional Ashkenazic sources from the twelfth and thirteenth centuries also mention the mother drinking from the wine. From the description of the ceremony proceedings, it seems that the mother drank from the wine at more or less the same time as the baby was sprinkled with it. The description of the ceremony does not differentiate between her and the baby receiving the wine. This would seem to imply that she was present at the ceremony and that a change occurred between the twelfth century, when *Mahzor Vitry* was compiled, and the fifteenth century, when the Maharil spoke of the mother being at home.

An alternative solution might be that the wine was brought to the mother at home. Many of the sources state that the wine was sent to the mother, using the verb *leshager*.[98] R. Jacob the Circumciser says the wine is sent to the mother (*lishloah*).[99] Both of these verbs could refer to the sending of the cup to the women's section or, alternatively, out of the synagogue. The Maharil's book of customs, for example, quotes R. Isaac Or Zaru'a and says that the cup is sent to the mother; we know that the custom in the period of the Maharil was that the woman remain at home.[100] This argument is strengthened by another halakhic issue. There is a discussion in the sources of what to do with wine used for circumcision ceremonies that took place on fast days.[101]

In such cases, the wine was saved until after the fast. This points to an accepted practice of drinking the wine, even if not necessarily in conjunction with the ceremony. It is hard to choose between this reconstruction of the situation and the possibility that the mother was present and drank the wine in the synagogue.[102]

Another issue related to the question of the mother's presence at the circumcision ceremony is that of ritual purity. Parturient women were ritually impure after birth. Some comments made in the literature that has reached us from Rashi's students mention that ritually impure women chose not to attend synagogue. Rashi himself, however, emphasizes that women who act in this way are especially pious and, moreover, that there is no reason for women who are ritually impure to refrain from coming to the synagogue.[102] In addition, the impurity of birth is different from other ritual impurities. Certainly, until the end of the thirteenth century, women who gave birth to a son were not considered ritually impure after a week. As Rashi explains, the circumcision ceremony was held on the eighth day because on that day the mother was no longer impure and could rejoice with her husband.[103] This custom changed at the end of the thirteenth century, when women started observing a longer period of impurity—forty days in the case of a boy.[104] Thus, purity practices prevalent until the late thirteenth century would have posed no barrier to mothers' attendance at synagogue circumcision ceremonies.

The evidence reviewed here is not conclusive, and it is impossible to determine the whereabouts of the mother with certainty. I would suggest that it is probable that mothers were present at the ceremony in many cases, at least until the end of the thirteenth century or the early fourteenth century. At that time, a number of changes took place: The ba'alat brit lost her active role, and, according to some of the sources, the giving of wine to the mother at the ceremony became a less integral part of the ritual; in some cases, it was not even mentioned. These developments correspond to a growing observance of a longer period of impurity after birth[105] as well as to a medical trend that advocated lengthening the lying-in period.[106]

In conclusion, our search for the mother during the ceremony revealed that the end of the thirteenth century was a time of change. Viewed together with the change in the role of the ba'alat brit, as well as in the permissibility of women acting as circumcisers that we saw earlier in this chapter, these issues seem to point to larger changes occurring in medieval Ashkenazic society.

THE COMMUNITY

The only participants in the ceremony that have not yet been discussed are the members of the community, the *kahal*, who took part in the ritual. As scholars have noted, the congregation was extremely important in the medieval ritual, and the ceremony usually took place immediately after the morning prayers. One can assume that the congregation was composed of the same group of people that participated in the morning prayers. The task of the participants was to respond to the verses recited by the father and the circumciser and to serve as a welcoming committee. These same people also participated in the two feasts — one the night before, and the other on the afternoon following the ritual.

The blessing chanted by the community, "as he has entered the covenant, so may he enter Torah, the wedding canopy and good deeds," symbolizes both the public aspects of the ritual and the connection between the circumcision and the baby's future life. If the blessing for a life of fulfillment of the commandments or the performance of good deeds is not connected to any specific stage of life, the other two blessings evoke two further status changes the boy will undergo — first, when he begins studying Torah and becomes part of the male world and, later, when he gets married. The community thus represents the society the infant will belong to, and presents, through the blessing, the stages of life the child will pass through in order to become a full member of the congregation.

The community in the synagogue is certainly the male community. There were probably a fair number of women at the ceremony as well — both because some women attended daily services and because such a celebration certainly drew others who did not attend daily. Sources from the fifteenth and sixteenth centuries suggest that some of the women remained at home with the parturient and that a celebration took place there while the men were in the synagogue. If, however, we accept the logic suggested in the previous sections of this chapter, it would follow that in periods when women had a larger role in the ritual, more would have been present in the synagogue.

Circumcision and Baptism: A Comparative Analysis

At this point, we may assemble the different pieces of the previous discussion. What similarities and differences can be revealed by comparing the Ashkenazic circumcision ceremony to the baptism rituals conducted by the Jews' Christian neighbors? How do they help us understand medieval Jewish social and ritual practices? There are many points of similarity between the circumcision ritual and the ritual of baptism: the white clothes worn by the infant; the carrying of the baby to and from the ceremony by a figure/figures other than the infant's parents; the importance attributed to the role of co-parents/ba'alei brit; the meals prepared before and after the circumcision ritual; and the washing of the infant and his preparation for the ritual. Even if, in some cases, these actions are ancient components of the ceremony, they took on new meanings in the medieval context, when a person was assigned especially to perform them. In other cases, we find new functions arising in the medieval circumcision ritual, such as that of the ba'alei brit. While we can expect any rite of initiation to involve persons who help and accompany the initiate, here we find shared features on many levels. For this reason, they require more detailed explanation.

The most apparent parallel in the two rituals is that between the ba'alei brit and the co-parents. This is also the most novel role within the medieval Ashkenazic community. Moreover, from a halakhic point of view, this role was not an essential component of the ritual. The ba'al brit was far less integral to the ritual than the baby, the circumciser, or the father who is commanded to circumcise his son. Hence, the roles of the ba'alei brit compared to those of the co-parents will be at the core of our discussion.

This comparison is suggested by the medieval sources themselves, in their choice of the term *ba'al brit*. As noted, this term is used in twelfth- and thirteenth-century sources, only to be replaced with the term *sandek* in late medieval and early modern texts. There are two other terms used in conjunction with these terms. R. Moses of Zurich explains that the sandek is the ba'al brit who is the *conpère*.[107] A different source, from fifteenth-century Germany, explains: "the ba'al brit, who is called *compère* and in my country *gevatter*."[108] These comments, using the vernacular term for the Latin *compater* as alternative terms for ba'alei brit, recount the terms the Jews used daily for this task.[109] Joseph Lynch, who investigated medieval co-parenthood in great depth, has commented on the vernacular and Latin forms of the terms. Arguing that the social function of co-parenthood was the most important, he has suggested that the terms *compater*, *commater*, and, *compaternitas* convey the importance of the spiritual parents acting together with the biological parents.[110] The Hebrew term *ba'al brit* conveys a similar idea, as the ba'al brit acts together with the person who is commanded to perform the circumcision, the father of the infant.

Over the past two decades, medievalists have turned their attention to the role of co-parents and especially to their social function. The work of anthropologists such as Eric Wolf and Sidney Mintz, mentioned at the beginning of this chapter, who studied contemporary co-parenthood practices in Latin America forty years ago, has also been central in historians' attempts at understanding medieval practices.[111] We will now investigate to what extent these explanations can be applied to medieval Jewish communities.

As mentioned at the outset of this chapter, one of the spiritual obligations the co-parents took upon themselves when sponsoring a child at baptism was the religious education of the godchildren. Despite the focus in ecclesiastical writings on the importance of co-parents as spiritual counselors and guides, this does not seem to have been the emphasis medieval Christians placed on the role.[112] In any event, this understanding of co-parenthood has almost no parallel in Jewish sources. While the ba'al brit was supposed to be a "good Jew," as R. Isaac b. Moses states,[113] there is no discussion of any future obligation of the ba'alei brit toward the infant.

This accords with another central difference between Christian and Jewish practice. While incest laws restricted co-parents' future relationships with the child they sponsored and his or her descendants, no such laws existed in the Jewish framework. From the Carolingian period onward, church authorities emphasized time and again that co-parents could not be relatives and that they could not be married in the future. As for Jewish society, we have no medieval registrar to inform us whether, as a rule, this honor was accorded to relatives or friends. From the rather sporadic accounts of circumcision ceremonies and their participants, however, I would suggest that both possibilities existed in Jewish reality. Although the parents of the baby were never ba'alei brit, grandparents and relatives were often ba'alei brit, as were friends. Since it was customary not to honor the same people as ba'alei brit for two children of the same parents, it is of course possible that any family with more than one son, or perhaps more than two sons, could distribute the honors to both family and friends.[114]

This difference between Jewish and Christian practices raises further questions. The first is why the Jewish institution of co-parenthood did not include the marriage restrictions that were part of the corresponding Christian institution of co-parenthood. The answer seems to be both social and ideological. From a practical point of view, in the medieval European world, Jews lived in small communities, often founded by a handful of families. Imposing such a restriction would have been nearly impossible. In addition, while medieval Christianity in general was marked by the development and expansion of restrictions on incest and marriage, medieval Judaism was not.[115] Thus, these differences between Jewish ba'alei brit and Christian co-parenthood were probably reflective of wider issues, which were only incidental to co-parenting *ba'alei brit* and the significance of each in the two communities.[116]

Recently historians studying co-parenthood in medieval Christian society have emphasized the social implications of sponsorship. They have suggested two main ways of understanding the function of co-parents. John Bossy has suggested that the role of co-parenthood was meant to mediate violence and aggression within medieval society. The connection forged between the natural parents of the baby and the co-parents neutralized tensions that might otherwise have been displayed in ways harmful to society. Ties of co-parents, forged between men and women of different social classes who were very unlikely to intermarry, facilitated more amicable relationships.[117] Bossy emphasized the cordial gestures that accompanied the ritual — the giving of a gift to the infant as well as the hosting of a meal by the co-parents. He also dwelt at length on the prohibitions that accompanied the honor. He was especially interested in the incest restrictions that such a connection introduced, and his analysis focused on the social-class differences between the co-parents and the natural parents. Bossy's approach is characteristic of a school of thought that sees ritual as a means of neutralizing tensions and fostering greater harmony within society.[118] The biological parents and the co-parents reached a higher level of affinity than they would have otherwise, while the restrictions that applied to this feeling of kinship helped supported the broader social hierarchy.

Over the past decade, another historian, Bernhard Jussen, has also dealt extensively with medieval sponsorship and baptism. Jussen has suggested that the ties of co-parents were not meant to reduce violence so much as to promote friendship. While his explanation is not very different from that of Bossy, he concentrates on how co-parenthood served political and strategic needs. He compares the understandings of co-parenthood and biological parenthood in medieval sources, suggesting that co-parenthood was both an expression of friendship and a means of gaining social status. As he says: "Sponsorship could either provide an official framework for useful relationships that already existed in practice or create such practically useful relationships in the first place."[119]

The work of Bossy and of Jussen is based to a large extent on Wolf's and Mintz's work on co-parenthood (*compadrazgo*) in Puerto Rico. Wolf and Mintz revealed different methods for distributing the honor of co-parenthood. Wolf, who studied middle-class society, found that parents chose to honor others of a higher social status. In this way, they hoped to protect themselves from future mishaps with more powerful persons, while furthering their relationships with people of higher social status. Mintz studied a poorer social group and discovered that they tended to honor close friends and even relatives (despite the religious restrictions), in order to strengthen their ties with their immediate surroundings. This poorer group believed that, in times of difficulties, only immediate family and friends could be trusted.[120]

Let us now apply these insights to the specific context of the medieval Jewish communities. As other research has shown, the small communities Jews lived in were often fraught with tensions. Honoring another member of the community might have been a declaration of allegiance or an attempt to make contact with a future partner. In a close-knit minority society, such as the medieval Jewish communities, the pattern outlined by Mintz, in which the immediate family and neighbors were most valued, seems to best explain the social practice.

Nevertheless, the differences between Jewish and Christian practices concerning the honoring of family members do raise questions concerning the function of ba'alei brit and problematize the borrowing of the anthropological interpretations suggested for medieval Christian society. While one could perhaps argue that the honoring of friends as ba'alei brit was part of the biological parents' networking and social-contact strategies, what was the social meaning of the honoring of grandparents and especially grandfathers as ba'alei brit? What function did honoring parents serve within the Jewish framework?

Bossy and Jussen pointed to the importance of co-parenthood in promoting goodwill and friendship in the often tense and violent urban environment. If we ignore the subject of violence within the Jewish community (which requires further research) and concentrate on the locus of families within the

Jewish community, we must ask: What tensions existed that the institution of ba'alei brit could alleviate? How could honoring a member of the family help in these situations?

Before answering these questions, we will compare the honor of serving as a ba'al brit to other honors distributed at rituals. This will improve our understanding of the role of the ba'al brit within Jewish society. Furthermore, in order to understand the tensions that were part of the workings of family dynamics, we cannot ignore the place of women in the circumcision ceremony. The changes in this area certainly attest both to the importance of the role of the ba'alei brit and to the social tensions surrounding it. By considering these different factors, I will try to explicate the function of the ba'alei brit in a comparative context.

Marriage

Marriage, as an agreement arranged by the parents of the bride and groom, was the ultimate attempt of families to coordinate alliances and cooperate financially in the premodern world. This was the case in both Jewish and Christian society.[121] Thus, an understanding of the workings of the marriage ceremony can help us understand the function of the ba'alei brit in the circumcision ceremony as well.

As in the circumcision ceremony, we find descriptions of the marriage ceremony along with instructions for its proper procedure already in the Mishna and the Talmud. As in the circumcision ritual, Jewish marriage rites underwent change throughout the centuries.[122] Unlike the role of the ba'al brit, which was newly introduced in the medieval period, the role of the *shushvin* is well known from the Mishna, the Talmud, and various Midrashim.[123] The shushvin, a role that some scholars have compared with the ba'al brit or the co-parents, provides a good example of some of these changes.[124] The shushvin was a figure whose task it was to help make the match between the bride's and the groom's families. In ancient times he also contributed, to a certain extent, to the financial standing of the young couple. In earlier sources, the shushvin played a number of roles: He gave the couple a gift, was an authority on all claims against the bride's virginity, and took part in the ceremony as well as in synagogue rituals on the Sabbath preceding the wedding.

The shushvinim are mentioned in twelfth- and thirteenth-century sources. There were usually two shushvinim, one from each side. They escorted the groom to the wedding ritual and were honored along with him on the Sabbath before the wedding, when they were called to the Torah.[125] The medieval sources do not provide any reference to their involvement in virginity claims, nor is there significant mention of financial involvement.[126] I have not found any evidence that might determine who the shushvin was — a relative or friend. Moreover, unlike the case of the ba'alei brit, we find no mention of complaints that a promise to serve as shushvin was violated. In one Ashkenazic source, however, we find the ba'al brit mentioned alongside the shushvin. The author of *Sefer Ḥasidim* says:

> Once a Ḥasid was asked to be a ba'al brit and to be a shushvin for a groom. He said to those who asked him: You would be better off buying yourself friends. Ask others and they will love you and I will consider it as if you had asked me.[127]

This source equates the two figures, as well as the honor of serving as a ba'al brit or shushvin. In both cases, the bestowal of the honor was considered a way to "buy friends." This interpretation seems to support Bossy's and Jussen's suggestions as to the function of the co-parents/ba'alei brit.[128]

We are still left with the difference between Jewish and Christian practice in bestowing the honor of ba'alei brit/co-parents on relatives. Even if we explain this difference, as I did before, as the result of differing Jewish and Christian understandings of incest, we must still determine the social function of having a grandparent serve as a ba'al brit. I would suggest that this may be linked to developments in the medieval marriage ceremony.

The twelfth and thirteenth centuries saw the emergence of new strategies of marriage negotiation in Ashkenazic society. One of the most noticeable changes was related to the monetary payments made by the families of the groom and the bride. Eleventh-century records show that marriage was an arrangement in which money changed hands. Up until the mid-thirteenth century, only the woman's family advanced money before marriage, in the form of a dowry, whereas the groom's family committed itself to funding by way of the sum promised in the ketubbah. A new ruling that originated in the twelfth century enhanced the position of the bride's family. Previously, once the marriage was contracted, the money was transferred to the husband's family, and, even if the bride died the day after the wedding, the money was not returned. In the twelfth century, a new ruling became accepted, whereby if the bride passed away within the first two years of marriage and no children had been born to the couple, the money was returned to the bride's family.[129]

In the mid-thirteenth century, double marriage payments seem to have become standard; thus, not only the bride's family, but also the groom's family, contributed to the young couple's economic position. Some scholars have suggested that this double marriage payment became necessary because the Jewish economy relied so heavily on moneylending. The new ruling was that if the bride or the groom passed away either before the birth of offspring or before two years had passed, the monies were returned to the respective families.[130] Although we have little information on this process, some of the issues regarding changes in marriage agreements are relevant to an understanding of the forces at work in the circumcision ceremony.[131]

This change in the dowry system was a response to existing social tensions; however, it also produced new frictions that the society had to cope with. I suggest that the role of ba'alei brit served to ease some of the tensions such negotiations must have generated. When honoring a family member or a friend, Jews were practicing what anthropologists have called "reproductive politics." As anthropologists such as Karen and Mark Paige have shown, ceremonies such as circumcision and baptism are often extensions of marriage rituals and can carry over tensions between the maternal and paternal families from the time of marriage to a later stage in the life of a couple.[132]

In medieval Jewish reality, the birth of a baby was the awaited outcome of all marriages. For young couples having their first children, the circumcision ritual was the first ritual after the marriage ceremony, if the firstborn was the coveted and hoped-for son. It was an opportunity for the hierarchy to proclaim its position. It is in this light that I propose that one of the keys to the social practice of having family members serve as ba'alei brit is linked to marriage arrangements in medieval Jewish communities.[133]

Women's Participation and Exclusion

In order to enhance this understanding, we must also examine the changes concerning the place of women in the ritual, emphasized in the first part of this chapter. In the response concerning the father whose mother and mother-in-law argued over the right to serve as ba'alat habrit, the justification provided for the choice of the paternal grandmother is the biblical commandment of honoring one's parent. As we have already seen, in all cases, the paternal choice was considered the most important.[134] Not only when deciding which parent to honor, but also in the case where the mother designated a ba'al brit of her choice who was not a relative, it was the father who decided, and the mother's appointment was invalid. The importance of the paternal family in this situation is striking. Although the patriarchal nature of Jewish society provides some explanation, nonetheless, this point requires further investigation. Why is the paternal family emphasized, and how does this connect to the ultimate exclusion of women from participation?

In the circumcision ritual, the families of the infant saw the connection they established in principle at the time of the marriage become actual. If the couple had a daughter, they of course would not conduct this ceremony, but in the case of the birth of a son, the circumcision ritual bestowed honor on others, and the paternal and maternal families once again asserted their relationship and status. In Jewish society, where children married young, and marriages were often arranged for them at an even younger age, circumcision was an event in which the couple was recognized as an independent unit with children of their own, and the connection between the families was reconfirmed and restated.

It seems significant that changes in marriage agreements occurred during the same period in which the role of the ba'al brit becomes significant. During this period, the paternal family, in fact, lost some of its previous power with respect to marriage agreements. I would suggest that we see here a symbolic reaction to this loss of power. While the maternal family demanded more for their daughters, some areas in which women had enjoyed relative freedom, such as the ritual front, were becoming more restricted. The tensions around the circumcision ceremony and the honor of ba'al brit reflect some of the strains that existed between the paternal and maternal families. The ritual honors granted to the paternal family compensated somewhat for the loss of their previous position.

The change in women's ritual experience connects in an additional way to "reproductive politics." Paige and Paige have argued that in patriarchal societies, rituals convey not only the communities' commitment to the infant, but also serve to display the place of women in society and the rights granted her.[135] If the function of the ba'al brit was to assert hierarchy, then the changes in women's roles reflect the struggles in this hierarchy. These struggles not only define the place of women (and their offspring) but also provide us with a prism of the society as a whole. As circumcision is an institutional practice, the social statement made by the performance of the ritual serves to reinforce its social message.[136]

Mary Douglas has also discussed rituals and change in similar contexts, placing special emphasis on the role of women. She suggested that conceptions of purity and impurity often underlie gender relationships and attitudes toward women within society.[137] While the participation of women in the circumcision ritual in the synagogue is not directly related to purity, their presence or lack of presence in the synagogue reflects prevalent gender interactions.[138]

It is in the ba'alat brit's function that the clearest change can be seen. While in the twelfth and thirteenth centuries (and perhaps even earlier), she is especially active — washing the baby, bringing him to the synagogue, holding him on her lap in the synagogue — after the thirteenth century, she was absent from the men's section during the ceremony. One must ask which part of this description represents the norm? Was it unusual for women to participate so actively in a ceremony at the synagogue or was the exclusion of women the exception to the rule?

When discussing the ba'alat brit earlier in the chapter, a central source dealt with R. Meir of Rothenburg's attempt to bar women from serving as ba'alot brit.[139] It is not surprising that this source, which tells us much about women's roles, is the source in which the practice was eliminated. By contrast, other references to the ba'alat brit, from the period after the practice was abolished, simply mention the ba'alat brit as the wife of the ba'al brit and provide few details. This is not extraordinary, since the role was no longer of great import. If the husband was chosen to be the ba'al brit, his wife automatically became the ba'alat brit.

I have argued that this change in women's role in the circumcision ceremony reflects tensions between families. However, it reflects additional tensions in society as well. The presence of women in the male section of the synagogue, an unusual occurrence in medieval Ashkenaz, must be further explained.

One reason for the active participation of women in the circumcision ceremony could be the nature of this specific ceremony. While it is a male ceremony, it is one that takes place while the infant is completely in his mother's care. In this aspect, the ritual differs from other rituals in which the initiate does not return to the same social space he left. In Ashkenaz, for example, Jewish boys who underwent the Torah initiation ceremony became part of a new social space, that of the male community. In the case of an infant, he was under the supervision of his mother both before and after the circumcision ritual. This factor, though it may account for female involvement in the ritual, does not explain the objections to women's participation or the changes in the ritual through time.

It seems that the best way to assess the change in the role of women in the ceremony is by examining R. Meir of Rothenburg's objections to this role. He mentions two main reasons: First, he says that it is inappropriate for women who are dressed and adorned with jewels to enter the men's section. Once again, we must ask what made this particularly inappropriate at this time, as we can assume that previously, female ba'alot brit entered the men's section adorned with jewels. In general, immodesty is an argument often marshaled to restrict women's activities in patriarchal societies. One has only to look at religious societies today to see living examples of this use of immodesty. It is important, however, to note the limits of this struggle. The objection is not to women's wearing of jewelry per se, but to their doing so in the men's section, where they could unintentionally cause men's thoughts to wander.

Second, he explains that the commandment of circumcision is the father's obligation and not that of women, and that women should not "snatch" the commandment from the men. The expression he uses "*laḥtof miẓvah*" (to snatch the commandment) is one that is not common in the medieval sources. It appears in the Talmud as well as in the Midrash in a completely different context, one far more positive than the context here.[140] The idea that a man, rather than a woman, should hold the baby makes sense if we think of the ritual as a male ceremony, a ceremony in which the baby becomes part of male society, even if only for a few short minutes. This would explain the importance of a man's holding of the infant. But this kind of explanation only increases our difficulties in understanding why women were allowed to be such active participants for a limited period of time.

I suggest that the context of R. Meir of Rothenburg's comment is far wider than that of the role of the ba'alat brit. What does R. Meir of Rothenburg mean when he accuses women of "snatching the commandment"? Clearly, one meaning of his comment is that women are taking over an area that is not meant for them. The barring of women from the circumcision ceremony alerts us to examine women's participation in ritual more extensively. We find that the case before us is not a unique one. In the eleventh, and especially in the twelfth, centuries, there is evidence that some women took upon themselves obligations that were traditionally male, such as time-bound commandments (*Mizvot aseh shehazman grama*) that only men are commanded to observe — among them, the donning of *tefillin* (phylacteries) and *zizit* (the ritual fringed garment). This practice was not supported by all in Ashkenaz, but was generally approval by figures such as R. Tam. During the course of the thirteenth century, the Hebrew sources begin to express discomfort with women's adoption of such practices, and the objections become more prevalent.[141] R. Meir of Rothenburg was one of the main figures objecting to women taking upon themselves some of these obligations.[142] The objections to women performing a variety of ritual activities — ba'alot brit, tefillin, and zizit — as well as the question of the kind of blessing they were allowed to make when performing the rituals, were all widely discussed during the twelfth and thirteenth centuries. While R. Tam allowed women to make the ritual blessing men made when performing these activities, fifty years later the permission he had given was being questioned.[143] During the second half of the thirteenth century and the fourteenth century, these objections became more forceful.[144]

Another example of an objection to women's performance of ritual functions was discussed above — the objection to women acting as circumcisers, which became accepted in the fourteenth century. This change seems to fit the development I am describing. In addition, as we discussed above, a more stringent approach toward impurity after birth was adopted at this time. These separate instances of objections to women's ritual participation, specifically in areas that are not traditionally female, seem to point to a broader social phenomenon. Even if each issue has its own inner logic and halakhic reasoning, the ensemble seems to be connected to a more general attitude toward women and ritual participation.

The restrictions on women's participation in public ritual as well as in their private devotion are evidence of a gender struggle within medieval Jewish society. These restrictions also accord with the struggle between the bride's and the groom's families, as well as changes that seem to have been part and parcel of the marriage economy of the time. The reality in Jewish society fits in with the European context as well. A similar development is evident in Christian society, where, following a period of relative religious freedom for women, as is evident in the growth of lay piety and female orders in the twelfth century, church authorities of the thirteenth century were determined to curb women's opportunities and especially their religious functions. Thus, for example, women who tried to preach were gravely reproached. Many of their religious practices, including fasting and other devotions, were criticized.[145] Women did continue to act as co-mothers, but as women had always played a more significant role in the baptism rite, this fact is not related to the restriction of recently obtained freedoms. These restrictions on women's ritual participation have a distinct parallel in thirteenth- and fourteenth-century discussions of children's ritual obligations. The appendix to this chapter outlines these changes as they deviate from the focus of chapter 2, but are central to a broader understanding of this topic.

Let us now return to the opening discussion of the co-parents and the ba'alei brit and summarize some of the issues raised in this chapter. The medieval Jewish community adapted the role of the ba'alei brit from their Christian neighbors. Like the Christians, they used it as a means of forming new relationships and strengthening existing contacts. Within the family framework, they chose to honor various members, in accordance with the status of the different members of their families. Among those honored were women—friends and relatives—just as women were honored as co-mothers in the baptism ceremony.

By examining these practices, we may obtain a better understanding of the tensions at work within Jewish society. As an institutional ritual, circumcision was a way for the community to strengthen and confirm its hierarchy. By following the development of this institutional rite during the medieval period, we can see how it reflects changes and tensions within Jewish society. Jewish women, like Christian women in the baptism ritual, took part in the circumcision ceremony. Their role is more surprising because, unlike baptism that was for female and male infants alike, circumcision was seen by many as an exclusively male rite.

By examining changes in the roles of women, we were able to point to a wider change in their ritual participation in Jewish society, as well as the broader transformations that were part of European society at large. The similarities between Jewish society and Christian society with respect to these two rites of passage are especially striking when one remembers that both ceremonies were definitive religious ceremonies. Although they were the ultimate symbol of difference, they reflect similar social strategies and changes.

Appendix

RITUAL OBLIGATIONS OF CHILDREN: CHANGING CONCEPTIONS

As we have seen in this chapter, the thirteenth century was a period in which women's ritual participation underwent substantial change. Figures such as R. Meir of Rothenburg were central in promoting this change and many of his recommendations were forcefully endorsed and gradually accepted. The chapter has focused on explaining some of these changes, first and foremost those concerning the circumcision ceremony. However, as we have seen, many of these issues have broader implications and contexts. One such example of a broader context that is central to this book's topic, although to a later stage of life, has to do with male children's ritual obligations. The obligations were discussed in the context of boys who were on the verge of or already at the age of education — ages five, six, or seven. Because these children have been studied extensively over the past years and because they are not included in the categories defined for this project, they will not be discussed at length.[146] However, awareness of the changes young children's ritual obligations were subject to enhances the historical conclusions of this study as well. This appendix will summarize conclusions of previous research.

In the medieval Jewish communities the question of how to educate children and what religious responsibilities they were to take upon themselves was a charged one. As a general trend one can see that during the course of the thirteenth century certain responsibilities were emphasized more and more as exclusively adult male responsibilities. During the thirteenth century, there are a number of instances in which the scholars debate the age at which children were obligated to perform certain duties. At this time, these obligations, required of all upon reaching age thirteen, were often taken on by children of younger ages, according to their abilities. Most of the obligations in question are traditionally male. During the second half of the thirteenth century and during the fourteenth century, understandings of these obligations changed.

While a thorough examination of this development is beyond the scope of this appendix, I will cite one example to illustrate this point. The precept of phylacteries, tefillin, worn on the arm during morning prayers, was not one that depended on the age of a child. Rather, tefillin were given to boys who were able to take care of them and to control their bodily functions. While eleventh- and twelfth-century scholars discuss boys not yet in school as donning tefillin,[147] thirteenth-century sources discuss tefillin in the context of boys who have started formal education. Yet there is a new twist to this discussion in the middle of the thirteenth century. R. Meir of Rothenburg emphasizes that only boys who can control their bodily functions and their thoughts may wear tefillin. These youngsters are defined as boys who have already received a formal education and even reached age thirteen.[148] This became standard practice in Ashkenaz, and by the fifteenth century, some even went so far as to say only married men should wear teffilin.[149] It would seem that a reevaluation of this religious obligation was taking place and that the age of taking on this precept was being raised. This is true of other religious obligations as well, such as having a child count as the tenth man needed for a *minyan*, a quorum, to pray in public.[150]

A somewhat parallel process in medieval Christian society has been outlined by scholars, most recently in the work of Kathryn Taglia. Taglia has discussed the evolution of communion and confirmation in France from part of the process of infant initiation to separate rites and has noted that during the thirteenth century communion was delayed to adolescence and was not held at age seven as was previously accepted.[151] Nicholas Orme has argued that this process went on in England as well, especially in regard to practices concerning confession and communion.[152] While the nature of observance of Jewish and Christian religious obligations was different, it would seem that a parallel process was taking place in both societies.

Even more important, during this same period, a reevaluation of women's responsibilities and participation was taking place. As we saw in this chapter, in the context of the same issue, tefillin, the same scholar R. Meir, and those who followed him, had new things to say about women and the precept. This case is different from that of male children since tefillin was not a female precept and women who wore tefillin were the exception, not the rule. However, during the Middle Ages, specifically in Ashkenaz, some women took this precept upon themselves. During the second half of the thirteenth century, sharp criticism of this practice was voiced and over time these objections became the norm. We have seen additional examples of such changes as well.[153] This attitude toward women's religious roles also has some parallel in medieval Christian society. I would suggest that this change of attitude toward both child and female participation in observances should perhaps be seen not as two separate issues, but rather as part of a whole. In Jewish society the religious responsibilities that had previously been those of young males and of some women came to be reserved for adult male society. I will return to this issue in the conclusions.

Chapter Three

ADDITIONAL BIRTH RITUALS

> R. Judah said: Three persons require guarding, namely a sick person, a bride groom, and a bride.
>
> Rashi: "A sick person: For his luck has turned bad and as a result the demons torment him. And also a woman who gives birth."
>
> — Berakhot 54b and Rashi

ALTHOUGH THE CIRCUMCISION RITUAL was the central birth rite celebrated in medieval Jewish society, it was not the only one. Circumcision was part of a ritual sequence that was designed both to usher the newborn into the community and to protect the baby from harm. This chapter will examine three birth ceremonies customary in the medieval Ashkenazic world: the Hollekreisch, the Wachnacht, and the Sabbath when the parturient first left her house (*Shabbat Yeziat haYoledet*). The exact details of these three ceremonies are not well known, as they are not treated as extensively as the circumcision ceremony. Indeed, they are only hinted at in sources from the High Middle Ages and are described in greater detail only in fifteenth-century documents. Moreover, unlike the previous discussion of the circumcision ritual and baptism, the Jewish rituals and their Christian parallels examined in this chapter were not an ancient or essential part of Jewish or Christian practice, nor did they determine Jewish and Christian identity. The differences between circumcision and baptism, on the one hand, and the rituals examined in this chapter, on the other, will enrich our analysis of the comparable elements in the ceremonies and provide a fuller understanding of the attitudes and beliefs about birth.

The Hollekreisch and Wachnacht rituals were ceremonies for the infant, and they will be discussed in the first part of the chapter. The Sabbath ritual was a ceremony for the mother after birth. However, since this ceremony is linked to the Hollekreisch, and since the analysis of this ritual increases our understanding of the ritual process of birth, I have included it in the discussion in the second part of this chapter. All three rituals will be compared to parallel Christian practices. The chapter will conclude with a summary discussion of the ritual birth process as a whole, as described in this chapter and in the preceding one.

Hollekreisch

This ritual, in which the infant was given a non-Jewish name, was customary for both boys and girls. In the case of boys, this name was in addition to the one given the baby at the circumcision ceremony. In the case of girls, no other naming ritual is mentioned in the sources. A ceremony called Hollekreisch is referred to in sources from the fifteenth century, such as the writings of R. Moses Mintz (1415–1483).[1] According to his description, the ceremony took place on the Sabbath on which the parturient first left the house. During the Hollekreisch ceremony, a number of children — girls for a girl, boys for a boy — gathered around the infant's cradle. The baby was lifted up and the participants recited a number of verses from the liturgy and the scriptures, especially the verses of Isaac's blessing of Jacob (Gen. 27), and then called out "*Holle, Holle*, what will this baby be named?" This was recited three times and, finally, the baby was given his/her name. Then cakes were served (figures 5a and 5b).[2]

Despite the fact that this ceremony, known by the name of Hollekreisch, appears only in sources from the fifteenth century and later, some earlier sources describe a custom that shares many aspects of the Hollekreisch. The earliest reference to such a ceremony can be found in *Mahzor Vitry*:

> It is a custom that at a convenient time, shortly after the circumcision ceremony, ten [men] gather. And they take a Pentateuch. And the little one is in the cradle dressed like on the day of his circumcision ceremony in grandeur. And they place a book on him and say "let this one [the boy] keep what is written in this [the Pentateuch]." And he says: "May God give you of the dew of heaven" [Gen. 27:28–29] and all the verses of blessings until "and only then you will be successful" [Josh. 1:8].[3] And they put a quill and ink in his hand so that he will be a scribe, adept in the Torah of God.[4]

While this custom is not identical with the Hollekreisch custom, it does contain some similar elements. This ceremony, like the Hollekreisch ceremony, took place around the baby's cradle and the verses recited during this ritual were the same as those recited during the Hollekreisch ceremony. However, in contrast to the Hollekreisch ritual, there is no mention of children participating in the ceremony or of any name-giving procedure. This custom, as it appears in *Mahzor Vitry*, is reminiscent of a custom practiced in Christian Europe. In order to protect children from demons and harmful elements, it was customary to place a New Testament in the baby's cradle under his head. The belief was that the Holy Scriptures could both chase away any evil spirits and ensure a bright future for the newborn.[5]

The custom of gathering around the cradle that appears in *Mahzor Vitry* has parallels in other contemporary sources. The author of *Sefer Hasidim* tells of a similar practice: "'This is the record of Adam's line' [Gen. 5:1]: From this we learn that they put the boy in a cradle and give him a name and place the book

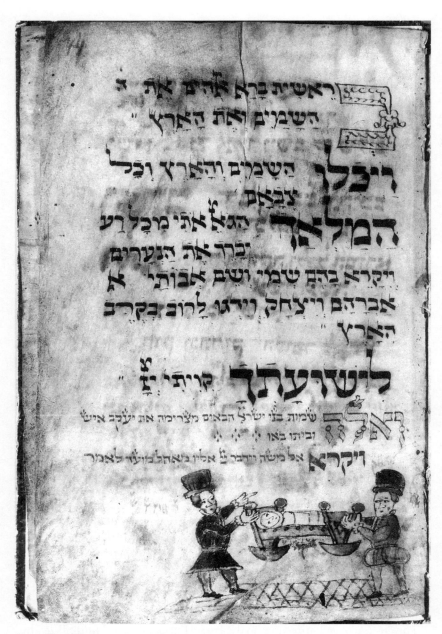

Figure 5. Hollekreisch. *Minhagbuch*, Nürnberg cod. 7058, fol. 43b–44b, from 1589. Photo courtesy of Germanisches Nationalmuseum, Nürnberg

כתב פאורייתא בכולת וכוות די עבה לכן או
לפת חביו כך פן שעישולה וכן יונה
או הדר להטות אל פתה מבול מועד

שאלו תלאידיו את ר' שמעון בן יוחאי. אמר מה משתה
תורה יולדת אכהות קרבן אחד לבן שבעת ערב
שטומאת ולד קוסבת ונשבתת שלא תקק טוד לכולה
לפיכן אמרת תורה הביאי קרבן.

תכא מנין שכה קדים במלאן כב קים סה היא אתבסרת
ועשה לו אטין שאחבן עתה כדרותא ביום שלים כשאתה
היולדת אבריסת והולך ישנא אטו נפל
בשוה הדי שכתאת שוכת אדיע/ אכן או לבת. ואתכסכה
רב לנקב. או בשלת בטורה. והשרים קדוין שם אבן
בתוא או בחמאויה. לכת בהה. וקרין לאותה שבת הוקראת
ואאסכ שבעה שם/ אכן ביום אלה. אטו שבעתי יקדוין אבן
ההוא שם קדים. שיצא כתב בתורה ואותה שם בתי
מדם להם שלשים. ובשין טמדת אדיעי. ואחרן
ברוא לנקב ה

וקורא שקראן הטער/ לאותו ילד בשאו הן שם כרכאב
או שם כנטי. מהצן לואר כל אילו הטסקים
שומר את להסורים ורבה ושמחת הלב

שגע כל אשה שהאשה מתכמרת עתה רבותינו
שהכנל אטר את שבוטא. או קרה נשונה.
ארוטת הורד. והאהלו של אשה על רכפה בעלה
היא טדרא אתף שהיא ברשות ה' טוף לה.

of Leviticus under his head."[6] As this description includes the element lacking in *Mahzor Vitry*, the naming of the child, it can serve to fill the lacunae in the other sources.[7]

Both the source in *Sefer Hasidim* and the source in *Mahzor Vitry* do not call the ceremony by the name Hollekreisch or by any other name. The timing of the ritual is also not clear. *Mahzor Vitry* mentions that this ritual took place around the time of the circumcision ceremony, while *Sefer Hasidim* does not mention a specific time for the ceremony, although we can assume that a naming ceremony took place earlier rather than later. Only in fifteenth-century sources do we find a specific name and time assigned to the ritual. They speak of a naming ceremony in which an additional name was given to boys and a name was given to girls. This name, at least in the case of boys was a *shem hol*, a name that was not holy (*kodesh*).[8] R. Moses Mintz explains that the Hollekreisch took place on the Sabbath that the parturient left her house — in other words, approximately four to five weeks after birth. The name given at the Hollekreisch is also sometimes called a *shem 'arisa* — cradle name.[9]

Some scholars have suggested that the act of naming the baby in the cradle gave the ritual its name. They explained that the word *Hollekreisch* was composed of two parts: *Kreisch*, meaning cradle or, in French, *crèche*, and *hol* from the Hebrew word *hol*.[10] This explanation, however, has no linguistic credibility. The medieval French word for *cradle* was not the modern *crèche*, but rather *brez* or *briç*, a word that became the modern French *berceau*. This word appears a number of times in Rashi's commentary on the Talmud.[11]

Another explanation commonly given for the name *Hollekreisch* is based on the comments of the fifteenth-century R. Moses Mintz. He said:

> For after the parturient who gave birth to a girl leaves her house, it is a custom to name the baby, and that naming is called *Hallekreisch*. I heard a reason from my father, may his memory be blessed, who heard from his mentors, that the meaning of *Hallekreisch* is that they cry out at that time to the [female] baby a not holy name and the same for a baby boy. For example if the "holy" name is Samuel and the hol name is Zanvil, they call him Zanvil at that time, etc. . . . And *Hallekreisch* is made up of two words, *Halle* from *hol* and *kreisch*, meaning "to cry out." In other words, the *shem hol* that is cried out and announced, for in the language of Lower Ashkenaz, they call a cry *kreisch*.[12]

This same explanation appears in the writings of other early modern authorities. One of them, R. Israel b. Shalom Shakhna of Lublin (d. 1558), explains that this custom is not the custom of the rabbis: "It is not the custom of Rabbis to give names to infants. Only children gather and lift up the baby and cry out his not-holy name. And all this is called *Hallekreisch*."[13] The same explanation also appears at length in R. Joseph Neurlingen's (1570–1637) book *Yosef Omez*.[14]

This suggestion, however, does not fit the ritual performance. If the meaning of the name *Hollekreisch* is the calling of the baby by a shem ḥol, why did the participants yell out "Holle, Holle"? How did yelling "Holle, Holle" help give the infant a name? At the end of the nineteenth century, two Jewish scholars hinted at what they saw as a solution to this question, and I will follow in their footsteps. Moritz Güdemann and Joseph Perles suggested in passing, that the cry "Holle, Holle" did not derive from the word *ḥol*, but rather from the name of a Germanic goddesslike figure by the name of Frau Holle.[15] This suggestion was greeted with dismay by some traditional Jewish scholars.[16]

In fact, folkloristic studies concerning the figure of Frau Holle strengthen the assumption that the Holle who is called upon is in fact this Germanic figure. Frau Holle was well known throughout northern Europe and was called by a number of different names such as Freyja, Stampa, Frau Rose, Perchta, and Befania, but principally as Frau Holle or Holda.[17] All these figures shared a number of common features and were closely associated with women. They were goddesses of the house and were held responsible for burnt baked goods as well as for improperly woven garments.[18] Most important, Frau Holle and her cohorts were closely connected with babies and fertility. Frau Holle was believed to wander the forests leading a group of babies whom she had snatched, especially during the winter months.[19] These kidnapped babies were susceptible to Frau Holle's machinations because they were as yet unbaptised. The children in her entourage were all tied to one another, and the last one, according to the legends, held a jug filled with tears, the tears belonging to his mother. One of the ways in which children could allegedly be released from Frau Holle's clutches or protected from her was by giving them a Christian name, as she did not kidnap baptized children.[20]

Frau Holle is mentioned in a number of medieval sources as part of a female religious practice that the church sought to abolish. The first source in which Frau Holle is mentioned is Burchard of Worms's *Decretum*. In the nineteenth chapter of this book, entitled *Corrector et medicus*, Burchard discusses the penance for women who followed Frau Holle. He warns of women who, "with a throng of demons transformed into the likenesses of women (she whom common folly calls the witch Hulda) ride on certain beasts on special nights and be numbered among their company."[21]

References to Frau Holle can be found in later sources as well. One thirteenth-century author laments the fact that some women pray to her daily, more than they do to the Virgin Mary herself.[22] As the folklorist Waschnitius demonstrated in the sources he collected on Frau Holle, her nightly travels were common knowledge. As mentioned, the principal strategy used to protect children from Frau Holle was baptism. However, in cases in which children had not yet been baptized, they were taken to church by women and picked up three times, while those present called out "*Holle, Holle, Holle,*" and gave the child a name.[23] Of course, once midwives and laypeople were given the authority to baptize babies in case of emergency (as was declared in a variety of synods from the thirteenth century onward), the need to trick Frau Holle into thinking a baby had been baptized was no longer as pressing.

In light of this discussion of Frau Holle and her position in medieval Christian culture, let us return to the Jewish Hollekreisch ritual. Is there any additional evidence that Jews were aware of and believed in figures like Frau Holle? It is well known that Jews in Germany and northern France believed in a wide range of demons and witches, as did their Christian neighbors. *Sefer Ḥasidim* contains many examples of discussions concerning werewolves and *streyas* (witches), and these figures were often associated with women.[24] In addition, there is a reference to Frau Holle herself in *Sefer Or Zaru'a*, in a discussion of a witch who has harmed a certain woman.[25] These shared beliefs should not surprise us, if we consider that the earliest Jewish and Christian authors concerning Frau Holle lived in close proximity. Buchard of Worms, the author of the first source mentioning Frau Holle, lived near a large Jewish community, and the Jews of Worms could certainly have been aware of Frau Holle, if belief in her was commonplace at the time. I would suggest that this ceremony is most likely one of a number of customs practiced by Jews that were designed to deal with these demonic figures, who were also feared by Jews.

Some common features are remarkable in both the Jewish ritual and the Christian practices concerning Frau Holle. In both cases, great importance is attached to giving the infant a name so as to protect the child. In both cases, the baby is lifted up and the participants call out *"Holle, Holle."* Even more important, in both cultures, the practices surrounding Frau Holle are not part of any official religious practice.[26] Rather, they accompany or precede an official birth ritual, such as baptism or circumcision. It is significant that the participants are women in the Christian case, and children in the Jewish case, as this seems to highlight the unofficial nature of the practice. This phenomenon serves as a fascinating example of how members of two religious groups can nonetheless adopt the same practice, each to serve its own purposes.

In the context of our discussion of birth rituals, the Jewish Hollekreisch ritual is yet another indication of the shared worlds and mentalities of Jews and Christians, particularly as they relate to the world of women. Members of each religious group chose to express their fear of Frau Holle in different ways. Christian children who were baptized at birth had no need for this ritual. Only children whose baptism was postponed for some reason needed protection from her.[27] On the other hand, it seems that every Jewish child, boys and girls alike, had a Hollekreisch. As they never received Christian names, Jews may have feared the consequences of lacking such. It should be noted that Frau Holle also had a Jewish equivalent, Lilith. According to traditions known centuries before the period under discussion, Lilith was a she-demon, extremely dangerous for newborns. Like Frau Holle, she would snatch them from their mothers and carry them off. Many Jewish amulets and incantations from the medieval period were designed to ward off Lilith, whom I will discuss later in this chapter.[28] We should note, however, that Jews chose to call out to Holle, rather than Lilith, when performing this ritual.

Wachnacht

The custom of holding a meal at the home of the newborn the night before circumcision, known as Wachnacht in early modern sources,[29] is frequently mentioned in medieval sources, where it is often called *Leili brit milah* — the eve of circumcision. I will begin my discussion of the Wachnacht by outlining its customs as described in these sources.

Our earliest description appears in *Maḥzor Vitry*, which discusses the meal on the eve of circumcision. As we saw in the previous chapter, this meal was the responsibility of the ba'al brit. The *Maḥzor* says:

> For the five kinds of grain like *oublies* and *cantelles*,[30] in cases in which these are the main foods at the meal, as is our custom on the eve of circumcision ceremony, recite the blessing "HaMoẓi Leḥem min ha'Areẓ."[31]

The *Maḥzor* goes on to describe the evening's events:

> The tradition of our fathers is Torah and a righteous man should adhere to it. On the eve of the eighth [day] the ba'al brit makes a feast in honor of the commandment.[32]

This meal on the eve of the circumcision ceremony was sponsored by the ba'al brit; special foods were eaten on the occasion.

Some scholars have suggested that this meal was a medieval development of the meal referred to in the Tosefta (Megilla 3:15) as *Shavu'a haBen* (lit., the week of the son). This ancient event is mentioned along with *Shavu'a haBat* (lit., the week of the daughter). We should not, however, connect the ancient Shavu'a haBen to the meal held in medieval times the night before the circumcision ceremony, as the ancient text seems to refer to the circumcision ceremony and the meal held after it.[33] Moreover, while medieval commentators also discussed the practice of Shavu'a haBen, they did not connect it to the meal held on the eve of circumcision. Rather, they thought this was the feast the father held *after* the circumcision ritual took place.[34]

The gathering on the eve of circumcision is mentioned for the first time in *Maḥzor Vitry*, and no explanation is given for it. The description in *Maḥzor Vitry* does not tell us where the meal took place, but, based on later sources, we may surmise that it was held in the house of the parturient, at her bedside. During medieval times, there is little mention of what went on during the course of the evening, other than the mention of the food served. Later sources, however, discuss card playing as well as the study of Torah.[35] They explain that the purpose of the meal was to ward off Lilith.[36] If this is so, then the Wachnacht fulfilled a purpose similar to that of the Hollekreisch.

The custom of holding a meal on the eve of circumcision is not unique to Ashkenazi Jews. It may be found in other communities in Provence and Spain as well as more distant diasporas. The fear of Lilith was widespread throughout the Jewish diasporas.[37] In medieval Germany and France, the existing beliefs and fears were connected to the common belief concerning Frau Holle. The holding of a vigil on the night before circumcision can be seen as a measure to protect the child, before circumcision, from lurking evil spirits as well as from other risks. Viewed in this manner, the Wachnacht is similar to the practice of leaving food out for Frau Holle on the nights after birth or to the vigil held to protect the infant on the night preceding the baptism ceremony. This vigil, which also included a meal, was meant to protect the infant from various evil spirits, such as Frau Holle, though she is not singled out. The vigil, like the Wachnacht, was hosted by the co-parents.[38]

One last detail mentioned in the sources merits further inquiry—the food consumed at the Wachnacht. *Maḥzor Vitry* mentions *oublies* and *cantilles* as the foods eaten during these festivities.[39] *Oublies* are wafers and *canesteles* or *cantilles* are little cakes. These baked goods were not made by the Jews, but were bought from their Christian neighbors, who ate them at their own feasts and celebrations.[40] They were considered festive foods, and Jews ate them not only at circumcision meals, but also on Purim. This fact comes up several times in halakhic discussions on the permissibility of eating *pat akum* (bread made by non-Jews).[41] It would seem that, at their birth ceremonies, Jews ate the same foods as were customary for Christian birth ceremonies!

As in the case of the Hollekreisch ritual, the information we have concerning the Wachnacht is not as extensive as that concerning circumcision. Both customs supported the birth and ritual process in Jewish society and dealt with the ever present fear of demons in the medieval world. As this fear was common to both Jews and the surrounding Christians, we find that parallel Jewish and Christian customs developed to overcome it; in the case of the Hollekreisch, we see how the Jews even adapted Christian customs.

The Sabbath of the Parturient

Like the Hollekreisch, the ritual for the parturient took place a month after birth. Unlike the customs discussed earlier, there is no mention of this or similar practices preceding the fifteenth-century source found in R. Moses Mintz's responsa, in which the Hollekreisch is mentioned as well.[42] R. Moses does not describe the ritual in detail, as his comment comes in the context of a discussion of divorce procedures. He mentions that the Hollekreisch took place on the Sabbath that the parturient left her house after birth to go to the synagogue.

If so, two birth rituals — one for the baby and one for the mother — took place on the same day.

The parturient's ritual has received scant attention in research over the years. Leopold Löw is one of the few scholars who devoted attention to this custom in his book *Die Lebensalter in der jüdischen Literatur* published in 1875. He suggested that this ritual was connected to both the biblical custom (Lev. 12) of bringing a sacrifice to the temple after birth and to the medieval Christian ritual known as churching (in German: *Aussegnung* or *Kirchengang*), in which the parturient went to church for the first time after birth. Löw argued that the late medieval Jewish ritual was an adaptation of the Christian churching ritual, which, in turn, was an adaptation of the biblical rite.[43]

My analysis will investigate Löw's suggestion concerning the connection between the Jewish parturient ritual and the Christian ritual of churching. After comparing the two, and the different interpretations attributed to the churching ritual by a variety of scholars, I will suggest an interpretation of both the Jewish and the Christian customs in a comparative perspective.

The Jewish Ritual

While the parturient ritual is mentioned in fifteenth-century sources only in passing, it is described in greater detail in the sixteenth- and seventeenth-century sources. The only Jewish source that includes a long description of the custom is the seventeenth-century book of customs written by Juspa the Shammes of Worms (1604–1678).[44] R. Juspa outlines the different stages of the lying-in period. He describes a ritual process, in which the Sabbath ritual was the last of three stages. For the first two and a half to three weeks after birth, the parturient lay in bed and was tended by her friends. Some of the information we have about this stage comes from descriptions of the circumcision ceremony. Although the mother did not attend this ritual, she helped prepare for it. Juspa reports:

> Three days before the circumcision, just before *minḥa* [afternoon prayers], the *shammes* calls: *Zu der jüdisch Kerze* [to the Jewish candles] up and down the street. And the women come to the parturient's house, and they wash the child and they throw coins into the bathing water, which are for the servant who is helping the parturient.[45] And they make the *jüdischen Kerzen* and twelve small wax candles that are lit during morning prayers on the day of circumcision in the synagogue.[46] And every time the baby is being bathed they call some women to come to the commandment [*miẓvah*] of washing the baby and they throw money into the bathing water for the maid.[47]

The preparation of candles mentioned here is not an early modern innovation. As we saw in the previous chapter, other sources discuss the preparation of twelve candles for circumcision but do not provide details on who prepared them or where they were prepared.

During this first stage, the parturient is attended to by friends and, in some cases, a maid. On the Sabbath about three weeks after birth, the parturient got out of bed, changed her sheets and clothing and hosted her friends who came to visit. This stage was called the *Pfühl* (lit. pillow). She then spent an additional week in bed. The third stage began a week later, on Friday. The parturient changed her clothes and put white sheets on her bed. She cleaned and dressed the baby. This was called *die weisse Pfühle*. That Sabbath morning, she proceeded to the synagogue, accompanied by her female friends and neighbors. She wore her Sabbath clothes covered with shrouds and on her head she wore a hat covered with a veil or scarf. The scarf and the shrouds were meant to trick any lurking evil spirits by suggesting that this woman was mourning rather than celebrating.[48] The woman's arrival in the synagogue was timed to coincide with the beginning of the morning blessings that preceded the recital of the Shema, and special tunes were sung in her honor.

If the baby was a boy, the woman gave the synagogue the embroidered *wimpel*. The wimpel was the cloth diaper from the circumcision ceremony that was embroidered by the mother and her friends. These wimpels were used to wrap the Torah scrolls in the synagogue (see figure 6). The father of the baby was called to the Torah and said a blessing for his wife. The parturient herself did not play any active role in the synagogue ritual. After services, she took off the scarf she had covered her head with and the shrouds she had worn and returned to her home accompanied by her friends. She prepared a meal for them and gave them small gifts of baked goods and fruit. That same afternoon, the Hollekreisch ritual took place. Aspects of this ritual process are illustrated in two illustrations from eighteenth-century books (see figures 6 and 7).

A different seventeenth-century source emphasizes the fact that every parturient, even those whose babies died immediately after birth, underwent this ritual. R. Yuda Levy Kirkhum's (d. 1632) book *Sefer Minhagot Wormeisa* states: "If the infant died within the first thirty days, the ḥazan (cantor) nevertheless says Kaddish in a special tune on the Sabbath that the women lead the parturient to the synagogue."[49] The parturient is such a central focus of this ritual, that even if the baby died she was still expected to undergo this ceremony. R. Yuda Kirkhum emphasizes that despite the death of the infant, services are to be held in a joyous manner. A different custom book from the sixteenth century supplies an alternative explanation for the ritual:

> It says in the Torah concerning a parturient: "On the completion of her period of purification, for either son or daughter, she shall bring to the priest, at the entrance of the Tent of Meeting, a lamb in its first year for a burnt offering, and a pigeon or a turtledove for a sin offering." R. Simeon b. Yoḥai was asked by his disciples: "Why did the Torah ordain that a woman after childbirth should bring a sacrifice?" He replied: "When she kneels in bearing she swears impetuously that she will have no more intercourse with her husband. The Torah therefore ordained

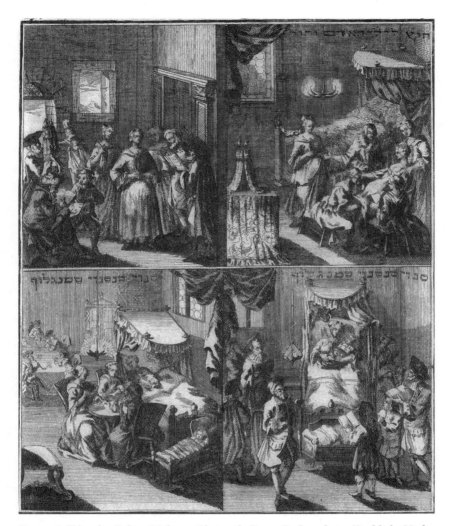

Figure 6. *"Von der Geburt."* Johann Christoph Georg Bodenschatz, *Kirchliche Verfassung der heutigen Juden*, Frankfurt-Leipzig, 1748–49). Photo courtesy of Hebrew National and University Library, Jerusalem.

that she should bring a sacrifice" [BT Niddah 31b]. This is a valid reason in the time that the Temple existed. But in our times, when the Temple does not exist, how is she atoned for? And I think that this is the basis for the custom in our generations, that on the thirtieth day when the parturient goes out and the baby is no longer in danger, the woman makes a festive meal and donates something to charity or her husband donates for her.[50]

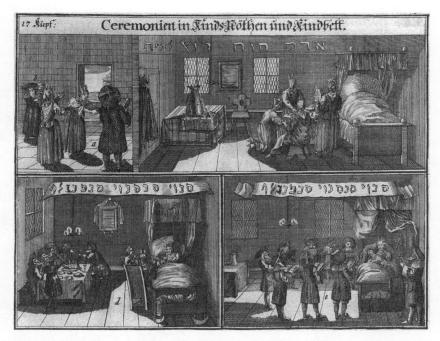

Figure 7. *"Ceremonien in Kinds-Nöthen und Kindbett."* Paul Christian Kirchner, *Jüdisches Ceremoniel oder dererjenigen Gebräuche,* den dieser neuen Auflage mit accuraten Kupfern von Sebastian Jacob Jungendres (Nürnberg, 1724), 149. Photo courtesy of Hebrew National and University Library, Jerusalem.

These two texts raise questions as to the purpose of the ritual — was it an atonement for sin at the time of birth? This would explain why a woman whose child died must undergo the ritual nonetheless. The festive elements of the ritual, however, are not related to the need for atonement. Thus, we must ask, why were they observed in cases in which the baby died at birth? Hamburger suggested that perhaps they were an expression of thanks for the mother's survival of childbirth.[51] This accords with what Glückel of Hamel wrote about going to the synagogue on the fifth week after birth. She comments that after she went to the synagogue and expressed her thanks to God for having survived childbirth, she dismissed her hired help and resumed her household chores.[52] Soreh bas Toyvim, in her *tekhine* (prayer) for women going to synagogue after birth, says that the purpose of this activity is both atonement and thanksgiving.[53]

If we accept that going to the synagogue on the Sabbath four to five weeks postpartum is an expression of the need for atonement after birth, then the synagogue ritual was an atonement for the vow the woman made during labor, when she vowed that her husband would never approach her again.[54] In the

Bible, the sacrifice was brought to the Temple forty days after the birth of a male and eighty days after birth of a female, and the ritual surrounding this event included atonement through sacrifice, and purification through ritual immersion.[55] In early modern Germany, this was not the case. Women went to the synagogue four to five weeks after birth, whether they had given birth to a son or a daughter. The immersion in the mikve, which allowed the parturient to resume conjugal relations with her husband, took place forty or eighty days postpartum (in some cases even later), depending on the sex of the newborn.

As discussed in the previous chapter, the practice of going to the mikve only forty or eighty days postpartum was relatively new. In medieval Ashkenaz, according to twelfth- and thirteenth-century sources, women immersed themselves twice, following Lev. 12 — once shortly after birth and a second time forty or eighty days after birth. Eric Zimmer has shown that, despite differing practices prior to the fifteenth century, after the fifteenth century, it became widely accepted for women to immerse only after forty or eighty days and, at times, even later.[56] For the purpose of this discussion, it is important to note that the ritual immersion was not timed to correspond with the Sabbath ritual and seems to have taken place at some later date.

The early modern sources thus distinguish between two separate processes. During the month or so after birth, the parturient refrained from her household chores, and her friends and neighbors took care of her. This period ended with her going to the synagogue, after which she resumed her duties. Whatever the reason for this practice, once this process was complete, the woman was still pending ritual immersion in the mikve. This immersion purified her from the impurity of birth and enabled her to return to her conjugal duties. In other words, two different timetables operate here. One timetable structured the return to the household and social roles, while the other shaped the return to the conjugal bed. If the timetable concerning the immersion in the mikve may be understood in light of the instructions in Leviticus, there is no clear explanation for the Sabbath ritual and its timing. This is so in spite of the attempt, in sixteenth-century ritual books, to connect the Sabbath ritual with Lev. 12.

The postpartum ritual of the communities in Germany is also attested to in early modern Polish sources. We can assume that German immigrants to Poland brought the custom with them.[57] In Italy, a similar custom was also common.[58]

Churching

The Christian ceremony known in modern times as churching, was known in Latin as "*Ordo intrandi mulieres in ecclesiam post partum*," and in German as *Kirchengang* or *Aussegnung*.[59] This ritual is known from the fourth century in Eastern Christianity, and became widespread in Western Europe from the seventh century on. Paula Rieder has argued that in Western Europe the churching ritual was reshaped during the twelfth and thirteenth centuries, when Marian devotion became prominent.[60] The Christian ceremony, like the Jewish one, was based on the biblical commandment of the purification in the Temple and on the description of Mary's purification after the birth of Jesus:[61]

> And when the time came for their purification according to the law of Moses, they brought him up to Jerusalem to present him to the Lord [as it is written in the law of the Lord, "Every firstborn male shall be designated as holy to the Lord] and they offered a sacrifice according to what is stated in the law of the Lord, "a pair of turtledoves or two young pigeons." Now there was a man in Jerusalem whose name was Simeon; this man was righteous and devout. . . . Guided by the Spirit, Simeon came into the temple; and when the parents brought in the child Jesus, to do for him what was customary under the law, Simeon took him in his arms and praised God, saying, Master, now you are dismissing your servant in peace, according to your word; for my eyes have seen your salvation, which you have prepared in the presence of all peoples, a light for revelation to the Gentiles and for glory to your people Israel.[62]

The medieval ritual was one aspect of the veneration of Mary and of the attempt to emulate her deeds (*imitatio Mariae*).[63]

The individual churching women experienced after childbirth was complemented by a public celebration of the Feast of the Purification of Mary that was commemorated every February in public ceremonies and processions. Recent research has emphasized the connections between these two rituals.[64] The Feast of Purification was celebrated in the Byzantine Empire from the third century onward and is well known in western Europe from the Carolingian period. It is called by a number of different names such as *Purificatio*, *Hypopanti*, and *Candalaria* as well as by the German *Lichtmess*.[65] The Jews living in Germany were familiar with this ceremony and were aware of its significance. A thirteenth-century source, *Sefer Nizahon Vetus*, mentions the Lichtmess celebration that commemorated the purification.[66]

The Feast of Purification was a day of great celebration for women in late medieval times. They wore white and walked in a procession carrying candles.[67] In the context of our discussion, we might note that Jacobus de Voragine in his famous *Legenda Aurea* (Golden Legend) suggested that these expressions were also modeled after an ancient pagan rite dedicated to Februa, the mother of Mars. He explains that:

> The Christians, converted from paganism, had difficulty giving them [the rites] up. Pope Sergius transmuted them, decreeing that the faithful should honor the holy mother of the Lord on this day by lighting up the whole world with lamps and candles. Thus the Roman celebration survived but with an altered meaning.[68]

The churching ceremony was the individual purification, the way in which Christian women imitated Mary and purified themselves from the impurity of birth. Christian women stayed at home for several weeks after birth. The duration of the lying-in period depended on custom and on the financial abilities of the family in question, and was usually one month long. Women usually did not wait the forty or eighty days mentioned in Leviticus 12 after birth. Rather, they went to church four or five weeks post partum.[69]

During the lying-in period, friends and relatives took care of the new mother and her infant. The lying-in period can be divided into three distinct stages: The first stage was about two or two and a half weeks long and began with birth. At the time of birth, the father called the midwives and the other women who had been asked in advance to attend the birth. Together, they prepared the room for birth, hanging amulets to protect the mother and the newborn. After birth, the new mother lay in bed and was washed and cared for by her caretakers. She did not change her sheets or get out of bed. Only close friends came to visit her during this period. In addition, women who could afford the expense hired a servant to take care of all the household needs. The lying-in chamber and the *Kindbett* in this chamber were surrounded by amulets meant to protect the mother and child from evil spirits. One of the main spirits from whom the mother and child were being protected, at least in Germany, was Frau Holle, who was known to harm unbaptized babies.[70] The infant was often baptized during this period, but the mother did not attend the baptism.

During the second stage after birth, one that lasted ten days to two weeks, the parturient was allowed to get out of bed, and her bedding was changed, but she did not leave her room. Groups of female friends came to visit her during this period, and, at times, a festive meal took place in her room. Following this period, the parturient remained in her home for an additional period of a week or ten days. During this period, she was allowed to leave her room, but not her house. At the end of this period, she left her home accompanied by her midwife and friends, wearing a veil and her best clothing. In Germany, women often brought the infant to church with them, while in England the custom varied. In some places, she then passed the child's christening cloth on to the priest. The parturient knelt in church, and the officiating priest or pastor read Psalm 121 ("By day the night will not strike you, nor the moon by night. The Lord will guard you from harm; He will guard your life. The Lord will guard your going and your coming now and forever" [121:6–8] as well as the postpartum blessing for women. All the women carried candles, a symbol of their devotion to Mary. After the ceremony, the parturient went back to her home and enjoyed a celebratory meal with her companions. This ritual was a rite of purification from childbirth and from the pollution of intercourse. After it, the women returned to their roles as wives and members of their communities. Until their churching, they did not return to the conjugal bed, nor did they resume their household responsibilities.[71]

Gail McMurray Gibson has recently studied the relationship between the churching ritual and the Feast of Purification of the Virgin Mary. She argues that they were both female rituals in which women played the central roles. In both instances, women wore white and paraded in the streets. She sees the two rites as instances in which women were able to express their femininity and their place in society as mothers.[72] Gibson also points to one of the issues that has troubled Christian scholars with respect to both the individual churching ceremony and the Marian ritual:[73] If Mary was a virgin at the time of the conception, why was she in need of purification? Some of the answers offered to this question in the medieval period enlighten the individual churching ceremony. Some theologians explained that if Mary, who was a virgin, needed to be purified, then all other women who give birth are unquestionably in need of purification.[74] Paula Reider has suggested that the way in which the medieval churching rite was conducted, displayed and emphasized the belief that the parturient had to be removed from society and purified before she could return to the normal social order. Women who gave birth in socially questionable circumstances often remained unchurched; this emphasized the breach of the social order.[75]

Other scholars have reminded us that medieval theologians often provided other reasons for the churching of women. Gregory the Great (540–604) and his followers objected to seeing churching as a rite of purification from birth. Instead, he and others argued that if the parturient was being purified, it was an act of purification from intercourse and the pleasures of the flesh.[76] They also suggested that churching was a rite of thanksgiving, expressing gratitude for the fact that the woman had survived childbirth. Still others argued that the purification of women after birth was a "folk custom," and that while the general public thought women had to be purified after birth, medieval scholars and clergy did not.[77]

These disagreements over the purpose of churching are clearly conveyed in the liturgy of the churching ritual. Most versions of the ritual from the twelfth and thirteenth centuries address the issue of purification and refer to the impure blood of childbirth, as well as to Mary as the inspiration for the rite. In the fifteenth century, a new version of the prayer for the service appeared, which presented a new blessing, omitting the New Testament references. The common name of the ritual then became the more neutral *Ordo ad introducendam mulierem*. Only in one case is the ritual referred to as *Ordo ad purificandum mulierem*.[78]

It is not clear if the churching of women was universal throughout the Middle Ages. Rieder has argued that, while in the early Middle Ages all women were churched, this was not the case in the High Middle Ages.[79] Other scholars have assumed that the churching of women was routine practice for most women and have suggested that this practice became especially important in the thirteenth century as part of the growing devotion to the Virgin Mary.[80] In fifteenth-century Germany, churching was common practice, though not considered an obligation; rather, it was a *consuetude* (custom).[81]

The ritual not only provided a benediction for the parturient, but was also considered a way of freeing the woman after birth from any lurking evil spirits.[82] Some considered this ritual so important that families requested that women who had died during childbirth be churched before burial.[83] At the same time, others, especially after the Reformation, saw the ritual, and purification in general, as unnecessary. The meaning of the rite, as well as its validity, was the topic of heated debates in England, as well as in Protestant Germany. While the Lutherans continued to allocate a divine place to Mary as the mother of God, they were not completely comfortable with a rite of purification. Part of their objection was that it was a Jewish ritual and that those who observed it were Judaizers. In spite of the objections of the clergy in Germany, however, the rite continued to be practiced at the insistence of women.[84]

While important differences exist between the rituals, especially in their institutional aspects, the similarities between them are striking. Among the differences between the two ceremonies, one element central to the Christian rite, the bearing of candles symbolizing the Virgin Mary, was obviously lacking from the Jewish custom. Not only did the Jewish ritual clearly distance itself from Mary, but candles could not have been carried at a ritual held on the Sabbath. An additional distinction is the place of the parturient in the ritual. The Jewish woman went to synagogue but stood in the separate women's section, while her husband and other men were active in the sanctuary—her husband recited a blessing for her during the reading of the Torah and the cantor sang special tunes in her honor. The only thing the woman did, in the case of the celebration of the birth of a son, was to pass the wimpel to her husband. By contrast, Christian women were more active. They answered questions posed by the priest and received the postpartum benediction (*benedictio post partum*); they knelt on a special churching stool and were the center of attention during the ritual.[85] It is possible that these differences are not all that significant, since we find similar distinctions between Jews and Christians in other instances. Jews lacked priests, and the husband and cantor seem to be filling in for them in this case.

The similarities between the churching ritual and the Sabbath ritual for the parturient are more obvious. The two rituals not only share the same underlying concept; they also possess many common features marking the entire postpartum period, from birth until the performance of the institutional rite. Both rituals were performed for the mother and not for the infant, and both shared a similar timetable for the process of her return to regular social functions. Another feature common to both rituals is women's involvement in the ritual process—watching the woman during and after birth, providing festive meals and accompanying her to church/synagogue. Although the men, at least in Jewish society, often helped draw and mount the amulets around the *Kindbett*, this was done before birth. After the onset of labor, they no longer entered the birthing chamber. In both Christian and Jewish society, the women remained in their houses, cared for by others, and did not resume their housework or leave their homes. In addition, this period after birth was characterized by a shared fear of demons who could harm the newborn.

There were similarities in the institutional part of this process as well. In both societies, the woman went to the place of worship on the day of rest. She wore her best clothes and a special veil on her head, which was removed only after the ritual. She brought the christening cloth or the wimpel with her to the ceremony and passed it on to her husband or to the priest. Furthermore, both Jewish and Christian mothers appeared in public for the first time since birth. In the case of boys in Judaism, and for both boys and girls in Christianity, the women had already missed their children's initiation ceremonies. Both rituals were explained in similar ways. Jewish sources explain the Sabbath ritual as providing a means of atonement for the vows the parturient took upon herself during birth and as an expression of thanks. Christian sources mention atonement, thanksgiving, and purification as reasons for the churching ceremony.

Birth Rituals and Their Social Context

The Sabbath ritual for the parturient, and the similarities between it and the Christian churching ritual, strengthen both the conclusions of the previous chapter, as well as our reflections on the cross-cultural influences of customs of the Hollekreisch and the Wachnacht. While the rituals discussed in the previous chapter, baptism and circumcision, like the synagogue and the church, remained separate and contrasting symbols, the social functions and the cultural values that were transmitted by these rituals are very much shared. The less "official" rituals discussed in this chapter emphasize the shared nature of these common social functions and cultural values. One of the key issues that came up when discussing the circumcision ritual was that of women's place in medieval Jewish society. The Sabbath ritual for women after birth furthers our possibilities for a better understanding of the construction of gender relations in medieval and early modern Jewish society. In the following interpretation, I have profited greatly from scholars who have employed the churching ritual as a key for understanding Christian society. The adaptation and discussion of these scholars' understandings of the churching process in the context of the Jewish ritual supports some of these explanations.

Some scholars, such as Keith Thomas and others, have argued that churching and the entire process undergone by women were deeply connected to beliefs in the impurity of women after giving birth. He believes that churching demonstrates the strength of these beliefs and that the objections to churching voiced in the early modern period are evidence of a gradual decline of the belief in magic.[86] The importance attributed to Lilith and other demons in the postpartum ritual, however, seems to belie this tendency.

Other scholars have focused more on the social significance of the churching process. Following Arnold van Gennep and Victor Turner, they have suggested viewing the churching process as a classic threefold rite of passage. First, the woman gives birth and is removed from her regular social order; subsequently, she remains in a liminal status during the period she spends at home; and, finally, she is reincorporated into society through the churching ritual.[87] This view of the ritual, however, has been criticized as male centered. In fact, the woman herself is not marginalized at this period; rather, she is enveloped by her female friends. While processional theory and liminality can perhaps outline the structure of the process, explaining this practice as a rite of passage does not do justice to its particularly female nature.[88] In addition, if this was a rite of passage — why did women undergo it with every birth and not just the first time they became mothers?

In the early 1990s, studies on churching, first and foremost by Adrian Wilson, suggested that churching was an expression of women's power in society. Following a suggestion made in passing by Natalie Zemon Davis in her article "Women on Top,"[89] Wilson suggested that the period from childbirth until churching was one in which the social order was temporarily suspended. While this moment served to strengthen the existing social order, during this period women were, according to Wilson, "on top." Wilson suggested that the rite should be understood mainly as a female collective ritual. During the weeks after birth, women did not perform their two most basic functions — conjugal and household duties. The involvement of other women in the house during these weeks was a form of "policing" meant to ensure this state of affairs. Women did not see themselves as impure, but rather as resisting patriarchal society.[90]

The weakest point of Wilson's argument concerns his understanding of the ritual of churching. He suggests that this ritual was a "woman's popular ritual" and that its practice exemplifies a logic that enhances women's position in society.[91] This idea seems questionable, however, if the churching ritual was commonly understood as a ritual of purification. If women were resisting patriarchy, why were they at the same time succumbing to it?

Susan Karant-Nunn has addressed this question in her work on churching. She has argued that while there was an element of extraordinary freedom from regular duties during the lying-in period for women, the churching ritual symbolized a return to the regular social order. While men perceived it as the end to this exceptional period, women saw it as an expressive rite in which they expressed their femininity and their identification with the Virgin Mary.[92] This approach has been suggested by others as well. Recently, Paula Rieder has discussed churching as a woman's rite, and has examined the social significance of this rite for women of different social strata. While the meaning of the ritual varied with its performer, there is no doubt that most women found great personal meaning in its performance. Furthermore, Rieder argues, the significance women attached to the ritual led the rest of medieval society to view it as important. The churching ceremony and the process that preceded it were a period in which women expressed themselves as women and identified with other mothers. Through this process, these women expressed their awareness of their bodies and their ability to give birth.[93]

These approaches, alone or in combination, expose the complexity of a society with many competing forces. The participants in the ritual process, the women who were so central to it, as well as the men, each understood it differently. From a male perspective, the period after birth was one in which the parturient was removed from society, while for the women this was a phase in which their female social experience was greatly enhanced. The arguments in early modern Europe over whether or not to do away with the churching ritual express these different perspectives and needs.

This suggestion, for an understanding of the postpartum process that includes the different needs and perspectives of men and women in the society, accords with our discussion of birth in chapter 1. We saw before how an attempt to explain churching as an expression of female power was complicated by the regulative aspects of churching. So, too, an attempt to explain birth as an exclusively female domain proved difficult. In both cases, we witnessed practices that created a unique niche for women, enabling them to express themselves in spite of the constraints of patriarchal societies. At the same time, we saw how male society regulated and supervised these processes.

The Jewish ritual can be better understood through many of our observations of the Christian ritual. If for the women this period was characterized by a different social order, while the churching ritual represented a return to the quotidian social order, the ritual in the synagogue also symbolized the return to mundane household and community responsibilities. As we have seen, the Jewish and Christian rituals share many features. The common interpretation of both the Jewish and the Christian rite strengthens the social explanations of the Christian rite proposed by scholars. Our insights into the Jewish rite can also explain why Christian women attributed such importance to this ritual. They help us understand why this was a ritual that women thought was worth fighting for. Our analysis also points to a social structure and framework of ideas common to both Jews and Christians. Because gender differentiations played such a crucial role in the functioning of the two societies, the common Jewish-Christian understanding implied by the temporary change in social order during the lying-in period is of even greater importance. The fact that the ritual was explained primarily in terms of impurity seems to correlate with other moments of breach in social order in which ritual impurity or the threat of ritual impurity leads to certain changes in the ordinary social hierarchy.

While I would not go so far as to suggest seeing the postpartum rituals mainly as a form of resistance to patriarchal authority, some aspects of this are hinted at in the sources. We saw a reference to this in the previous chapter, when

R. Jacob Mulin spoke of the custom of women pestering men who came to pick the baby up for a circumcision. We also saw an element of resistance in the story of the men who became upset as they waited for women who did not show up for a circumcision ceremony.[94] The women were busy celebrating with the mother of the infant and neglected to come to the synagogue on time.

Certain authors seem to hint at the idea that the postpartum period was one in which women saw themselves in a position different than their usual one, and took advantage of this atypical status. For example, R. Joseph Juspa Hahn Neurlingen of Frankfurt (d. 1637), author of the compilation *Sefer Yosef Omez*, comments on the practices observed during the lying-in period — such as the amulets that surrounded the Kindbetterin's room and the knife she held in her hand to ward off Lilith at all times. He says that these practices were observed until the women went to the synagogue. But he also reprimands the women, reminding them that although they are not following their routine, they are still obligated by some aspects of it. He reminds them that they are to wash their hands and recite their prayers, even though they are at home.[95] It seems that some women argued actively or believed that they could not perform mundane religious observances until they were ritually pure, and this was indeed an issue in question in the early modern period. Other books, such as *Sifrei Ḥannah*, a genre of instructional manuals for women, also scold women for not praying during this period.[96] R. Juspa Hahn Kashman suggests the opposite, that some of these women ignore these restrictions and try to perform certain commandments too early.[97] It would seem that some women, as well as some legal authorities, saw this period as beyond the normal restrictions of society.

We have demonstrated that the lying-in period was a unique time for women, and that the institutional rite terminating it was a forum for women's self expression, as well as a symbolic return to the social order. The explanation in social terms that we have advanced for both the Jewish and the Christian ritual facilitates a better understanding of both societies. Without the comparison with Christian ritual, making sense of the usually terse references to the ritual, as they appear in the varied Jewish sources, would be a difficult task indeed. This comparison, however, not only provides us with a better understanding of the parallel rituals, it also raises central questions as to the place of theology and religious institutions in ritual development and practice.

In the context of churching and the Sabbath ritual, one can see clear connections between practices, and Jewish and Christian religious ideologies. One possible reading could lead us to conclude that the Jewish ritual was adapted from surrounding Christian society. In the spirit of what Ivan Marcus has called "inward acculturation,"[98] I suggest that Jews adapted these postpartum customs and birth rituals to fit their social and ritual needs, and that eventually, they became an integral part of Jewish practice. In the case of the Hollekreisch and the Wachtnacht, the rite provided protection against a demon that was neither part of mainstream Judaism nor of officially approved

Christianity. In the case of the postpartum ritual, we must learn how Jews related to the Marian elements so central to Christian practice, even after the Reformation. Were the Jews aware of these Marian elements and, if so, how did they contend with them?

The Virgin Mary was a central figure both in medieval devotion as a whole and in female devotion in particular. Recent research has emphasized how central the Jews were in Marian piety. William Jordan has argued for the centrality of Marian elements in the Talmud trials against the Jews, and scholars who study medieval and early modern England have discussed the anti-Jewish elements in Marian devotion even, or perhaps especially, after the expulsion of the Jews from England.[99] Finally, scholars of medieval Germany such as Mary Minty and Heidi Röcklein have noted the interesting phenomenon of synagogues turned into churches dedicated to the Virgin in certain locations after their Jewish communities were exiled.[100] This seems to point to a little-examined topic that requires further investigation.

Here, I wish to discuss another aspect of this same issue. Rather than examine how Marian piety related to the Jews, this discussion focuses on the Jews' awareness of Mary and of practices related to her. Polemical comments show that Jews were well aware of Marian devotion and of some of its practices. It is not improbable that Jewish women became aware of the details of the churching ritual, including the Marian elements at its core, through their frequent daily contacts with Christian women. The contact between Jewish and Christian women was especially common around birth. They may have shared medical information and practitioners, and non-Jewish servants frequently attended Jewish households, especially after birth.[101] Jewish women were probably well aware of the belief in Mary's role as a protector at birth, and they most certainly were familiar with statues of her in the cities, which were often shrines of pilgrimage and devotion.

In fact, a legend from the early modern period accredits Jewish women with a certain belief in the Virgin. This legend has a Christian hero exclaiming that he, unlike Jewish women, really believes in the Virgin. The accusation against Jewish women is directly related to birth and practices surrounding it:

> Do not banish me from your presence, for I am not like those Jewesses who invoke the Virgin's aid in giving birth and then go through their homes with white napkins crying: "Be gone Oh Mary from this Jewish home."[102]

I do not wish to question the historical veracity of the charge made in this tale against Jewish women who called on the Virgin Mary for help during birth and/or chased her out of their homes afterward. I would like to suggest, however, that the Jewish ritual suggests an awareness of Marian elements.

Earlier, we noted that the Jewish ritual designated two separate timetables. The synagogue ritual structured the return to household and social roles, while the immersion in the mikve shaped the return to the conjugal bed. I also noted the difference between Jewish and Christian explanations of the postpartum ritual. While the Jews explained their ritual as an act of atonement and thanksgiving, Christians explained churching as a ceremony of purification, atonement, and thanksgiving. In my opinion, the difference here is telling. Purification, an element clearly related to Mary, and devotion to her, was unconsciously separated from the atonement and thanksgiving of the Jewish ritual.[103] The timing of the ritual immersion was, of course, based on biblical instructions in Leviticus, but the break between the Sabbath ritual and the immersion created a distance between the Jewish and Christian ritual. The most visible difference between the two was the absence of a candle-bearing procession in the Jewish ritual. Of course, Jews could not have included candles in a ritual conducted on the Sabbath, but the exclusion of candles contributed to the distinction.

An alternative argument might be that, as our earliest information on the developed Jewish Sabbath ritual dates only from the fifteenth century, this custom might have gained popularity in Jewish society mainly after the Reformation and after Marian devotion lost some (though far from all) of its importance. This argument is for the moment inconclusive. Although we have no sources concerning the Jewish Sabbath ritual before the fifteenth century, it is impossible to determine when the ritual began. It may well have had antecedents in medieval times. The first descriptions of the ritual appear before the Reformation and at about the same time as the texts on changes in the observance of the laws of impurity after birth and the discussions on the question of the presence of the mother at the circumcision ritual. When they are first mentioned in fourteenth- and fifteenth-century documents, all three issues — the appearance of the postpartum ritual in the sources, the change in postpartum purity laws, and the clear evidence that the mother of the infant was not at the circumcision ritual — seem to have been fairly new. The evidence, however, is far from conclusive. In addition, although historians have pointed to changes in the view of Mary after the Reformation, Mary was still central in Protestant theology. As Susan Karant-Nunn, who studied churching in Germany, has argued, this component cannot be easily dismissed.[104] Further study of medieval Jewish attitudes toward Marian devotion, as well as components of Jewish practice related to Marian devotions are fascinating subject that that remain, however, beyond the scope of this study.

Chapters 2 and 3 have demonstrated how a careful analysis of birth rites can facilitate a better understanding of the social context in which they were performed. Furthermore, our study demonstrates the benefits of studying Jewish and Christian rituals together. The Sabbath ritual, as well as the Hollekreisch and the Wachnacht, were part of a complex of rituals that demonstrate the importance attributed to birth and the social process undergone by the family of the newborn. They also attest to the practices of the community in accepting a new member into their midst and in receiving the mothers back into the regular social order. Unlike studies of customs that have focused only on the Jewish tradition, the comparative approach employed here reveals the shared mentalities of Jews and their Christian neighbors. This comparison has great potential for social interpretation. Whereas the theological and religious differences were most prominent and all encompassing in theological writings, a comparison of these rites reveals the gender codes of a common society in which both Jews and Christians lived. Whether studying the co-parents/ba'alei brit, the rituals to protect the baby from demons, or the customs of the parturient, these shared codes and beliefs demonstrate the joint social structures of Jews and Christians in medieval and early modern Europe.

At the same time, religious and theological tensions were ever present. Whether in the case of baptism and circumcision, each ritual symbolizing the separate identities of Jews and Christians, or in the case of Marian devotion, these same rituals symbolized the difference between Jews and Christians.

Appendix

THE DESCRIPTION OF THE PARTURIENT'S RITUAL ACCORDING TO R. JUSPA SHAMMES OF WORMS

—R. Jousep (Juspa) Schammes (1604–1678), *Minhagim deKehilat Kodesh Wormeisa (Wormser Minhagbuch)*, no. 288

The Custom of Parturients Who Give Birth to Males or Females

Immediately after birth they make a circle with a *neter* [chalk] in the room of the parturients and write on it "barring Lilith" and underneath this: "Adam and Eve." In this way, they write all around that circle, as is the custom everywhere. And some write on the entrance of the room like this: "Adam, and Eve, barring Lilith, Sanoi, and Sansoi and Samengloff,"[105] and this is a fitting custom. . . .

From the *jüdische Windel* [cloth diaper], after the third day after circumcision [*shlish hamilah*], they make the *wimpel*,[106] and they write on it the signatures of the child—when he will be called to the Torah, and also the day of his birth, the month of birth, as well as the year of his birth—and they draw on it the horoscope of that month. And the parturient does not go out of her house of birth until the fourth Sabbath after the birth and sometimes the fifth Sabbath.[107] How? First, I will inform you that each woman who gives birth needs to be in her house until the end of *der Kreis aus ist*. In other words, each night beginning with the day of birth, the woman who waits by her bedside to serve her takes a drawn sword[108] and turns the parturient with it several times and recites some chants that the women know. And so they do every evening, for four weeks from the day of the birth. . . .

The Sabbath preceding the Sabbath that she goes out of her [house of] birth [that is, the Sabbath that is called *sie geht aus der Kindbett*],[109] on that Sabbath, during the morning prayers, she wears fine clothing and beautifies her bed and beautifies the child and his bed and cleans the room she is in very, very well and beautifies it. And the women come to visit her and they see her clothing and her bed and the child's bed, and this is called *Pfühl* [pillow or bed]. And the Sabbath afterward, that is the same Sabbath on which she leaves her house of birth to go to the synagogue, on that Friday night, as the Sabbath arrives, she beautifies her bed with white sheets and pillows and the women come and visit her, and this they call *die weisse Pfühle*. It is also customary for neighbors and relatives to send food to the parturient. And most of them send cookies that are called *Brezel* and some send *Zucker Konfekt* [sugar candies] and some send whatever they wish and they honor the parturient with them. And she wears a pretty scarf and a *Sturz* on the *Schleier*[110] and she wears a *Röckli* [skirt or dress], a garment of shrouds underneath her outfit, when she goes from her house of birth to the synagogue on Sabbath morning. And after she goes out of the synagogue she wears a beautiful *Schleier* and she takes off the *Sturz* and the *Röckli*.[111] . . .

During the morning prayers on that Sabbath, it is obligatory to call the husband of the parturient to the Torah and they make two blessings for him, one for his promise to donate one liter of wax. And while he is still standing in front of the Torah scroll, his wife sends him the wimpel, because here they put the wimpel in the synagogue immediately on the Sabbath on which the parturient leaves her house for the synagogue.[112] . . .

On that Sabbath, each parturient, whether she had a boy or a girl, sends small bowls filled with fruit and sugar to her relatives and neighbors and especially to those who honored her with the portions that are regularly sent to a parturient, as described above. For the three meals [of the Sabbath], the parturients invite female neighbors and relatives, whomever they want, and they eat, drink, and rejoice with the parturients.

Chapter Four

MATERNAL NURSING AND WET NURSES: FEEDING AND CARING FOR INFANTS

> Most women have compassion for their children and nurse them.
> —Jacob Mulin, *Shut Maharil*

IN MEDIEVAL JEWISH SOCIETY, as in all premodern societies, infancy was fraught with danger. Disease and malnutrition resulted in a high rate of infant mortality; many children did not survive the first year of their lives.[1] This chapter will focus on the care given children during infancy, and especially on breast-feeding, a practice crucial for children's survival.[2]

At the outset, a word about the sources is in order. The available sources provide only brief glimpses of the way infants were fed, bathed, and clothed. As a result of our lack of information, it is impossible to document many aspects of their care. Furthermore, Jewish sources are very limited in comparison with those available on medieval Christian society. In thirteenth-century Christian sources, we find descriptions of appropriate methods of caring for infants. Encyclopedists such as Bartholemæus Anglicus described how wet nurses and parents were to attend to their offspring.[3] Another source, used extensively in studying the lives of Christians in medieval Europe, is art—illuminations and sculptures that depict child care.[4] By contrast, few such descriptions and depictions have survived from medieval Ashkenaz, and most of our knowledge is gleaned from details mentioned in passing in various texts.[5]

There is one exception: The discussion of breast-feeding practices in medieval Ashkenaz had many halakhic implications. This chapter will use the information provided in halakhic sources on breast-feeding and wet-nursing practices to present the social context in which infants and young children were cared for. As a result of this wealth of sources, this chapter (unlike others in this book), is based primarily on halakhic material and is framed around a number of important halakhic issues. As we shall see, although these sources are abundant, their legal nature imposes its own limitations.

The theme of breast-feeding, although more pronounced in the Jewish halakhic sources, is also prominent in medieval sources that discuss Christian children. Since children who were not breast-fed had almost no chance of survival during the Middle Ages, feeding an infant was the most central issue pertaining to his/her care; all other questions pertaining to an infant's well-being were marginal compared with this cardinal concern.[6] A mother who chose not to nurse her children did not have adequate milk substitutes, especially since, in the period before the pasteurization of animal's milk, the child's chances of surviving substitutes were slight.[7] Consequently, most families had two options: either the mother herself nursed the infant or a wet nurse was hired.[8]

Nursing was understood as a "natural" task and an obligation of women. This understanding had implications both for daily life and for women's and children's place in the social order.[9] As anthropologists studying a wide range of societies and historical periods have demonstrated, patterns of breast-feeding and wet nursing differ from place to place and among different historical periods.[10] For example, studies of eighteenth-century Iceland have demonstrated how a negative understanding of breast-feeding caused many parents to avoid nourishing their children with breast milk, preferring to feed their children animal milk. Although this approach resulted in the death of many children, it was continued as a result of deep cultural beliefs.[11] Other, less radical cases, prove this point as well. For example, in medieval Spain, women were instructed not to breast-feed their children during the first eight days, a belief that harmed children who did not receive the nutritious milk that characterizes the first days after birth.[12] This aptly demonstrates how specific cultures shaped and reshaped attitudes toward the biological female ability to nurse. As in the discussion of birth in the first chapter of this book, this chapter will seek to expose some of the cultural codes and understandings that existed in the Jewish communities of medieval Europe.

Examining breast-feeding practices illuminates women's roles as mothers and wives as well as attitudes toward children. The picture that emerges from discussions concerning breast-feeding is one of competing interests. For example, the interests of the mother and of others concerned with the baby's welfare were not always identical. The father of the infant and, given the nature of Jewish society, Jewish communal institutions, were relevant third parties in this matter. Hence, the interpretations assigned to the various interests and practices surrounding breast-feeding often expose the gender hierarchies of the society. Furthermore, the employment of Christian wet nurses was common practice in medieval Jewish Europe. Thus, discussions of wet nursing reveal not only the hierarchies within the nuclear family and community, but also the relations between Jews and Christians within the household and the relationships between Jewish employers and their employees.

Nursing practices also provide a unique opportunity for comparison between Jewish and Christian practices in medieval society. As described in the introduction, breast-feeding was treated by some scholars of medieval childhood as an issue of utmost importance, and even as a marker of the extent of parental love for their children.[13] One approach to this question is demographic. David Herlihy and Christiane Klapisch-Zuber examined the *castato* of Florence and analyzed the records concerning the employment of wet nurses, the duration of children's stays with wet nurses, and the statistics concerning infant death.[14] Others, who objected to Ariès's suggestion concerning the emotional attachment between mothers and children, surveyed a wide range of literary evidence, from belles lettres to canon law, for evidence of the concern for children's welfare.[15] These issues and debates have brought to light many details concerning the care of infants and the nature of the relationships between parents and children in medieval society.

These questions have received little attention in Jewish studies. Only a handful of articles have discussed the relationships between parents and children, and breast-feeding practices in medieval times have received little notice. A preliminary article was written by Ephraim E. Urbach investigating a very specific topic — crib death. This topic is one that illuminates nursing practices, as discussions of cases of infant death often provide details on child care. In addition, the halakhic sources that discuss crib death convey the rabbis' understandings of motherhood and of mothers' interactions with their children. Urbach's article analyzes numerous halakhic responsa concerning this topic, but only one of his sources is dated to the medieval period.[16] Other articles that discuss nursing practices do so only in passing, as their main focus is on attitudes toward children and childhood.[17] A basic premise of these studies is that Jewish families, unlike Christian families, did not send their children out of their homes to wet nurses' homes. Consequently, scholars have argued that Jews were more preoccupied than Christians with their children's welfare.

My discussion will posit the existence of childhood and infancy as distinct stages in medieval society, and will examine the strong emotional ties between parents, particularly mothers, and their children.[18] I will outline the social and cultural aspects of breast-feeding practices in the Jewish communities of Germany and northern France. The central part of the chapter will examine the social practices connected to breast-feeding and wet nursing: How long were infants nursed? If the mother did not nurse her children, did the wet nurse come to the house or were Jewish children sent out to live in other homes? Were wet nurses characteristic of a certain social class and how was their employment viewed? Was the wet nurse Jewish or Christian, and what were the concerns when hiring a wet nurse? In light of this discussion, I will examine the implications of these practices on the medieval Jewish communities and their relationships with their Christian neighbors.

In contrast to the first parts of the chapter that focus on the household at large — the Jewish family and its employees — the final part of the chapter will discuss the social consequences of a topic of major concern in the responsa literature: women's commitment to feed their own children. Most of the cases discussed in the medieval literature concern instances in which the nuclear family has fallen apart. What was a woman's commitment to nurse her child in cases where she was widowed or divorced during the period she was nursing her child? As we shall see, these events were of central importance to medieval Jewish society, and a topic of heated debate and change during the High Middle Ages. The conclusions point to the wider implications of breast-feeding for our understanding of Jewish-Christian relations and the construction of gender in medieval society.

ANCIENT FOUNDATIONS
Jewish Legal Rulings

We cannot approach this topic without a brief survey of the literature from pre–medieval times. Most of the medieval Jewish sources that discuss breast-feeding are legal sources that assume familiarity with the ancient discussions that served as the basis for the medieval halakhic rulings. In addition, the Mishnaic and talmudic rulings concerning nursing were not merely legal precedents that served as the basis for the decisions of medieval rabbis; these sources also instruct us on medical theories about nursing as well as cultural understandings of the obligations of wives and husbands toward each other.[19]

Most of the ancient sources discuss the mother's obligation to nurse her children. The ancient sources see breast-feeding as a natural attribute of women: "Whatsoever gives birth, gives suck."[20]. The general assumption was that all women nurse and that women, naturally, want to breast-feed their children.[21] According to tradition, Hannah is presented as praying for a child as follows:

> Sovereign of the Universe, among all the things that Thou hast created in a woman, Thou hast not created one without a purpose: eyes to see, ears to hear, a nose to smell, a mouth to speak, hands to do work, legs to walk with, breasts to give suck. These breasts that Thou hast put on my heart, are they not to give suck? Give me a son so that I may suckle with them.[22]

Nevertheless, despite the natural inclination to nurse that, it was assumed, all women possessed, nursing was neither dependent solely on the desire of the mother to nurse, nor was it understood as a mother's obligation toward her child. Breast-feeding is mentioned in the Mishna and the Tosefta as one of the obligations women have toward their husbands:

> These are the tasks that a wife must carry out for her husband: she must grind corn and bake and do washing, cook and suckle her child. . . . If she brought him one bondswoman, she need not grind nor bake nor wash; if two, she need not cook nor give suck to her child.

Furthermore, if she nursed her child herself, her other tasks were reduced.[23]

This connection between biological attributes and social expectations was part and parcel of all halakhic discussions of nursing. We can see how breast-feeding is, legally, a responsibility a woman owed to her husband (rather than to her child). This legal construction is indeed telling, since breast-feeding could well have been constructed as an obligation of mothers to their children, just as education, according to Jewish law, is an obligation that fathers owe their sons. This ancient formulation, which remained integral to medieval Jewish society, prescribes a Jewish family in which men, as the heads of their households and of the community, were those who determined the orders of nursing.

The obligation to breast-feed, as well as the benefits that women who nursed were entitled to, were part of the marriage agreement. A defined period of nursing, twenty-four months, was the legal time period discussed in the sources, and a nursing mother was assigned unique legal status as a *meniqa*. Due to her special circumstances, a mother nursing a child under twenty-four months of age was exempt from fasting on fast days, and special laws of purity and impurity related to menstruation applied to her.[24] In addition, as nursing was part of the matrimonial agreement, and out of concern with the welfare of infants, a nursing mother who was widowed was not allowed to remarry until the baby was over twenty-four months of age:

> "A nursing mother whose husband died — she should not be betrothed nor should she wed until twenty-four months have been completed," the words of R. Meir. And R. Judah says: "Eighteen months." And R. Jonathan b. Joseph says: "The House of Shammai says twenty-four months and the House of Hillel says eighteen months." Said R. Simeon b. Gamliel: "In accord with the opinion of the one who says twenty-four months, she is permitted to be wed in twenty-one months. In accord with the opinion of the one who says eighteen months, she may be wed in fifteen months, for the milk deteriorates only after three months of conception."[25]

These categories are repeated in the Talmud, and the House of Shammai's opinion became the accepted one.

The Talmud also discusses cases in which the child was given to a wet nurse, or was weaned or died before age two and his/her widowed mother wished to remarry. According to the Babylonian Talmud, if the child died, the mother could remarry. If, however, a mother had weaned her child after nursing him/her herself, or had hired a wet nurse after nursing for a while, she still could not remarry before the end of the allotted period.[26] One of the explanations for this law, an explanation offered by the Palestinian Talmud and suggested and rejected in the Babylonian Talmud, is that the widowed mother who wishes to remarry is suspect of having caused the death of her own child in order to improve her value in the marriage market.[27]

Most discussions concerning remarriage and nursing mothers in the Mishna and Talmud distinguished between widows and divorcées. Since breast-feeding was an obligation women owed their husbands, it was not the duty of divorcées to nurse their children. Divorced women were to be paid by their ex-husbands for nursing their children, but if they chose not to nurse, they had no obligation toward their child or toward their ex-husband.[28] By contrast, widows were viewed as obligated to their deceased husbands; in that capacity they had to nurse their children until they reached the age of twenty-four months and were not allowed to remarry earlier. As we shall see, these laws were central to medieval discussions.

Cases concerning the remarriage of nursing widows and divorcées are discussed with great frequency throughout ancient and medieval times. The concern for the welfare of children and women in these situations is a central factor in these discussions. The crucial question was how to treat marriages contracted during the period of nursing. The standard opinion was that these couples must be divorced.[29] While most discussions distinguished between widows and divorcées, some opinions equated both situations and ruled that divorcées, like widows, could not remarry during the twenty-four months of nursing.[30] As we will see, this opinion was very influential during the Middle Ages in Ashkenaz.

An additional problem concerned the law if a woman (divorced or married) refused to nurse her child. This case is of great importance, since it demonstrates the awareness that, even if breast-feeding was considered the natural role of mothers, not all women wanted to nurse their children. In such cases, the determining factor was whether the baby had already nursed from his/her mother and recognized her. In cases in which the baby recognized the mother, she was obliged to continue nursing and was not allowed to hire a wet nurse. The reason for this ruling was the fear for the infant's life if the mother stopped nursing. These laws pertained to both boys and girls.[31] An additional measure, designed to help protect the life of the infant, was birth control. According to Jewish law, a nursing mother was permitted to use a *mokh*, a cervical sponge, throughout the twenty-four months of nursing, so as to prevent the conception of a new child who would endanger the existing infant's milk supply.[32]

A central figure in these discussions is the wet nurse. Since she was hired to take the mother's place, she was also bound by the same obligations. At least in theory, she was responsible for the child for the full twenty-four months and was not supposed to get married or become pregnant during this period.[33] Her obligations are not outlined at length in the ancient sources, as she was not the focus of the legal rulings; they are implicit, however, in many of the discussions. The lack of discussion on wet nurses is also a consequence of the fact that they were, in many cases, non-Jewish. Although we find no negative assessment of the practice of employing non-Jewish women, some precautions were applied. The Mishna states: "The daughter of an Israelite may not give suck to the daughter of an idolatress, but an idolatress may suckle the child of an Israelite woman in her [the Israelite woman's] own domain."[34] The reasoning for this ruling was that a non-Jewish woman must be supervised when caring for a Jewish child, in order to protect his life. At the same time, a Jewish woman should not, according to this understanding, aid in providing sustenance for a non-Jewish child.

Jews, Christians, and Muslims

The Jewish approaches to breast-feeding were based on Greek medicine and on foundations the Jews shared with their neighbors, Christian and Muslim. From a medical perspective, breast milk was seen as part of the blood system.[35] When women nursed, they often did not menstruate. Therefore, according to ancient medicine, breast milk was menstrual blood that turned into milk, and when a woman became pregnant again, the milk turned back into blood.[36] This idea, as well as the belief that pregnant women could not nurse, were at the foundation of the legal principles concerning breast-feeding.

On the whole, the baby's father and his power are at the center of these discussions. By law, only in exceptional circumstances could someone other than the father decide how his child would be fed and cared for. In Roman society, for example, the father was responsible for employing a wet nurse.[37] As we saw above, according to Jewish law, the father was responsible for the nursing of his son or daughter. The halakhic principles were meant to protect the life of the infant as well as provide a clear-cut division of labor between both parents.

Early Christian law does not contain any discussions of nursing or of who is obligated to nurse. In what some see as one of the great accomplishments of early Christianity,[38] infanticide was strictly forbidden. There were, however, no guidelines concerning nursing such as those found in Jewish sources. Research on the first centuries of Christianity has suggested that many Roman women breast-fed their own children, although women of the highest social and economic status hired wet nurses. Despite the evidence of this social reality in which wet nurses were frequently employed, it seems there was no legislation concerning the social arrangements made, nor was there legislation concerning the remarriage of nursing mothers.[39]

Medieval families shared similar characteristics. In some cases, the mothers nursed their infants themselves, while in other households, especially in the wealthier ones, wet nurses were hired. The medieval compilers of canon law were concerned with nursing mothers in a number of instances, but were mainly interested in the implications of nursing on correct marital relations; hence, they do not discuss the welfare of children or the remarriage of mothers. Rather, they forbid nursing women to have sexual intercourse with their husbands. The reason for this prohibition, however, was not to prevent an additional pregnancy, but rather, because they realized that a nursing woman's chances of conceiving were not good, and they did not want good Christians to have sexual relations for nonreproductive purposes.[40] Despite this difference, the social circumstances of breast-feeding in Jewish and Christian societies contained many similarities, as I will demonstrate later in this chapter.

The Koran, on the other hand, presents a legal system that is much closer to the Jewish legal principles outlined above. As in Judaism, Islamic law defined twenty-four months as the period of breast-feeding. A woman who was divorced during this period and continued to nurse her child received full support from the infant's father for the duration. In contrast to Jewish law, however, a widow was not forbidden to remarry during this time. Moreover, Islamic legislation was far more flexible with respect to the sending of an infant to a new wet nurse, even after it was used to its own mother or wet nurse. Islamic law differs substantially from Jewish and Christian legislation with respect to the implications of breast-feeding. Islamic legislation developed a system of complicated kinship connections defined through wet nursing, that were expressed through marriage prohibitions. Children who were not biologically related but who were the "milk children" of the same woman were not allowed to marry each other. This complex system shows how one of the medical beliefs outlined above was interpreted by Muslim lawmakers. Since milk was understood to be blood that had turned into milk, two children who nursed from the same woman shared this milk-blood. Consequently, marriage between them was understood as a form of incest.[41]

This short survey of the different laws related to nursing and of the relationships between the three monotheistic traditions exposes a complex structure embracing many possible conflicts. Mothers and fathers could differ on the manner of feeding the child, whether the child nursed from a wet nurse or the mother herself. Concern for the child's welfare was sometimes at odds with the mother's own wishes to remarry. In addition, the employment of wet nurses brought an additional element into the family. As we turn to the Middle Ages, I will seek to describe how medieval Jewish families functioned within this framework.

Medieval Nursing Practices

Medieval Jewish society, which saw itself as adhering to ancient talmudic principles, manifested continuity with the ancient world while reinterpreting some of the ancient rulings. The two most important principles continued to be the duration of breast-feeding and women's obligation toward their husbands to breast-feed their children. I will briefly examine the first principle and demonstrate the second principle throughout the rest of the chapter.

As noted above, the ancient recommendation was that infants should be nursed for a period of twenty-four months, and medieval legal decisions manifest the attempt to enforce this rule. Nevertheless, contemporary sources contain little information about the length of the period of breast-feeding in medieval Jewish society. A variety of sources refer to women's nursing of their children for a period that ranged from two to four or five years. For example, the author of *Mahzor Vitry* discusses the Mishna, "at the age of five one is ripe for Bible" (Avot 5:21), and explains why it is appropriate to wait until age five to start schooling. He explains that a child is like a tree.[42] According to Jewish Law, the fruits of a tree growing in Israel may not be eaten during the first three years of the tree's growth. The fruit of a tree of this sort is known as *orlah* (lit., uncircumcised). He explains:

> And so a child should be weaned in his third year, after two years have passed by, as it is the way of infants to nurse twenty-four months. . . . And in the fourth year he will place a book before him or teach him a little by heart like "Moses commanded the Torah to us" (Deut. 33:4), so that he will grow accustomed to it. And in the fifth year, he will teach him Bible.[43]

In a different source, one of the Tosafists comments that a healthy child nurses for four years and an unhealthy child for five years.[44] This idea is repeated in a fourteenth-century treatise from Christian Spain as well.[45] Other sources suggest that some women did not breast-feed their children even for the duration of the required two-year period. R. Judah b. Nathan (Riban, twelfth century) mentions the Talmudic passage in Tractate Yevamot, which discusses situations in which a nursing mother discovers she is pregnant during the twenty-four-month nursing period. It is clear from his discussion that, in such a case, the woman had weaned her child before the age of two.[46] In a discussion of women who were widowed or divorced and wished to stop nursing, eighteen months is mentioned as an acceptable age.[47]

It seems that the age of formal education is a terminus ad quem for the duration of nursing. It is likely that most children nursed until age two (and at times even less); this also accords with the use of nursing as a method of birth control in premodern times. While breast-feeding was not considered a reliable form of birth control (as we see from the permission given to nursing mothers to use birth control), it often delayed additional pregnancies. Hence, women who wanted to give birth to additional children as quickly as possible often gave their children to wet nurses.[48]

A comparison of the material that emerges from the Jewish sources with what we know of Christian society reveals similar recommendations and practices. Among Christians, two years was also the prescribed period of breast-feeding, but there is little information as to how closely this recommendation was followed. A study of wet-nurse contracts, mainly from fifteenth-century Italy, has revealed that officially wet nurses were hired for a period of thirty months; in practice, however, most infants were weaned at the age of eighteen months; following this period, the wet nurse remained with the infant as a nanny.[49] Evidence from Christian society demonstrates that many infants experienced frequent change of wet nurses. The frequent death of infants following such changes is evidence that this practice posed a serious threat to infants' welfare.[50]

Manuals written for parents in Christian society suggested weaning girls about six months before boys, and this seems to have been the practice.[51] In contrast, almost none of the Jewish sources mentions discrepancies between the duration of nursing for boys and for girls, whereas some sources emphasize that both girls and boys should be nursed until age two.[52] It may be, though, that the souces' emphasis hints at the more favorable treatment of boys in practice.

In summary, it seems that the Talmudic directive to breast-feed infants for twenty-four months was observed in medieval Ashkenaz, at least when mothers nursed their own children. In some cases, children were nursed for even longer, until age four or five. This duration fits Jewish guidelines and was common practice in medieval Christian society as well. This practice varied, however, since often the mothers did not nurse their children themselves and wet nurses were hired for them. Wet-nursing practices created a new set of circumstances, since the wet nurse was not a member of the infant's family, and her circumstances could change and influence the duration of her employment. We shall now turn to examine the wet nurse and the details of her job.

Wet Nurses

Although the care of infants was the responsibility of their mothers, in many cases, especially in the cities, the mother was assisted by a wet nurse. The wet nurse's position in the house varied from place to place and among the different social classes, but she was always an employee bound by contract to her employers. In medieval Jewish society, as in Christian society and according to the Mishna, the wealthier a woman was, the more likely she was to employ a wet nurse.[53]

Studies of Christian households have outlined the terms by which wet nurses were contracted. They demonstrate that, although the wet nurse was usually supervised by the infant's mother, she was hired by its father. In cases in which the wet nurse was married, the contract was made between the infant's father and the wet nurse's husband.[54] The fact that the responsibility of hiring the wet nurse was the father's, despite the female nature of the job, is an important feature of medieval life and of the control patriarchy exercised over women in society. This was also the case in Jewish and in Muslim society. This arrangement accords with the halakhic understanding of the duty of breast-feeding, as described above. These cultural understandings created social circumstances in which the infant's mother worked with the wet nurse on a daily basis, but usually played little or no role in the formal agreement between the infant's family and the wet nurse.[55] From a legal point of view, there were only two instances in which a woman was responsible for hiring a wet nurse herself—if she gave birth to an infant out of wedlock, or if she was a widow. Otherwise, the father of the infant—whether husband or ex-husband—was supposed to take care of these issues.[56]

Research on wet-nursing practices in medieval Christian society has identified a number of guidelines regulating the terms of employment of wet nurses. First of all, wet nurses were hired for a defined period of time and were expected to remain for the full allotted period. In addition, they were expected not to become pregnant until the end of this time. To this end, part of the wet nurse's salary was withheld until the agreement had been fulfilled. The Jewish sources prescribe the same set of terms when employing Jewish and Christian wet nurses. For example, Ra'avan (R. Eliezer b. Nathan, c. 1090–c. 1170) reports the excuses a Jewish woman could offer to object to her employment in a Christian home as a wet nurse, because of the implications of the promise not to become pregnant.[57] Some of the monetary terms of employment are specified in a case from medieval Germany:

> Leah who lives in Ashkenaz hired [a wet nurse] to nurse her son for twenty dinar plus expenses for half a year. After she had nursed the boy for four or five weeks, she decided to go to France and demanded four dinars from Leah according to the terms of her employment, which were twenty dinars plus expenses [for the full period]. And Leah responded, "I hired you for half a year, and I won't give you anything [unless you serve] until the end of the period."
>
> Now, Rav said [in the Talmud] that a laborer is entitled to withdraw even in the middle of the day.[58] So, if Leah can find another wet-nurse [who will work] until the end of the period for sixteen dinars, she should give Rachel the four dinars. But if she cannot find anyone who will work for the remaining time period for less than twenty dinars, then she should not give her anything, since the employer has the advantage.[59]

In this case, "Leah" has the advantage over "Rachel" and she must be satisfied with the new wet nurse before "Rachel" can be released from her contract. It is possible that "Rachel" was hired after a different wet nurse backed out of her contract, as wet nurses were usually hired for twenty-four months or more, and according to this source, she was hired for only six months.[60]

Further illustration of the terms of employment can be found in a question that appears in the responsa of R. Asher b. Yeḥiel:

> "Rachel" was pregnant by "Reuven" and he married her and she gave birth to a son [Baby A] and he gave the son to a wet nurse and left her and went to another city and married another woman. And she ["Rachel"] hired herself out as a wet nurse to a different master in order to support herself in the house of the infant [Baby B] and she agreed to nurse him for a set time with a great forfeit [if she ruptured the contract], and eight or nine months have passed by, and the baby [B]

recognizes her and refuses to nurse from anyone else. But now, the wet nurse who nurses her ["Rachel's"] son [Baby A] refuses to nurse him, as the father of the child left for to a different city and no one is paying her salary. And the courts tell her ["Rachel"] that she should nurse her son. But she says that she can't, because she is obligated to nurse the son of her master. And her master says he will not allow her [to leave] because he has already paid her salary, and also because his son will not nurse from anyone else, and one soul may not take precedence over another.

Answer: The law sides with the father of the infant [Baby B], because she committed herself to nurse him. Thus, she is obligated to nurse him [Baby B], so as not to kill the infant. She is not commanded, however, to nurse her own son, even if she was married. And since the father of the infant [Baby A] does not provide her maintenance, [we] cannot [let her] die of starvation, especially in this case, as she isn't married and isn't obligated to nurse his son. Moreover, her son [Baby A] is already accustomed to nursing from another woman, whereas this infant [baby B] is used to her milk and won't nurse from anyone else, and one soul does not take precedence over another. Rather, let the court hire a wet nurse for him [Baby A] and force the infant's father to pay. And if the court cannot force him, let the court pay the salary [of the wet nurse].[61]

This responsum, like most written by R. Asher, is in answer to a question he was asked during the period he lived in Spain. In this case, despite the differences that existed between the Jews of Spain and the Jews in Ashkenaz, I would argue that the practices concerning the employment of wet nursing were similar. R. Asher himself uses precedents from Ashkenaz and points to similarities between Ashkenazic and Spanish practice.[62]

These two sources, the case of "Leah" and "Rachel" in Germany and of "Rachel" in Spain, illuminate the extent of a wet nurse's obligations and the absolute importance of breast milk to children's survival. The Spanish case emphasizes the importance attributed to having the wet nurse feed only one infant. The wet nurse must deny even her own child's well-being and prefer the baby she was hired to nurse over her own child. Incidentally, this responsum also shows the extent to which the law exempting a mother from the obligation of nursing her own child could be applied. In addition, both cases illustrate the desire of the infant's parents to avoid switching wet nurses. R. Asher's response highlights the importance he saw in ensuring that the child would not be harmed by replacing a wet nurse he was familiar with. The many cases in the literature that discuss wet nurses who broke their contracts are an indication of the frequency and severity of the difficulties faced by parents.

Scholars who have studied wet-nursing practices in Christian society have discussed the contracts wet nurses or their husbands signed when taking on new employment. In many cases the agreement was that the wet nurse would lose part of her salary if she left her job before her contract allowed her to do so. Many of the women who left their jobs early did so because of an additional pregnancy that prevented them from continuing to work. One of the ways employers tried to ensure that wet nurses would not leave their employment was by obtaining securities that would guarantee their stay. In other cases, they had the wet nurse, or her husband, swear that she would not break her contract.[63]

We find some mention of this practice in Jewish sources as well, although no contracts from the medieval period have been found. The Mordekhai mentions three different ways of ensuring that a wet nurse would remain with an infant throughout the entire period she was needed or, at least, minimizing the potential damage of her leaving. He mentions vows/oaths, guarantees, and the option of hiring two wet nurses so that at least one of the two will stay on.[64] Other sources provide further details of these practices. Oaths seemed to have been common. Women who swore not to leave their position usually committed themselves not to marry if they were single, and not to conceive, if they were married.[65] In the case of married women, this promise came under the category of vows by which a woman denies herself something. Since (according to Num. 31:10) such vows may be annulled by the husband, some legal authorities saw this oath as not sufficiently binding.[66] However, it should be noted that in the case of a Christian wet nurse, the Jewish legal authorities were not willing to accept her oaths as valid. The rabbis argued that because Jews feared that gentiles would harm their children, no Jew would risk his child's life and continue to employ a Christian wet nurse who wished to terminate her contract.

Monetary guarantees or securities were another matter. As in Christian society, the wet nurses (Jewish and Christian) often agreed to forfeit a part of their promised wage if they left early.[67] As for employing two wet nurses, this was a costly as well as a risky business. After all, both wet nurses could decide to leave, and then the infant would be no better off. This point does come up, however, in another Spanish responsum, written by R. Solomon Ibn Aderet (Rashba, thirteenth century). He discusses a case in which two wet nurses were hired, and the question addressed to him is whether one of them may be allowed to get married, as the child is used to nursing from two women, and if one of them cannot continue she may be replaced.[68]

In addition to their wages, the wet nurses received clothing and food.[69] Moreover, it seems that it eventually became customary to provide wet nurses with gifts at certain times of the year. The Jewish sources discuss this custom in connection with non-Jewish wet nurses, but it is likely that this was the prevailing custom when employing Jewish wet nurses too, as it was between Christian employers and their wet nurses.[70] The practice that raised the most concern was that of giving Christian wet nurses gifts on the holiday of Purim. This custom is mentioned in the literature written by Rashi and his students, as well as in later literature.

One of the traditional obligations of Purim is the giving of gifts to the poor.[71] But the intent of the commandment was the giving of gifts to the Jewish poor, and rabbis raised objections to giving Christian wet nurses money intended for Jewish purposes. Examining the sources that discuss this practice, one notes a change that took place over time. Rashi states:

> We have seen people who distribute [gifts] on Purim to servants and maids in Jewish homes. And this infuriated my rabbi, as it says "and presents to the poor" (Esther 9:22) — [gifts] to Jews and not to non-Jews. . . . As at first, those poor who were ashamed [to beg] sent their children with their gentile wet nurses to make the rounds of the Jewish homes, the [people] grew accustomed to giving [money] to the maids and wet nurses[72] for their own benefit as well, and not only for the needs of the children.[73]

Rashi and his contemporaries seem to have regarded this practice as flawed and forbidden. By contrast, thirteenth-century literature takes a very different approach. R. Samson b. Zadok, the student of R. Meir of Rothenburg says:

> The monies that we are accustomed to give to the maids on Purim — they [the maids] should not become accustomed to this in a city where it is not the practice. And R. Ephraim [probably R. Ephraim of Regensburg, in the second half of the twelfth century]: "I who lavished silver on her and gold — which they used for Baal" (Hos. 2:10). But in a place where they have already become accustomed, one should not cancel this practice in the interests of peace [*darkhei shalom*], as it says, "We support the poor of the heathen along with the poor of Israel in the interests of peace, and heathens may be assisted in the sabbatical year and greetings may be addressed to them, in the interests of peace (Gittin 61a)."[74]

Another thirteenth-century source states that wet nurses stipulate this money as part of their conditions of employment. R. Menahem b. Jacob of Worms (turn of thirteenth century) explains that one should put aside special money for the Christian servants before Purim since "they work for us all year for Purim and make clear conditions about the money they receive on Purim; therefore, it is [considered part of] their salary."[75] His comment indicates that terminating this custom would have caused great anger and resentment.

This custom raises some questions concerning the social class of the wet nurses in general, and those who came to work for Jews, in particular.[76] While no wet nurse came from a high social standing, and all the wet nurses undoubtedly belonged to the lower class, we may wonder to what extent Christian women who worked for Jews differed from other women employed by Christian families. Perhaps these extra presents, given, not by the employer, but by the employer's community on days such as Purim, are evidence of the low wages these wet nurses received. Another detail in this source reinforces this impression: These wet nurses are said to have gone with the children of poor Jews to collect presents for the poor on Purim. If poor Jews, who were themselves in need of charity, had wet nurses, then these wet nurses surely could not have earned much.

Mother or Wet Nurse?

We have examined some of the terms that regulated the employment of wet nurses in medieval society. These detailed terms, as well as the frequency with which wet nurses are mentioned in the sources, demonstrate that wet nursing was a widespread practice. It is impossible to assess to what extent Jewish families hired wet nurses, especially since halakhic responsa are our main source for examining this issue. These sources discuss cases in which there were problems; it is impossible to evaluate to what extent they represent the quotidian reality. Nevertheless, the many discussions of difficulties that arose when employing wet nurses demonstrate that hiring a wet nurse was a widespread practice.

Other than the general guidelines described above, many of which are based on talmudic principles, there is little discussion in the Ashkenazic sources of whether or not the practice of hiring wet nurses was a good or desired one. Explicit instructions that maternal breast-feeding is superior to hired help appear only in Jewish sources from Spain and Italy. This is not surprising, as this advice is found in medical tractates written in Italy and Spain; such tracts were almost nonexistent in medieval Ashkenaz.[77] Although we have little unequivocal evidence in the sources, I would suggest that the Jews in Ashkenaz, like their counterparts in Spain and Italy, and like their Christian neighbors, believed that maternal breast-feeding was preferable.[78] The importance attributed to maternal nursing derived from the common belief that breast milk not only gave nourishment, but also passed on personality traits. Therefore, in theory, when hiring a wet nurse, it was important not only to ensure that she was healthy and that her milk was plentiful, but also that she was of solid character. Nevertheless, wet nursing was quite common, and, in reality, more attention was paid to the nutrition of wet nurses than to their personalities. R. Isaac b. Moses, for example, quotes the Talmud, which emphasizes the importance of proper nutrition and provides a list of foods considered unhealthy for wet nurses. These include pumpkins, quince, unripe dates, small fish, lichen, and earth.[79]

Another way to learn about the importance attributed to maternal breast-feeding is by examining stories popular among Jews and Christians that discussed the employment of wet nurses, as well as cases in which infants refused to nurse from them. Many of these stories discuss the births and lives of heroes and saints. For example, the Jewish sources discuss the infancy of Moses. According to the Talmud and the Midrash, Moses refused to nurse from Egyptian women: "Then his sister said to Pharaoh's daughter: Shall I go and get you a Hebrew nurse to suckle the child for you?" (Exod. 2:7). The medieval Jewish commentators explain: "Why did Miriam say 'a Hebrew nurse'? Couldn't

Moses have nursed from a non-Jewish wet nurse?" Their argument is that since according to Jewish law a non-Jewish woman is permitted to nurse a Jewish child, Pharoah's daughter could have hired an Egyptian wet nurse. Why, then, did Miriam search specifically for a Jewish wet nurse? The answer given by the commentators is as follows:

> She suggested [hiring] a Jewish wet nurse because Moses had already been brought to Egyptian wet nurses and had refused to nurse from all of them. And why did he refuse? God said: "A mouth that will converse with me, shall it nurse from an impure woman?"[80]

This literary topos of a child who refuses to nurse from a foreign woman is also well known in medieval Christian literature. Narratives of the Virgin Mary's infancy also discuss her refusal to nurse from anyone except her mother, as do tales of Jesus' infancy.[81] Nicholas Orme relates one such story that reflects national pride, rather than sanctity. In it, an English child, the son of royalty, refuses to nurse from a French wet nurse. Stories of saints also emphasize the fact that their mothers nursed them, and that they were not given to wet nurses. For example, Bernard of Clairvaux (1090–1153) and Catherine of Sienna (1347–1380) are both mentioned as having been nursed by their mothers.[82] Some medieval stories emphasize the importance mothers accorded to nursing their children themselves. The Duchess of Bourlon, who lived during the eleventh century, is said to have been especially careful that her children not be nursed by anyone other than herself. One day, when she was at church, her son cried until a wet nurse was brought to pacify him. When she discovered this, she tried to force him to throw up what he had nursed, but did not succeed in doing so. The legend held that, as a result of this incident, this son was not as successful as his brothers.[83] This story and others helped promote maternal nursing. The beliefs promoted did not, however, restrict the practice of hiring wet nurses; in many cases, the mother herself nursed along with a wet nurse.[84]

While one could generalize from this topos and view it as a directive for motherly nursing, at least in the case of Moses, the commentary focuses more on the fact that he refused to nurse from an Egyptian woman than on his insistence on his mother. This focus on the consequences of nursing from a non-Jewish woman seems to be relevant for medieval Ashkenaz, where Jews frequently employed Christian wet nurses.

Jews and Christians

As noted above, there was no legal prohibition against Moses' nursing from an Egyptian woman. The Midrash's author's concern was for his own purity. While this concern could, theoretically, have influenced Jewish practices related to employing non-Jewish wet nurses, in reality, the employment of non-

Jewish wet nurses was widespread, and medieval Jewish sources express no discomfort with the practice of hiring them.

In medieval Christian society, wet nurses were employed in one of two ways: Either the wet nurse lived in the infant's house or the infant was sent to the wet nurse's home. Families that could afford to employ a wet nurse in their home opted to do so, whereas poorer families resorted to sending their infants to the wet nurse's home. According to Jewish law, the first option was the preferred one, if the wet nurse was not Jewish. The Mishna in Avodah Zara states clearly that a gentile woman may nurse a Jewish child only when she is on the Jewish woman's premises.[85] While it seems that most of the women employed by Jews as wet nurses were Christian, there were some Jewish wet nurses as well.

It is impossible to generalize about the patterns of employment of Jewish wet nurses. Most of the sources that discuss their employment, like many of the sources that discuss the employment of Christian wet nurses, talk about Jewish women who worked in the homes of their employers. It seems that many of these Jewish wet nurses were single women who had given birth, poor women, and/or women who were widowed or abandoned by their spouses.[86] R. Isaac b. Moses quotes the case of such a woman in his compendium *Sefer Or Zaru'a*. This woman began her career as a wet nurse as a divorcée after the birth of a child. It is unclear what the fate of her child was. Perhaps it died at birth and perhaps she gave him/her to a wet nurse. In another case, that of "Rachel" and "Leah" from Germany, examined above, we saw another example of a Jewish wet nurse whose marital status was unclear, but who, I suggested, was widowed, as she was conducting her own business negotiations.[87] It is interesting to note that the patriarchal responsibility over choosing a wet nurse can be found throughout the Middle Ages in medieval Ashkenaz, despite the tremendous freedom Jewish women enjoyed in business negotiations.

The sources do not allow us to determine whether there were more Jewish or Christian wet nurses employed in Jewish homes. However, the extensive discussion of the employment of Christian wet nurses demonstrates that Christian wet nurses were commonplace in Jewish households. The little known to us on the demographics of the Jewish community also supports this conclusion: There were more Jewish women in need of wet nurses than Jewish women who could provide this service. Consequently, the Jews had to look outside their communities for women who could fill this need.

Our knowledge of the employment of Christian wet nurses in Jewish homes stems from a variety of sources, written by both Jews and Christians. One important source of information is the papal documents that address the employment of Christians by Jews, which make it clear that Christian wet nurses lived in Jewish homes.[88] Warnings against this practice were issued repeatedly during the Middle Ages, especially from the end of the twelfth century on.[89] Based on the frequent reissuing of this prohibition, it seems that the employment of Christian wet nurses by Jews was widespread. This practice is also attested to in charters given to the Jews, in which it is clearly stated that Jews may employ non-Jewish wet nurses.[90] The practice was clearly forbidden in the edicts issued by Alexander III in 1179, which stated that Jews and Muslims could not own (Christian) slaves or servants in their homes in order to nurse their children, serve them, or for any other purpose. The bull stated that any Christian living in a Jewish home would be excommunicated.[91] The reason for forbidding Christians to live in Jewish homes is clearly stated:

> And we command . . . and forbid the tending of Jewish children by [Christian] midwives and wet nurses in their [the Jews] homes. For the customs of the Jews and ours are completely dissimilar, and [motivated by their hatred for the human race], they may easily influence the simple souls to come to their faith and heresy through extended contact and familiarity.[92]

Jewish sources also point to the common practice of employing Christian wet nurses in Jewish homes.[93] Most authors do not feel the need to justify the presence of a Christian woman in the house, and she is simply mentioned when relevant. These references manifest a major difference between the Christian sources that discuss Christian wet nurses who work for Jews and the Jewish sources on this issue. While the Christian sources forbid this practice completely,[94] the Jewish sources are more matter-of-fact about the practice, and only a small number of sources voice any opposition to it.

A source from *Sefer Ḥasidim* that discusses this practice illustrates the general approach to employing Christian wet nurses and the fears Jews had in this context:

> A man had two non-Jewish wet nurses in his home and they were at strife.[95] People said to him, "Why are you creating arguments in your home?" He said: "If they live in harmony, perhaps they will steal from me. But now each one fears the other." They said to him, "About you it is said: 'So that you do not bring bloodguilt on your house' (Deut. 22:8), and it is written: 'And do not rely on your own understanding' (Prov. 3:5), since your [actions] cause that one might kill the infant that the other wet nurse is nursing or the other the child of the first wet nurse."[96]

This story documents the presence of non-Jewish wet nurses in Jewish homes. Although the sources mention the fear that the wet nurses would kill their charges, this fear stems from the animosity between the two wet nurses, rather than from hostility related to Jewish-Christian relations. The advice to the protagonist of the story is that the Ḥasid should not cause disharmony in his own household, not that he should not employ non-Jewish wet nurses.

Other cautions against employing Christian wet nurses discuss specific issues, but do not forbid or censure the actual practice of their employment. *Sefer Ḥasidim* mentions the possible dangers of having a Jewish child hear a

Christian lullaby sung by his or her wet nurse. R. Judah the Pious does not recommend, however, firing the wet nurse, but rather that the wet nurse not sing.[97] The same tendency is illustrated in discussions of the danger of wet nurses teaching children improper behavior.[98]

An additional problem mentioned in the sources was the nonkosher food wet nurses introduced into Jewish households:

> Non-Jewish wet nurses and servants ate impure things in the house, and the young children would eat them too. Also, the adults could not guard [the kashrut] of the dishes. Therefore one should not remain in the same city.[99]

The context of this comment is a discussion in *Sefer Ḥasidim* of cases in which a Ḥasid who fears for his soul and for his Judaism should leave the city, rather than live in a state of danger (of conversion). The advice given to the Ḥasid in this case, leaving the city, is unrelated to the employment of wet nurses. This practice was an aspect of medieval Jewish life: The specific circumstances in this city, including the practices of wet nurses, endangered the Ḥasid and his devotion.

Other sources discuss the nonkosher food that was part of a non-Jewish wet nurse's presence in the house. Since it was her responsibility to feed the infant, the fear was that she would feed the infant improperly. One approach was that the young children's eating of the wet nurse's food posed no problem, since a minor is allowed to eat nonkosher food. There is ample evidence that, in certain cases, for example, if the child's health required it, parents fed their children foods that adults did not eat because of dietary restrictions. At times, this violated both the laws of kashrut and the laws of the Sabbath.[100] Moreover, nonkosher substances could be found regularly in Jewish homes, even if they were not meant to be eaten. For example, sores and boils were often treated with lard and the fat of other animals; these substances were used, not only for children, but also as cures for adults. Children are said to have eaten lard both for medicinal purposes and at the table, even when adults were sitting at the same table eating.[101] As such, it would seem that, although modern practice instinctively rejects this notion, medieval Jews often had these nonkosher substances in their homes and on their tables.[102]

As opposed to those who sanctioned bringing the food of non-Jewish wet nurses into the Jewish homes and, in some cases, even permitted the mother of the child to feed her child this food herself, there was a second approach hinted at in the source from *Sefer Ḥasidim* examined above. This source discussed elements that could induce Jews to convert and mentioned the wet nurses' impure food as one such temptation. While the text does not explain how moving to a different city would solve the problem, it does demonstrate that contact with impure food can serve as an impetus for conversion.

This fear is mentioned in other sources as well. For example: R. Isaac b. Moses, the author of the compendium Sefer Or Zaru'a, discusses this concern.

He explains that one can give young children nonkosher food. Yet he stipulates some precautions:

> Despite this, one should warn the wet nurse not to eat impure meat or pork and certainly not to feed them [the infants] impure substances, as it is written: "What caused [Aḥer to apostasize]..." And some commentaries on the passage explain, that some say that when she [his mother] was pregnant with him, she would pass in front of idolatry, and she smelled something of that *min*[103] and they gave it to her and she ate and that *min* bubbled in her body.... For everything that a woman eats, the infant eats. And this caused him to turn to evil ways in his old age.[104]

R. Isaac's comment expresses the belief, discussed above, that the food a wet nurse eats influences the infant she nurses, just as any food a person eats influences who they are. His objection is not commonly found in the sources and, on the whole, the halakha does not discuss this issue.

Another objection to children's eating of nonkosher food from wet nurses is provided in one of R. Meir b. Barukh's responsa. R. Meir discusses the educational effect of this practice. His concern is that children will learn to obey their wet nurses rather than their fathers. After all, their fathers forbid them to eat nonkosher food, so if they eat the food their wet nurses provide, they are acting against his will. Despite this concern, Maharam allows children to eat the food of their wet nurses.[105]

It is noteworthy that despite their objections — whether they be fear for the soul and future Jewish character of the child, or concern for the parent's educational authority, none of the sources state outright that Jews should not employ Christian wet nurses. It is also of note that those who raise oppositions to Christian wet nurses and their practices are German, whereas northern French authorities seem to find less to criticize in these practices.

In contrast to the attitudes voiced in the Jewish sources, I have already noted the fierce objections expressed by church authorities to Christian women working in Jewish homes. The church authorities objected to this practice for ideological and practical reasons related to the social context of hired Christian wet nurses. How could Christian women be under the authority of people who are inferior to them? In addition, the church feared that these Christian women would be exploited sexually, harassed and humiliated, and, even worse, convinced to convert and adopt a Jewish way of life.[106]

One example of such humiliation appears in accusations raised by both Pope Innocent III (d. 1216) and Henricus Segusio (1200–1270). Both accuse the Jews of forcing the wet nurses who worked in their homes to spill out their milk for three days after receiving communion. There is no hint or mention of this practice in any of the medieval Jewish sources.[107] However, this belief is further evidence of medieval understandings of the influence of the food eaten by a nursing woman on the feeding child. Since this accusation appears only in these two sources, it is hard to determine whether or not this was common, or even occasional, Jewish practice. In any case, its appearance in Christian sources is further evidence of Christian sensitivity to possible insults to their religion by Jews. In addition, frequently reissued edicts regularly mention the fear that Christian women working in Jewish households would learn the Jewish ways of life and ultimately convert. It would seem, though, that these protestations were overcome by the needs of everyday life that compelled Christian women to seek such employment and Jewish families to hire them.

IN AND OUT OF THE HOUSE

Both Christian and Jewish sources discuss at length cases in which Christian women nurse Jewish children in Jewish homes. This discussion confirms that the instructions in the Mishna and Talmud in tractate Avodah Zara, which state that gentile women should only be employed on Jewish premises, were applied in practice. Scholars have assumed that, because Jews followed the laws prohibiting idolatry (concentrated in tractate Avodah Zara), Christian wet nurses who nursed Jewish children always did so in the home. Most medieval sources seem to confirm this. Rashi, for example, explains the Talmudic injunction that a non-Jewish woman nurses Jewish children *bir'shuta* — in her own domain — in the following way: "In her own domain — the domain of the Jewess, but she should not give [the baby] to be taken to her [the non-Jewish wet nurse's] home, so that she [the wet nurse] will not kill him."[108] His comment echoes the talmudic explanation for this ruling. The fear of infants dying at the hands of their non-Jewish caretakers outside the home features throughout the discussions of this practice, although it is not considered a reason to stop the practice. It would seem that while Jews felt they could supervise the Christian wet nurses sufficiently within their own homes, they felt they could not do so outside them. While most scholars have attributed this fear to the distrust that existed between Jews and Christians in medieval society, it should be noted that this concern is not solely an expression of religious tension. As Klapisch-Zuber and Herlihy have shown, in fourteenth-century Italy, Christian children sent to the homes of wet nurses (as opposed to having live-in wet nurses) suffered from higher mortality.

The argument that Christian women were employed only within Jewish homes ignores one well-known source that suggests otherwise. In the Paris disputation of 1240, R. Yeḥiel of Paris comments on the practice of sending Jewish children to Christian wet nurses in Christian homes. As part of his argument for the good relations and trust that existed between Jews and Christians, he states: "Go to the streets of the Jews and see . . . and they place our children in their homes to be nursed."[109] Some scholars have dismissed this comment as an apologetic attempt of R. Yeḥiel's to depict a more trusting relationship between Jews and Christians than existed in reality. I would suggest, however, that we accept his comment as testimony of a regular practice, since a number of other sources from France corroborate it.

An investigation concerning whether Jewish children were sent to the homes of Christian wet nurses requires an excursus into the legal literature of the period. The Tosafist commentary on Tractate Avodah Zara discusses the same passage that Rashi discussed, regarding nursing infants on Jewish premises. Unlike Rashi, who explains that the fear that the gentile nurse will kill the child determines the location in which the wet nurse cares for her charge, the Tosafist says:

> If so, one must be careful not to let a Jewess who is going out of town leave her son alone at home in the hands of a non-Jewish wet nurse, if there are no other Jewesses in the city who come in and go out at all times. And even in such cases, from the time the baby is put to sleep, he should not be left alone. As for a young boy or girl left alone at the home of an idol worshiper to be cured, R. Isaac said this is not allowed for a number of reasons since they [the idol worshipers] are suspected of spilling blood. And even if they [the children] are grown, they may be lured to *minut* [Christianity].[110]

This source describes a situation in which the mother of the infant goes out of town and leaves her child alone with the Christian wet nurse, who is clearly responsible for the child's care. The discussion, as presented, does not clearly indicate where the wet nurse is physically taking care of the child — in her own home or in the child's home. Permission is given only if a Jewish friend of the mother checks on the wet nurse frequently; there seems to be a special concern for the baby's welfare during the night.[111] The second part of the Tosafist's comment discusses a different issue raised in the Talmud, concerning leaving sick children in the homes of non-Jewish healers to be nursed back to health. In this case, it is clear that the children are in the non-Jewish home. R. Isaac (R"i haZaken of Dampierre, d. end of twelfth century) forbids this practice, but it clearly does take place in spite of his objections.

The mention of the practice of sending sick children to Christian healers' homes, makes it likely that the Jewish infants referred to in the previous lines of the same text were those who stayed in Christian wet nurses' homes. The Tosafist's comments are further explained in an additional source. Commenting on the same passage in tractate Avodah Zara, R. Elḥanan, the son of R. Isaac of Dampierre (who objected to the practice) explains:

> "Not if she is on her own." Therefore one should be careful not to place a Jewish infant in the home of a non-Jew to be nursed. And even in a Jewish home, one cannot leave them [the infants] if they do not come and go, which is like having others standing by her. . . . And this applies to nursing and also to children who need to be cured. It seems from this that they should not be left alone in the house of the non-Jew without any Jews present for a month or two months. And even though we are not afraid that she will apply poison to her breast [one of the fears in the case of nursing], they [the non-Jews] are suspect of spilling blood.[112]

R. Elhanan's warning against sending an infant to the wet nurse's home or even leaving him/her in a Jewish home alone with the wet nurse at night manifests a fierce objection to this practice. We see from this source, that the rabbis were not discussing a mere overnight stay, but a much lengthier one. It follows from this that some Jewish children were sent to the homes of wet nurses for extended periods, at least during the day. In summary, these sources seem to indicate differing attitudes toward these issues. The more lenient approach allowed Jewish children to be cared for in Christian homes, certainly during the day, and, in some cases, at night as well. The more stringent approach required them to remain at home and under constant Jewish supervision.

Other sources that discuss the employment of Christian wet nurses also relate to the presence of Jewish children in Christian wet nurses' homes. The basis for these discussions is the thirteenth-century composition *Sefer haTerumah* written by R. Barukh b. Isaac of Paris (d. 1211).[113] As Simha Emanuel has demonstrated, R. Barukh was a French scholar, and not of German origin as thought in previous research.[114] R. Barukh says:

> "A gentile woman may nurse an Israelite child if others are standing by, but not if she is on her own." This ruling implies that one may not give the son of an Israelite to a non-Jewish woman unless others are standing by her or, at the very least, if there are Jews coming and going. But it does not seem that having an Israelite woman standing by her is a requirement. This applies to the domain of the heathens. But in the domain of Israel, it is allowed in any case. . . . And if the Israelite woman goes out of town, she should not leave her son alone with a heathen woman. But if there are Israelite women in the city, it is permissible, since they are used to coming there and making sure that the Israelite's son is not alone. And at the very least, at night it is forbidden to leave him with the heathen alone after bed time.[115]

This source seems to point quite clearly to the practice of sending children to Christian wet nurses' homes, as R. Yehiel of Paris himself suggested. R. Barukh suggests that these children stayed at the wet nurse's home during the day. He did not permit the child to stay in the Christian home without supervision, and it is clear that he expects Jewish women to drop by and check on the child's welfare. The reality he describes is, in any case, not that of a live-in wet nurse. His attitude toward the question of whether the infants could stay at the Christian wet nurse's home at night is less clear. May a child never sleep in a Christian home, or is this the case only when his mother is out of town? This question remains unresolved, but, in any case, the passage clearly documents the practice, mentioned by R. Yehiel of Paris, of sending Jewish children to Christian homes.

R. Barukh's opinion is quoted by other halakhic authorities in the thirteenth century. For example, R. Moses of Couçy, who was the youngest of the participants in the Paris disputation, mentions this issue in his *Sefer Mizvot Gadol*:

But a gentile nurses the son of Israel while others are standing by her. And R. Barukh wrote that it seems that even if there is no Jew at home, it is allowed if the Jews in the city come and go; but if all the Jews left the city and the wet nurse remained, it is prohibited.[116]

R. Moses' quote of R. Barukh is again unclear as to whose house is being supervised. A possible explanation can be found in the comments of a third halakhic figure, R. Jacob Ḥazan of London. He explains that R. Barukh said that "even if there is no Jew in the house, if there is a Jewish home in the city or someone coming in and checking, it is allowed. If all the Jews have left the city, then it is prohibited."[117] It seems he is saying that as long as there was another Jewish household in the city, the child would be considered adequately supervised in the Christian home.

On the basis of these texts, I would suggest that there were parents who left their children in Christian homes to be cared for during the day and, at times, even overnight. Some objected quite fiercely to this practice, and called for more stringent behavior. Among the reasons they gave for their objection was their fear that the Christian women might kill the children while working in the house, and their fear that the children themselves might be influenced by the Christian family with whom they were living.[118] The sources examined above, however, reflect mainly the practice of the Jews living in Paris and northern France. They demonstrate that, in spite of their fears, Jews sent their children to Christian wet nurses' homes.[119]

R. Barukh's opinion featured prominently in much of the literature of the subsequent generations.[120] Yet one caveat is in order. While R. Barukh's ruling was accepted in France, it is not often quoted in the German sources and seems to meet with objections on the part of German rabbis. While northern France and Germany shared a common heritage, as we have seen previously, this would seem to be one of the issues on which they differed. Some twelfth-century German authorities state clearly that Christian wet nurses worked only in Jewish households.[121] One thirteenth-century source, however, discusses this issue in a vein similar to R. Barukh's ruling, and declares that during the day children could be left in the home of the Christian wet nurse.[122] This source is R. Eleazar b. Judah (Rokeaḥl's *Sefer Rokeaḥl*. As this is perhaps a later addition to the Rokeaḥ, we cannot be sure to what extent this quotation reflects the reality in R. Eleazar b. Judah's place and time. His opinion is definitely not the only one in thirteenth-century Germany, and other sources fiercely object to the practice. For example, R. Isaac b. Moses, the author of the *Or Zaru'a* repeats Rashi's assertion that Christian wet nurses are to be feared, and states specifically that even if a Jew comes in and out to supervise the infant's care, this must take place in the home of the Jew and that children cannot be left in Christian homes.[123]

This long discussion of the legal texts points to a dimension of Jewish-Christian relations that has not yet been taken into consideration. If Jews in northern France and perhaps, in a more limited fashion, in Germany, were sending their children to non-Jewish homes to be nursed, we should see this as an important component in the daily contacts between Jews and Christians. If Jewish infants spent time every day in Christian homes, then their parents, or at the very least their mothers, were in these Christian homes on a daily basis and were exposed, even if unconsciously, to elements of Christian daily routine. It is not surprising that given the choice, Jews — like their Christian neighbors — preferred employing wet nurses in their own homes. As discussed above, employment in the home ensured lower mortality rates and better supervision.[124] This was, however, also more costly, and I would suggest that economics played a crucial role when families decided how and where to employ a wet nurse.[125]

The sources examined reveal the creative interpretations the medieval halakhic authorities provided for the instructions given in tractate Avodah Zara. The purpose of this reinterpretation was to construct a framework that fit the medieval reality and its constraints. We should note, however, that tractate Avodah Zara contains instructions regarding another relevant set of circumstances: Jewish women were forbidden to serve as wet nurses for non-Jewish children under any circumstances. The reason for their absolute and complete denial of permission was theological — a Jewish woman who nursed the son of a gentile idol worshiper was helping to raise a future idol worshiper, a practice no Jew should abet.

Finding such cases in medieval sources is difficult. Considering all the practical problems that might arise from such a situation, it is hard to imagine a situation in which Jewish women would work in Christian homes. One can assume that such women, if they existed, were on the margins of Jewish society. Some Jewish women did work as wet nurses in the homes of other Jews[126] and, given the legal guidelines discussed above, might have been preferred over Christian wet nurses. An examination of the medieval sources, however, does not reveal a single case of Jewish women who nursed Christian children. In addition, the canonical sources that discuss the employment of Christian women in Jewish homes do not make much mention of this possibility.[127] The medieval Jewish sources that discuss wet nursing devote little attention to this situation, and, with one exception, they quote the talmudic discussion without any further comments or additions.[128]

We do find one interesting exception to this rule, although it pertains less to contracted wet nursing than to neighborly relations. Some medieval Jewish sources discuss a problem that occurred on Sabbath. In some cases, Jewish women suffered from a surplus of milk on Sabbath. The ruling in such a case was to allow this woman to nurse as much as possible until the pain subsided. On weekdays, these women often expressed the excess milk. But on the Sabbath, expressing milk was forbidden. The halakhic ruling was that Jewish women could nurse Christian children if such a necessity arose, in order to ease their pain. R. Mordekhai b. Hillel, in his comments on tractate Avodah Zara states: "And on the Sabbath, if the Jewish woman has too much milk and she is in pain, she is allowed to nurse the child of a non-Jewish woman."[129] This ruling, in combination with those considered above, concerning the sending of Jewish children to Christian homes, provides evidence of the intimacy of the daily contacts between Jews and Christians. If Jewish children were cared for on a daily basis in Christian homes, then Jewish women must have been somewhat familiar with the way these homes functioned.[130] If a Jewish woman could nurse her Christian neighbor's child when she had a surplus of milk, then their relationship must have been a familiar one.[131]

These relationships between Jewish and Christian women, even if they were tinged at times with hostility and suspicion, cannot be dismissed as inconsequential. Recent work on the anthropology of breast-feeding has demonstrated that giving a child to a wet nurse of a different religious or ethnic group has important social significance. In some cases, when the practice is reciprocal, this is a way of furthering the relationship between the two groups.[132] While it is not a formal connection between the groups, it is an informal link that enhances the contacts between them.[133] This idea was certainly not foreign to Jews or Christians in the Middle Ages. It is the basis for medieval (and ancient) Jewish laws governing employment of Christian wet nurses, as well as Christian objections to this practice. Jewish and Christian women who conversed daily, whether as employers and employees or as neighbors helping each other out in a bind, had ample opportunity to exchange opinions and information. This shared knowledge was probably connected to child care, a topic of mutual interest and concern. Although this kind of connection certainly did not eliminate the fears we noted above of Jewish children being hurt or even killed by Christian wet nurses, it does point to a relationship between Jewish and Christian women that has received little attention to date. These opportunities for contact illustrate the constant communication that existed between Jewish and Christian women, as we saw in the case of the birth practices examined in chapter 1.[134] The close quarters of the home certainly allowed Jewish and Christian women many intimate moments for the exchange of opinions and information.

Nursing Mothers, Small Children: Regulating Interests

Our discussion so far has dealt at length with wet nurses, their responsibilities and lives. Investigating the world of wet nurses has also directed our attention to the fathers of the infants, who were legally responsible for ensuring their well-being. However, except for a brief discussion regarding the superiority of maternal breast-feeding over hired wet nursing, we have only touched on the mothers of the children who gave their offspring to be nursed. The remainder of this chapter will be devoted to these women and their dilemmas.

Note that the emphases of my discussion reflect those of the medieval sources. As such, this case is a superb example of the difficulties the extant sources pose to learning more about medieval women and their lives. I began this chapter by stating that at times mothers and their children had conflicting interests. These conflicts are at the crux of the legal literature. Consequently, we have no information about routine practices. The legal assumption was that if the family unit was harmonious and complete, any problems that arose would and could be worked out within its framework. The sources that discuss wet-nursing practices allow only a very partial glimpse into the lives of these families, at the instances when problems with wet nurses required outside intervention.

As the authorities assumed that families could usually solve whatever problems arose in connection to breast-feeding within the framework of the family, there are few discussions of married women who chose to breast-feed or to not breast-feed their children. Discussions of this subject come up in one context only — contraception. Subsequent pregnancies, especially when a woman was breast-feeding, endangered the life of the nursing infant.[135] While modern medical research has suggested that, due to poor nutrition in the past, fewer women were able to conceive while breast-feeding, apparently, conception during this period was not an uncommon experience,[136] and medieval Jewish sources discuss the issue at length. Permission to prevent conception, mentioned already in the Talmud, was also discussed in medieval texts.[137] Unlike Christian society, in which church directives indicated abstention from sexual relations during the entire period of nursing, as mentioned above, some Jewish legal authorities allowed nursing women to use a form of contraception known as a *mokh* — a cervical sponge; no legal authority recommended abstention.[138]

While the legal sources discussing these issues cannot shed much light on the daily lives of mothers whose lives were not fraught with difficulties (such as wet nurses who quit and husbands who did not want them to breast-feed), the medieval attitudes toward contraception can enhance our understanding of family planning, as well as the circumstances surrounding the employment of wet nurses. If contraception was forbidden, then the need for a wet nurse was greater. In families where, for religious reason (such as fulfilling the commandment of procreation),[139] the couple wished to have more children as quickly as possible, women would surely hire wet nurses. In other cases, however, whether because of poverty or out of a need or desire to space children, the permissibility of contraception was important, and Jewish women regularly employed this method of birth control. Indeed, some authorities argued that nursing women must use some form of contraception to prevent an additional pregnancy in order to protect the life of the existing infant.[140]

One such discussion about the spacing of children and the use of breast-feeding as a method of family planning can be found in *Sefer Ḥasidim*:

> It is said: "After weaning Lo-Ruhama" (Hos. 1:8). Once she had given birth to a son and a daughter, she weaned her. For his wife had already given birth to a son and a daughter and there was a waiting period. But after the birth of the first son, there was no delay, because he had not fulfilled the obligation of procreation. And if a man has one son or one daughter and the mother nurses that son or that daughter, as long as she nurses, she cannot conceive. Furthermore, she is too poor to hire a wet nurse[141] or she is concerned that the child will not nurse [from a wet nurse] because he already recognizes his mother. In such a case, she should not refrain from nursing the infant because of this danger. For the claim is that one existing life does not supersede that of another possible life (Ohalot 7:6) that may come into being if she conceives. But if the woman, the mother of the child, nurses, and another woman nurses the child with her, since the other wet nurse, who is not the mother of the child, provides for him, the mother of the child can stop nursing so that she may conceive. And if she is poor, then they said, "the Holy One, blessed be He, said: My children, borrow on my account and I will pay" (Beẓah 15b), especially since, in this case, the mother of the child does so in order to become pregnant, as she cannot conceive while she nurses. Only [be sure] that the wet nurse has abundant milk.[142]

Although this case does not discuss contraception at length, it does demonstrate the general belief that a breast-feeding mother cannot conceive. We see here that even when the Ḥasid clearly seeks to fulfill the commandment of procreation, in this exceptional case, the health of the existing infant takes precedence.

This discussion in *Sefer Ḥasidim* illuminates the ways in which attitudes toward contraception are directly related to the understandings of procreation, as discussed in chapter 1. As in the case of the commandment to procreate, there is a clear difference between the roles men and women are expected to play. Because men are instructed to procreate, they are not allowed to prevent procreation. As a result, contraception was women's business.[143] Despite the ostensible differences between Jewish and Christian understandings of procreation,[144] it is well known that in Christian society contraception was women's business as well, often called *arte muliebri*.[145] Thus, both in Jewish society (with the explicit permission of male legal authorities), and in Christian society (despite the official prohibition of the practice), women practiced forms of contraception, and this is an instance in which one can see how women could control their fertility.[146]

On the whole, medieval Jewish authorities do not discuss the issue of contraception at length; they merely repeat the sanction of the practice as it appears in the Mishna. One can only speculate on the reasons the issue is not debated at length — it may be that, since contraception was seen as women's business, and that men had an interest in letting them do as they saw fit, they refrained from passing legislation. In any case, they may have felt that women would ignore their rulings.[147] Whatever the case, the few legal authorities who do discuss the issue permit breast-feeding mothers to use some form of contraception. One opinion, that of R. Tam, one of the most prominent legal authorities of the period, stands out in its decisiveness. R. Tam, took a very firm position on the question of contraception. He said that a nursing woman *must* use some form of contraception, in order to ensure the life of her living child, who was dependent on her for his/her nourishment.[148]

R. Tam allows breast-feeding mothers to use contraception only in severely restricted circumstances — if it is necessary to protect the life of the nursing infant. This authorization could be applied, however, only in the context of an intact family. The assumption was also that if an additional pregnancy did occur during the two years of lactation, the father would care sufficiently about his existing offspring to ensure his/her well-being (BT Yevamot 42a). The situation became much stickier when the family was no longer together, whether as a result of divorce or widowhood.

I have already outlined the legal restrictions concerning the remarriage of divorcees and widows with children under the age of two. In these cases, the authorities feared that the mother might neglect the infant out of a desire to strengthen her relationship with her new partner. The stepfather was not expected to have any special sentiments toward his stepchildren or to show any special compassion or concern for their welfare. In addition, the sources suggest that other relatives on the deceased husband's side, at least in the case of widows, could not be trusted to look out for the infant's welfare, since these relatives often had interests connected to inheritance that would be threatened by the survival of the infant.[149]

The authorities' concern for the infant's welfare is reflected in the frequency of cases dealing with widowed or divorced mothers of small infants. These occupy a prominent position in the discussions concerning breast-feeding. Although there are no statistics concerning the percentage of women who became widows or divorcées before their youngest child reached the age of twenty-four months, this was not a rare phenomenon. Recent research has shown that divorce was widespread in medieval Ashkenaz, and that the dangers that travel and disease posed in medieval times caused many women to become widowed at an early age.[150]

When examining the talmudic laws regarding wet nursing, we saw that according to Jewish law widows were not supposed to remarry until their youngest child reached the age of twenty-four months. In the case of divorcées, women were not officially obligated to nurse their children after their divorce, and, if they did, their husbands were supposed to pay them for their labors. Although in theory they could remarry after three months, in practice, they were often forced to wait longer, out of concern for the infants' welfare. These laws were discussed and redefined in medieval Ashkenaz.

Twelfth- and Thirteenth-Century Scandals

The question of the remarriage of widowed and divorced women during the period of their nursing was subject to intense scrutiny during the second half of the twelfth century; these discussions still echoed vividly during the first part of the thirteenth century. During the course of the twelfth and thirteenth centuries, legal attitudes toward divorced or widowed women with infants under twenty-four months of age underwent marked change. In almost all the cases brought before the courts or that required the ruling of individual rabbis, the mothers wished to remarry, and the legal restrictions of their status as nursing mothers posed barriers to their newly proposed marriages. These cases are sometimes brought by the men who wish to marry these women, sometimes by the women themselves, or their families, and, at times, by their ex-husbands or the deceased husband's family.[151]

The sources from the period preceding the mid–twelfth century closely follow the talmudic rulings. Divorcées and widows were treated differently, and the more lenient legal authorities allowed nursing women to remarry when their children reached the age of eighteen months, rather than wait until the end of the twenty-fourth-month period. For example, R. Samson of Falaise, who was a student of Rashi's, and was R. Tam's teacher and brother-in-law, is said to have ruled that a divorcée could remarry three months after her divorce if she had never nursed her infant.[152] While R. Samson agreed that it was better if the woman waited longer before marrying again and stated that "if she acts stringently, she should be blessed," he seems to recognize the need some of these women had to remarry.[153] In addition, some sources report that R. Samson followed Beit Hillel's opinion, ruling that a woman who was nursing her child could remarry after fifteen or eighteen months,[154] rather than waiting the full twenty-four months, as was generally accepted.[155]

R. Tam set about changing these legal norms. His central ruling had to do with the status of divorcées. In vehement opposition to his brother-in-law, R. Samson, and contrary to the opinion of many of his contemporaries and predecessors, R. Tam held that both divorcées and widows must wait the full twenty-four months before remarrying, without any exceptions to the rule. Even if the woman had never nursed her child, and could transfer it to a wet nurse without problem, she was not allowed to remarry until her child reached the age of two.[156] R. Tam adapted two different discussions of divorced and widowed women, which appear in the Mishna and the Talmud, as his precedents. One precedent was a Mishna in Tractate *Sotah* that discusses how to treat pregnant or nursing women who are suspected of adultery. Women who were accused by their husbands of extramarital affairs were subjected to an ordeal that included the drinking of "bitter waters" (Num. 5:27). According to the Mishna, however, pregnant women and nursing mothers should not drink this water.[157] R. Tam deduces from this that since a pregnant woman and a nursing mother are placed in the same category, the same rules should apply to both. Therefore, divorcées and widows should be bound by the same legal obligations concerning remarriage and should be treated in the same way from a legal point of view.

The more central reason R. Tam gives for his ruling is related to his fear that if the child's mother remarries, she may become less devoted to ensuring the child's well-being, and consequently, the child may die. This concern concurs with his ruling discussed above, concerning contraception. He explains this fear in two ways — one worry is, as discussed above, that if the mother becomes pregnant again she will not be able to nurse her child. The other concerns the talmudic understanding of how a divorced or widowed woman ensures her own financial support. According to the Talmud, a widow is embarrassed to claim her welfare in front of the court, and because she is afraid to appear in front of the court, her embarrassment can lead to the death of her child.[158] R. Tam argues that if a widow has this fear, then surely a divorcée, whose husband is alive, shares this feeling.[159] Since, as we saw above, there is no expectation that the new husband provide for the child's needs, it is imperative not to allow the mother to become part of a relationship that might lead to her neglect of the child's welfare.

This argument is presented in the Tractate Yevamot to explain why a widow must wait before she remarries.[160] Yet these reasons do not make sense in the medieval context, where women frequently went to court, and so one would not expect them to be embarrassed to sue anyone.[161] In addition, not only did Jewish law allow divorce, but, as marriages were arranged and children were often wed at an early age, many seemed to have chosen divorce. Some scholars have recently estimated that the rate of divorce in medieval Ashkenaz was high.[162] In this cultural setting, women were not embarrassed to confront their ex-husbands in court. R. Tam's position presented a tremendous obstacle to young divorcées with children under age two who wished to remarry. His opinion became the dominant one in both Germany and northern France during the century that followed,[163] although other opinions, such as that of R. Samson of Falaise discussed above, were still considered.[164]

One issue, however, remained unresolved. What should be done in a case where a widow or divorcée remarried without seeking permission? Should they be forced to divorce or was their marriage validated post factum? One of R. Tam's students, R. Joseph Bekhor Shor, quoting a ruling by R. Tam, claimed that the couple need not divorce; they were merely obliged to live separately until the waiting period was over; others did not agree.[165] In the thirteenth century, attitudes toward women who remarried became even stricter. A famous case was discussed throughout Ashkenaz and became a precedent for the generations that followed. A woman from Krakow, who is called the widow of Krakow in the halakhic literature, married a well-known Polish rabbi, R. Jacob Savra of Krakow. Before she remarried, she hired a wet nurse[166] and had her swear in front of witnesses that she would not leave her post before the infant was twenty-four months old. In spite of her attempt to assure the infant's well-being, when the marriage was publicized, some rabbinic authorities thought R. Jacob should be forced to divorce the widow. This case, however, had some unique circumstances. R. Jacob was a Cohen, the descendant of Aaronic priests. Hence, according to Jewish law, he could not marry a divorcée. Therefore, had the couple been divorced, they would not have been able to remarry when the infant reached the age of twenty-four months.

As part of the attempt to resolve this case, scholars throughout Europe were contacted and asked to express their opinions. This case is mentioned already in R. Isaac b. Moses's *Sefer Or Zaru'a* and is continually discussed for many years afterward.[167] Although there are numerous accounts of this story, many details concerning the case are unclear, and Israel Ta-Shma even suggested that over time the details of the case were censored by copyists.[168] Questions were sent to many scholars, and only one scholar, R. Tuviah (Tobias) of Vienne, was willing to allow the couple to remain married. R. Tuviah, a thirteenth-century French scholar, argued that since the wet nurse had sworn she would remain in her post, the couple should not be forced to divorce.[169] All the German scholars, on the other hand, were of the opinion that R. Jacob must divorce his wife, and they even threatened to excommunicate him if he did not do so. They refused to accept the oath of the wet nurse or the securities she gave as binding, arguing that the wet nurse's husband could easily annul her vow.[170] This stringent ruling became the normative one and had far-reaching consequences.[171]

In examining the response to this trend, it becomes clear that many medieval women and their families felt that these laws, and especially the stringency with which they were enforced, were unnecessarily harsh. For example, in a twelfth-century case from France, a young woman named Frieda, the daughter of R. Isaac of Rouen, wishes to obtain permission to remarry although she is pregnant. As a young divorcée who had not yet given birth, Frieda could surely have decided not to nurse her child and obtained a wet nurse for him. Her father and his colleague, R. Moses haDoeg b. Nathan, present this argument in their suit for permission for her to remarry.[172] Frieda's family, arguing on her behalf, contends that it is of utmost importance for her to be able to remarry as quickly as possible. The opposition argues for enforcing R. Tam's ruling.

We can assume that many of the women who were divorced and widowed with small infants were fairly young, as they were in their childbearing years. Probably, in many cases, as in the case of Frieda, their families supported, or perhaps even encouraged them to remarry quickly. This is supported by studies of widows in medieval Christian society. Scholars have demonstrated the need young widows often had to remarry quickly after their husband's deaths, even if they had two or three small children. The reality that widows faced in medieval Jewish society has not yet been studied extensively. Yet the situation described in the sources examined here, concerning the issue of breast-feeding, points to a similar need to remarry.

The stance of the legal authorities here is fascinating, if we compare their position concerning widows to their position on wet nurses. In the case of single Jewish wet nurses, they voiced great concern that the women not commit themselves to service, as this would automatically hinder their ability to marry. Thus, in the case of a Jewish wet nurse who committed herself to a twenty-four-month contract, but later regretted her commitment, R. Isaac b. Moses ruled:

> And I think that certainly a woman who vowed in public . . . if she came before a wise man and said "I swore in front of many to nurse for twenty-four months and not to marry and now I regret this because I am afraid I will sin carnally, as I thought I could suffer twenty-four months without a husband, but now I cannot suffer any longer . . . she is to be permitted [to marry and break her contract], since it is certainly to accomplish a good deed.[173]

One can see from this comparison how great the concern for the infant's welfare was, since the authorities do not raise the possibility of the promiscuity of divorcées and widows during the period they were not allowed to remarry, as this consideration is minor in comparison to the concern for the infant's life.

Furthermore, if we compare the legal rulings concerning remarriage of mothers of infants to those concerning the remarriage of their fathers, we see a marked difference. Widowed men with small children were allowed to remarry much more quickly than other men, even within the week of the *shiv'a* (the week of mourning following the burial) that immediately followed their wives' deaths, so that there would be someone to take care of the family.

The central factor in all of these rulings is the infant's welfare. This concern is illustrated in the differing attitudes and laws concerning mothers', fathers', and wet nurses' obligations to the children, as well as in discussions of contraception. This concern seems to have been even greater in the twelfth and thirteenth century, when R. Tam's ruling became accepted. One must ask why R. Tam and the generations that followed him were so strict with nursing widows and divorcées, barring opportunities that legal authorities of previous generations had allowed.

Israel Ta-Shma suggested a halakhic answer to this question. One of the reasons R. Tam quotes is the fear, mentioned and dismissed in the Babylonian Talmud, that women might kill their children in order to remarry. Hence, the prohibition on remarriage, even in the event of the death of the child, was to ensure that no mother would purposely kill her child.[174] This reason was accepted in antiquity by Palestinian Jews, and Ta-Shma suggested that R. Tam's quoting of this reason is related to his revival of some of the Palestinian rulings.[175] While this suggestion has a certain halakhic logic, one cannot ignore the tremendous influence R. Tam's ruling had on the daily lives of families. In light of this, Ta-Shma further suggested that perhaps this strictness was linked to a growing concern with infant abandonment in twelfth- and thirteenth-century Europe. This issue will be investigated in the next chapter.

Breast-feeding and Medieval Society

This chapter has examined breast-feeding practices and regulations in two different contexts. The first context was that of medieval society at large. Here we looked at the implications of wet nursing as part of the complex Jewish-Christian relations in medieval Germany and northern France. Our study revealed how the social construction of breast-feeding can throw new light on gender and, especially, on social relationships. The daily exchanges between Jewish and Christian women surely led to an intimate knowledge of each other, even if these women were not always on friendly terms, and even if their relationship was largely determined by their respective status as employer and employee.[176] Such informal relationships, as both the church and Jewish law were well aware, were crucial in defining the relationship between Jews and Christians and represented complex forms of socialization of both mothers and their children.

At the same time, these relationships had other, more hostile, aspects. On the one hand, the Jews, as members of a minority society, bore certain fears of the consequences of employing a Christian woman in or out of the house. On the other hand, as employers, Jews could, at times, exploit and harass their Christian employees, a situation feared by the church, and that did nothing to increase goodwill between Jews and Christians. The particular juncture of complex power relations and great intimacy made the employment of wet nurses an important site of Jewish-Christian relations.

From a gender perspective, we saw how in medieval Ashkenaz, as in many other societies, although mothers and their children were intensely involved in the politics of breast-feeding, it was the fathers and other men who generally decided who should be breast-fed by whom and how and they usually controlled the hiring of wet nurses. The restrictions on Jewish women that prevented them from remarrying were unique to Jews in medieval Christian society, since Christian law contained no such limitations.[177] The position of men as those obligated to ensure their child's well-being, and the consequent commitment of their wives, divorcées, and widows to this purpose, produced a complex situation in which women no longer protected by marital frameworks were not free to contract new relationships. As we saw, a notable change in Jewish attitudes, severely restricting the remarriage of divorcées and widows was the ruling of R. Tam, in the second half of the twelfth century, which was accepted and vehemently enforced by the generations that followed. Over and above concern for the welfare of the infant, R. Tam's ruling is based on the division of child care in medieval society and its understandings of parenting and its responsibilities. We will now turn to examine these understandings in the medieval context.

Chapter Five

PARENTS AND CHILDREN: COMPETING VALUES

> That is why a person is called a miniature world: because he resembles the whole world and in his wisdom he can rule and know all things created by his wisdom, "because she was the mother of all the living" (Gen. 3:20) to provide for them and lead them in wisdom as a mother for her child.
> — R. Judah Ḥasid, MS Oxford Bodl. Opp. 540

THE PREVIOUS CHAPTER DISCUSSED some of the social consequences of breast-feeding and sketched an outline of the division of labor and child-care responsibilities between men and women in medieval Jewish society. The example of breast-feeding, along with other examples discussed throughout the book, demonstrates the cultural understandings of biological attributes. We saw how Jewish-Christian relations, as well as hierarchies within the family and the community, were shaped by ideology and by the constraints of everyday life in the medieval cities. When discussing Jewish women, we saw how societies' values and needs bound women to their children and determined their responsibilities. Underlying these discussions, we found that these practices were oftentimes the result of competing interests within society; these competing interests led to legal and practical decisions that were, in some cases, at odds with religious beliefs or with earlier legal practices.

The nutrition of children and the social construction of breast-feeding are just two components of medieval understandings of parenthood. This chapter will focus more broadly on the social conceptions of parenting and especially on motherhood in medieval Ashkenaz. Understandings of gender and family as well as practical needs and religious precepts all combined to shape the medieval understandings of parenthood and the division of child-care responsibilities between men and women in Jewish society. The first part of the chapter will discuss theories of parenting in Jewish society, and the division of labor and the nature of parent-child relationships that resulted from these understandings. These will be compared and contrasted with contemporary Christian writings on these topics. The second part of the chapter will show how these theories were translated into reality, in a realm of competing interests within the family and the community.

Theories of Parenthood

As is the case with manuals on nursing or infant care, no instruction manuals on parenthood were composed in medieval Ashkenaz. Moreover, since parenting has few medical aspects, there are no instructions concerning parenting in medical manuscripts. As we saw in chapter 4, even the few instructions that were recorded in the Jewish sources concerning care for infants are usually concerned with the employment of wet nurses and do not provide instructions to parents. Perhaps the assumption was that women, who were the main caregivers of young children, instinctively knew what they were supposed to do and did not need further instruction, while men, who employed wet nurses, needed advice.

As noted above, some manuals of this sort existed in Christian society, although such compositions were more plentiful in the late Middle Ages.[1] Books that were written in the thirteenth and fourteenth centuries such as Bartholomeus Anglicus's (d. 1250) *Liber de Proprietatibus Rerum*; Phillipe de Novarre's (1195–1265) *Les quatres ages de l'homme*, and Konrad v. Megenburg's (1309–1374) *Das Buch der Natur*, all devoted attention to parental roles; there is no equivalent of these compositions in medieval Ashkenazic culture. In addition, information about parenting can also be gleaned from stories about saints' lives and from instructional letters written by parents for their children and by husbands for their wives.[2] These sources, which have no direct parallels in medieval Jewish society, also discuss parenting relatively briefly and seem to share the assumption of some of the Jewish texts, namely, that parents know naturally how to raise their children. Hence, the lack of attention devoted to parenting in both the Jewish and Christian sources does not necessarily indicate that these issues were unimportant, but it does pose a challenge for historians who wish to describe and analyze these issues.

We will start our investigation with a common source, which was interpreted and commented on by both medieval Jews and Christians—the fifth commandment: "Honor your father and your mother" (Exod. 20:12) and other related verses. Most commentators write about the main focus of the commandment—the obligations of children toward their parents, and do not discuss the responsibilities of parents toward their children, which is the flip side of this commandment. In specifying the obligations of children toward their parents, the verse in Lev. (19:5) is frequently quoted as well: "You shall each revere his mother and his father." A variety of topics emerge from the discussion of these verses: children's obligations to obey and honor their parents, to support them in their old age and fulfill their wishes, and their duty to bury their parents after their death.[3] Most of these duties become relevant when parents reach old age and can no longer fend for themselves.[4]

Some commentators also discuss what parents do for their children, at times in the context of an explanation of why children must honor and tend to their parents. R. Joseph Bekhor Shor (twelfth century) explains:

> "Honor your father and your mother": Even though I said you should only honor and worship me, honor your father and your mother! "And do not forget all his bounties" (Ps. 103:2), for they brought you to this world and sustained [weaned] you well until you grew up. And they worry for you and all their efforts are only for you. And if you honor them and recompense them for their efforts, I will know that you will honor me.[5]

This source instructs us that parents deserve to be honored because they brought their children into this world and took care of their needs.

The sources and commentators do not distinguish between the obligation of honoring mothers and fathers. A close reading of the commentaries, however, reveals gender differences between the honor merited by each parent. Although parents are mentioned together in the Ten Commandments, there is a clear hierarchy between them. Most medieval authors follow the Mishna and the Talmud, where it is stated that in cases where both parents compete for an honor, one must "leave your mother's honor and fulfill the honor due to your father ... for both you and your mother are bound to honor your father."[6] This idea is repeated with slightly different emphasis in a thirteenth-century commentary on the Book of Exodus: "'Honor your father' (the father is mentioned first because he is the mainstay of the home) 'and your mother' (who gave birth to you)."[7] This hierarchy points to a still higher authority, God, who is to be honored above both parents.[8] This commentary, designating the father as *ikar habayit* (the mainstay) is striking, since traditional Jewish sources often present women as the center of the home. This comment, however, also accords with other understandings of the father's role in procreation, as we saw in chapter 1.

The commentators also remark on the nature of relationships of children to their parents. The classic explanation for the different order in which the mother and father are mentioned in the verses in Exodus ("Honor your father and your mother") and in Leviticus ("You shall each revere his mother and his father") concerns gender differences. As fathers are "naturally" more feared, mothers are mentioned first when speaking of fear. On the other hand, since mothers are honored more, fathers are mentioned first in that context.[9] In this way, one can learn to honor and respect even those who are not instinctively respected and honored. The thirteenth-century scholar R. Moses of Couçy rephrases the talmudic distinction as follows:

> And when speaking of honor, [Scripture] mentioned the father's honor before the mother's, because his [the child's] heart is more prone to honor his mother because she cajoles him [with her] words. And the fear of the mother is mentioned before fear of the father, because [the child's] heart is more fearful of his father's scolding. This teaches us that both are equal in honor and in fear."[10]

This explanation relies on the popular belief that women are weaker and thus provoke less fear than men.

Another reason for the difference in attitudes and in emotional attachments to mothers and fathers can be found in a comment of one of the Tosafists on Lev. 19:3: "R. Abraham wrote: The reason for mentioning the mother before the father is that a young child knows his mother first and then his father."[11] This explanation expresses the division of labor in the medieval family. Mothers cared for young children; fathers did not. *Midrash Aseret haDibrot*, a story compilation of the Ten Commandments that was popular in Ashkenaz during the Middle Ages, expands on this idea. In it, God says:

> Fathers who you were born from, honor them like you honor me. He who is Blessed said: The belly that gave birth to you, honor. The breasts you nursed from, cherish. For they were with me when I created you for it says: "You shall each revere his mother and his father."[12]

This explanation for why mothers deserve to be honored emphasizes the mother's role in taking care of her children and, especially, physically bearing and feeding them. Fathers were to be honored because of their paternity, but unlike mothers, no actions of theirs are mentioned in this context.[13]

Medieval Christian authors commenting on the same verses outlined a similar gender hierarchy and placed fathers before mothers; they also presented a gendered division of labor, and provided two reasons for honoring each parent, both reminiscent of those mentioned by the Jewish authors. The first explanation for the honoring of fathers more than mothers was the woman's obligation to honor her husband. Like their mother, children were obligated first to honor their fathers, and only then, their mothers.[14] The other reason for giving precedence to fathers was related to medieval medical theories of embryology and conceptions of birth and infant care. While the mother provided the surroundings for the fetus in utero and protected it while its body parts were forming, the father was understood as contributing the brains and the spirit of the infant.[15] For example, Thomas Aquinas (1225–1274), much like the author of Midrash Aseret haDibrot, suggested that children were to honor their fathers in gratitude for their creation and their education, and their mothers in recognition of their sorrow and pain in birth and their devoted care.[16]

This approach to parenthood and, in this specific case, to parents' fundamental merits, was shared by both Jews and Christians in the Middle Ages. The idea expressed in Jewish sources is also found in Christian commentary on the verse: "But we were gentle among you, like a nurse (τροφός) taking care of her children" (1 Thess. 2:7). The commentators explain that mothers naturally provide care for their children, and that this care is the reason for honoring and respecting them.[17] These merits of women are often mentioned when discussing the Virgin Mary and the reasons for honoring her. In some sources, a comparison is made between the honor deserved by parents to that due the Virgin:

We owe her honor because she is the mother of our Lord. Indeed, one who does not honor the mother, without doubt will dishonor the son. So it says in the Scriptures "Honor your father and your mother" (Exod. 20:12). Therefore what shall we say, brothers? For she herself is our mother. Indeed through her we are born, through her we are nourished, through her we grow. Through her we are born, not in this world but with the Lord.[18]

These understandings of the honor owed by children to their parents, and the consequent division of labor and the responsibilities among the two parents, support perceptions in both Jewish and Christian culture that identified women with physicality and corporeality. These conceptions, defining the contribution of each parent to their children's being, as well as what they were entitled to receive from their children in return, both explained and justified the medieval way of life and the ideal constructions of family relations.

A unique source, the piyut *Oraḥ Ḥayim*, written by R. Simon b. Isaac b. Abun in the early eleventh century in Ashkenaz, discusses the fifth commandment and describes in great detail the care parents were expected to provide for their children.[19] This is one of the few sources that actually describes men as caring for young children. R. Simon describes the father and mother as nurses—*Omen uMeneqet*, an image that points to the devoted care the children receive from their parents.[20] Although the two terms *omen* and *meneqet* may be rendered in English as nurse (and in Latin as *nutrix*), they are two separate terms. The term *meneqet* comes from the verb to nurse/breast-feed, and refers only to women who cared for infants, whereas, in the biblical context, *omen* refers to men and, in the female form, *omenet* refers to women who do not breast-feed the child but who care for the child like a caretaker.[21] Rashi, however, explains that the omen cares for the child, employing the French term *nourriture*—the same verb *nutrire* from which the Latin *nutrix* is derived.[22] R. Simon b. Isaac refers to both the mother and the father by these names. In addition, he provides a detailed list of all the things parents do for their children, without distinction between gender roles. Most of these deeds are related to the first stages of a child's life. Both parents pray for the birth of a son,[23] bring him into the covenant, nurse, feed, clothe, educate, and pray for the infant. In addition, parents teach their child a profession and marry him off. This piyut is one of the few sources that provides a detailed list of what child care entailed. It is unique in that it attributes some of the actions related to early child care to men; most of the other sources treat the care of young children as the sole responsibility of women.

Parental Love and Care

The sources see mothers' love for their children as "natural," unique and special to women. The author of *Sefer Ḥasidim*, in discussing how society should treat the handicapped, comments on mothers' care for their children:

For He created people whole in body so that they can assist those who are missing limbs. Just as the infant is born and does not walk and his mother cares for all his needs, so the Holy One, blessed be He finds them [the cripples] people who will fulfill their needs. For all of Israel are fathers and mothers to each other as it is said: "You stand this day all of you before the Lord your God — your tribal heads, your elders and your officials, all the men of Israel, your children" (Deut. 29:9). It does not say "and your children"; rather, it says "your children" without an "and" — to teach us that you should consider all the people of Israel your own children and tend to all their needs.[24]

This source points once again to women's role in caring for infants. The same idea is expressed in another source written by Ḥasidei Ashkenaz:

That is why a person is called a miniature world: because he resembles the whole world, and in his wisdom he can rule and know all things created by his wisdom, "because she was the mother of all the living" (Gen. 3:20) to provide for them and lead them in wisdom, as a mother for her child.[25]

This devotion and subsequent responsibility is expressed in legal rulings as well. Jewish laws convey this idea, for example, when discussing custody in cases of divorce. According to the law, all children remain with their mothers until age six, and girls always remain their mothers' wards.[26] Other examples have to do with smaller, more mundane details. For instance, certain laws of the Sabbath assume that mothers were the main caretakers. For instance, a mother is permitted to feed her child food that was prepared by hired help on the Sabbath, although from a strictly legal standpoint, it would be preferable to have the servants themselves feed the child. However, if the child insisted that s/he would eat only if fed by the mother, the mother was permitted to do so. In his *Sefer Miẓvot Gadol (Semag)*, R. Moses of Couçy explains:

And if the infant does not have what to eat, he can tell the Canaanite to cook pap [for the child] on the Sabbath. And if the child wants to be fed only by his mother, the master from Couçy explained that the mother may feed it, even a milk dish that was milked and cooked by the Canaanite on the Sabbath.[27]

Similar legal exceptions are made on Yom Kippur, in discussing the special permission given to women to prepare food for their children and wash their hands.[28] Another example of special permission given to women is that of washing clothes soiled by children on the Sabbath.[29] Although in legal literature, general examples are usually addressed to men, all these instructions were addressed specifically to women and, as such, can be seen to exclude men. In addition, in a discussion of one of these halakhic topics, one of the legal authorities comments that R. Isaac of Dampierre, who objected to allowing women to wash the clothes of children soiled on the Sabbath, heard from the *women* that R. Tam had allowed the practice.[30] This reference to women reporting on what a legal authority instructed them indicates that the matter under discussion is a woman's issue. As a rule, women are cited as authorities for the transmission of halakhic opinions of important rabbinic figures only in the context of commandments and deeds performed specifically by women.[31]

There is one similar case, in which the issue discussed concerns men's care for children; this discussion is in many ways the exception that proves the rule. When discussing soiled clothes on the Sabbath, a case is brought in which a father is dirtied by his child while holding him in the synagogue.[32] The source provides explicit instructions, specifying the circumstances under which this man can clean himself. For our study, however, we should note that this case of men caring for young children (in the synagogue) is a singular exception.[33] More important, certain groups, such as Ḥasidei Ashkenaz, discouraged men from taking an active role in caring for children if it might in any way interfere with their obligations of worship.[34]

Young children and their relationships with their fathers are usually mentioned in discussions of the noise and dirt generated by them. For example, when discussing the customs of R. Judah b. Isaac, one of Rashi's teachers who died during the First Crusade (1096), it is told:

> Once a child was sitting on Rabbi's shoulder in the synagogue. When the time came to read the *Shema*, he asked that the child be removed since children are frequently in the dirt and it is improper to read Shema near them.[35]

The idea that toddlers were dirty is found in other references to young children as well.[36] A source in *Sefer Ḥasidim* discusses the problem of dealing with a child who urinated on his/her father's lap in the synagogue.[37]

These sources indicate that while young children were present in the synagogue, the tendency was to remove them and the dirt they made. This accords with the division of labor between the parents. Women were considered responsible for caring for small children. Until the boys reached the age of education, fathers were expected to devote themselves to more important tasks. At the same time, it is clear that many fathers were drawn to tend to their children, and the instructions that they must not do so were designed to restrain them.[38] In part, this was an expression of respect for the synagogue and its sanctity. The complaints voiced by the rabbis are no different from those of preachers and pastors concerning young children who attended church services.[39]

Taking care of children was considered part of women's wisdom, just like birth and its complexities. This understanding was shared by Jews and Christians alike.[40] A case brought before Gregory IX in 1229 exemplifies this shared Jewish-Christian understanding of the nature of parenting. The pope was asked about a couple from Strasbourg who argued over the religious education and identity of their four-year-old son. In this case, the father had converted to Christianity while the mother had remained Jewish. The reasons the mother provided for retaining custody of her son, arguments she hoped would im-press the church authorities, evoke her efforts during the early years of her son's life:

> Since the boy is still an infant, he needs the care of a mother more than that of a father. Furthermore, the burden of bearing and the pain of giving birth to him, and the toil of the time after his birth, are known to have been hers; this is why the lawful union of husband and wife is called matrimony rather than patrimony. Thus, it is more fitting for the said boy to remain in the care of the mother, rather than go to the father who had recently become a Christian.[41]

The mother's description of her dedication to her child repeats the common theme of mothers as worthy of credit and respect because of their role in nurturing infants. She does not mention her role in the child's upbringing, probably because it would have been disadvantageous to her plea. Gregory IX certainly did not want to hear of her role in educating her child.

The ages mentioned in this story are significant. Although the boy is four, the mother emphasizes how close to infancy he still is and suggests that it is more fitting that the boy remain with her. In a similar vein, the papal ruling also refers to his age, in arguing that the boy is old enough to be taken away from his mother, "to the greatest advantage of the Christian faith." It seems from the text that had he been less than three years old, the decision in the case might have been different. One can only wonder what the ruling might have been had the case been that of a daughter rather than a son.

Besides dividing responsibilities between the two parents, the sources also distinguish between mothers' and fathers' love for their children. The care mothers provided their children was seen as an expression of "natural love." Fathers, on the other hand, were expected to do more for their children, and especially, for their sons, and the emphasis was on their care for their older children. If they were concerned only with their children's physical welfare, they were reprimanded, whereas women were praised for tending to infants' needs. *Sefer Hasidim* provides advice on this topic as well:

> "The fear of the Lord is the beginning of knowledge; fools despise wisdom and discipline" (Prov. 1:7). How is discipline and wisdom connected to the beginning of knowledge? It says "My son, heed the discipline of your father and do not forsake the instruction of your mother" (ibid., 8). According to the letter of the law, one need not love children before they begin to fear and love God for it says "Those who love me I love" (ibid., 8:17). For if a man loves the bodies of his children as a dog loves his pups, and as all other creatures [love their offspring], of this it is said: "Man is in no way superior to the beast" (Eccles. 3:19). But if a man loves for the sake of Heaven, [he should love] their souls more than their bodies. For example, if he leads his sons and daughters in the dark or in a place that he sees is not safe for their bodies, he summons his male and female servants, or he himself walks with them, lest they be harmed in body or be pained. How much more,

then, should he guard his sons' and daughters' minds, lest they sin toward He who created the world; thus, he should be more concerned lest they sin in their deeds, their bodies, and their thoughts. Witness[42] how many fasts and abstentions and cries and pleas a person performs when his son falls ill, because his soul is concerned for the body of his son. He should certainly do at least as much if he [his son] sins, for the well being of the soul is eternal.[43] Hence, he should take guard lest they sin in their deeds, bodies, or thoughts, for it says: "For Job thought, 'Perhaps my children have sinned and blasphemed God in their thoughts' (Job 1:5)."[44]

This admonition is directed to fathers. Women's love for their children is seen as natural, perhaps like the love of a female dog toward her pups. In contrast, the emphasis here seems to be on fathers' love for their children at an age in which they should fear God, but may stray outside in the dark and think harmful thoughts. Medieval Christian preachers suggested similar ideas, encouraging their listeners to foster spiritual love and not love that resembles the love of animals for their offspring.[45]

The same idea is expressed in a case that is, in many ways, exceptional. *Sefer Hasidim* brings the case of a dying father, discussing the future of his children, who would become orphans upon his death:

> A man was very ill. When he cried, they said to him: "Why are you crying? If it is for your little children, your brothers will take your place." He said: "My brothers will take care of their worldly needs. I am only crying, because, had I lived, I would have reproached them and tormented them so that they could attain the world to come, by teaching them and directing them in the path of righteousness." The guardian he appointed for his son said: "I will replace you [be under you], and serve in your position."
>
> He said to him: "No. Serve, rather, to replace me [be under me], but from *your own* position—[that is], if they were to cause you sorrow or steal from you, you would beat them so they do so no more. Thus, you will be in the place of their maker: Educate them to perform the commandments, and if they sin toward the Creator, torment them and don't say, 'How can I hit an orphan?' Rather, if they say: 'If our father were alive, he would have pity on us and would not allow us to be beaten,' tell them: '[Your father] would have hit you even more. It is he who commanded me to torment you . . . and they will be loyal like a dog, for a dog is beaten and he is loyal to his master, because he gives him food. So do to my children. Give my sons food, and let your fear be upon them when they sin, and show them love when they do the will of the Creator, as you command them.'"[46]

The responsibility this father wants his friend to take upon himself as guardian is a harsh one. He does not discuss his children's physical welfare at all. He is concerned solely with the children's piety. This father sees himself as solely in charge of the one aspect of his children's education, begun only once they reached the age of five or six.

These two passages clearly address the responsibilities of fathers toward their children once they reached the age of education. Another passage in *Sefer Ḥasidim* discusses the proper attitude of fathers toward young children in the context of a father who wants to do penance. The passage suggests that a man who does true penance does not tend to his children, but rather lets his wife take care of them; if he feels deep sorrow whenever he hears them cry, but does not approach them because he wishes to continue studying Torah, he will be greatly rewarded.[47]

All these sources distinguishing between spiritual love and natural love are from *Sefer Ḥasidim*. As discussed in the introduction, Ḥasidei Ashkenaz have often been portrayed as a distinct social group that held a more stringent and ascetic worldview than other groups within the medieval Jewish community.[48] However, this distinction between fatherly spiritual love and motherly natural love can be found in contemporary Christian sources as well. I would suggest that the particularities of the genre of *Sefer Ḥasidim* enable us to hear ideas that are muted in other genres. This conclusion is supported by other sources. Parallel Christian writings express the expectation that mothers would display natural affection for their children, while fathers were expected to foster spiritual love.[49] Another commonly expressed theme, discussed at length by Shulamith Shahar, was that women find it easier to feel close to their children during the first years of their lives, while fathers find it easier to communicate with them once they grow older. We saw this idea echoed in the first part of this chapter when examining the reasoning for the wording of the fifth commandment.[50] Hence, this division between "natural" love and spiritual love was a feature of medieval life, and was not merely characteristic of *Sefer Ḥasidim* and its milieu.

Although the medieval texts generally assume that women would have compassion as well the instinctual need to care for their children, they also discuss cases in which women act in ways contrary to those expected of them. The details of these instances reaffirm the belief that a mother "naturally" cares for her child. For example, when discussing the two women who came before King Solomon, R. Judah the Pious remarks:

> "Later, two women came to the king" (1 Kings 3:16). My father (R. Samuel the Pious) asked, "What were these two women arguing about? When the first said, 'The live one is my son' (3:22), the other should say: 'I am glad you are saying so. Give him money and I will give him money, and he will inherit your money and my money.' Furthermore, she was mad (crazy), for she said, 'Cut the live child' (3:24), and even an infant could sense that she was not his mother." Rather, this is the way he (R. Samuel the Pious) interpreted the verse according to the simple meaning of the text (*p'shat*). Both women were widows of a rich man, and it was

the custom that when a man died, his mother would take only 200 *zuz* from her ketubbah and she would become the custodian of the child's money and support herself from it until the child grew up. For who is loyal to a child like its mother? So Solomon said cunningly to the women: "'Disputed money of doubtful ownership should be divided among the disputants' (BT Bava Mezi'a 2b). I will divide the child and the money." And the woman whose son was alive said to the king, because she pitied her son: "Give her the live child," and the other woman said: "You are being deceitful so that all will say that you are merciful and therefore are his mother. . . . Since this dispute exists, let us act by the law of the Torah and divide." Then Solomon said: "From the words of the first woman, I cannot tell if she is telling the truth, but I can tell from the words of the second. Since she cruelly said, "Cut him," and did not pity him, she is clearly not his mother."[51]

R. Judah clearly expects a woman to be merciful and loving toward her children, as he says: "For who is loyal to a child like its mother?" In addition, he calls the woman who suggests cutting the child "mad." This approach is echoed in a Tosafist commentary on Exod. 2:2:

"And when she saw how good he was . . ."[52] It should not be understood that she hid him [in the basket] because she saw that he was good and beautiful. Because all women who give birth to sons/children[53] show compassion for their children, whether beautiful or ugly, we should explain in this manner: "And God saw all he had made and found it was very good" (Gen. 1:31) . . . in this case because Moses was born at six months of age, and she looked at him when he was born [to see] whether he was a stillborn [in which case] she wouldn't trouble to save him. [But] she saw he was good and beautiful, and his hair and nails were formed, and she knew he could live.[54]

This understanding, that women show "natural" compassion for their children, comes up in a discussion of breast-feeding as well. R. Jacob Mulin discusses the case of a woman who gave birth to a child out of wedlock and her obligation to nurse the child. He explains that the sages obligated this woman legally to nurse her child so as to protect the child but that "most women have compassion for their children and nurse them."[55] As we have already demonstrated, although they held a basic belief that most women would choose to nurse their offspring, medieval Jewish authorities made provisions to ensure infants' well-being.

This attitude—asserting, on the one hand, that women possessed an instinctive compassion for their children, while attempting to assure children's welfare by law—is not unique to the medieval Jewish sources, or to medieval society. The sources in Christian Europe that support each side of this issue have been thoroughly explored by scholars who have argued for and against theories proposed by Philippe Ariès.[56] The next sections of this chapter will examine some of the issues raised by Ariès's followers and his opponents, such as expressions of sorrow concerning the death of children, infanticide, and abandonment, within the still unexplored context of the medieval Jewish world.

Death and Mourning

Attitudes toward death and mourning customs for children have been investigated by scholars in an effort to discern the attitudes of parents regarding infant death in the Middle Ages, and the strength of parental attachment to their children. While Ariès and his followers argued that in the Middle Ages, parents did not mourn the loss of their children, others have worked intensively to demonstrate parents' grief at such deaths. The Jewish sources, like the contemporary Christian ones, show that death was greeted with sorrow. Within Jewish sources, however, we find many exceptional instances, in which the sorrow and grief is not as straightforward. As we investigate this topic in the Jewish sources, a number of gender distinctions concerning the death of children as well as medieval attitudes toward death will be examined.

Both medieval Jewish and Christian sources warn parents, and especially mothers, not to mourn the death of their children excessively and inappropriately. Medieval Jewish commentators, like their Christian counterparts, discuss the importance of accepting God's judgment and the death of their children and not wallowing in grief. A story from BT *Mo'ed Katan* was often cited as a model:

> R. Judah said as citing Rav, Whoever indulges in grief to excess over his dead will weep for another. There was a certain woman that lived in the neighborhood of R. Huna; she had seven sons, one of whom died, and she wept for him rather excessively. R. Huna sent [word] to her, "Act not thus." She heeded him not [and] he said to her: "If you heed my word, it is well, but if not, are you anxious to make provision [shrouds] for yet another?" He [the next son] died, and they all died. In the end, he said to her, "Are you fumbling with provision for yourself?" And she died.[57]

This story of the mother and her seven sons is found in a number of variations.[58] One, that of the mother and her seven sons who were killed as martyrs during the Maccabean era, will be discussed in the final section of this chapter. Other versions, such as that attributed to *Sefer Ḥasidim* explained that the woman mentioned in this story sinned when her first son died by refusing to recognize God's judgment and will. Her refusal led to the eventual death of all her sons.[59]

The death of children is also explained as the result of other sins committed by parents. For instance, *Sefer Ḥasidim* discusses those who sin by lamenting the death of their children excessively, while failing to mourn the death of a righteous leader (Zaddik) sufficiently. The author of *Sefer Ḥasidim* links the response to the death of the Zaddik to the death of children, explaining that the grief parents feel after the death of their children helps such people atone for their sins, including that of their improper response to the Zaddik's death.[60] The claim that children's deaths are a consequence of the parents' sins is a common one in medieval literature. For example, R. Eleazar b. Judah of Worms explains that his loved ones died because of his sins after the death of his wife and daughters.[61]

The anguish and sorrow felt by parents upon the death of their children is said to atone for their sins.[62] For example:

> There are people of whom it is decreed that their children will die without successors, and they [the children] die at ten years of age and older. And why did they not die young, at age one, so that he [the parent/father] would not be so sad? Because it is known to the Creator of the world at what hour a person will experience great sorrow and be condemned to die, and the son dies so that the father or the mother will live. This is why the child lived until age ten, so that the father will be deeply sorrowful, and he will be atoned for [by the sorrow] and live.[63]

In this case the child dies for his parent's sin, and his death is not only a punishment, but also an atonement.[64]

Another passage in *Sefer Hasidim* describes the great sorrow felt by parents upon the death of their children and the atoning power of that sorrow:

> The students were sitting in front of their rabbi. One said: "May it be [God's will] that my wife will conceive, if the infant is born alive; if not, may she not conceive." His friend said: "May my wife conceive." His friend [the first speaker] said: "And if it [the baby] dies, it would be better if it were never born, for it says: 'Do not delude your maidservant' (2 Kings 4:16) and 'Don't mislead me' (4:28). And when the baby is born I will pray that it will live." The wise man said: "There are infants, boys or girls, that redeem their father or mother from death or troubles as it says: 'Jacob who redeemed Abraham' (Isa. 29:22).[65] Some are ordained to death or sorrow for the father's or the mother's sake; the child dies and the father or mother are sad, and this sorrow redeems him, for 'from all sorrow there is some gain' (Prov. 14:23).[66]

Nevertheless, this grief was supposed to remain within bounds. There were times when mourning was not appropriate. For example, parents were instructed to not be too sad about their children's death on the High Holidays, days that were considered days of judgment:

> On the Judgment Day, those who are worthy and equal stand together. And the father should not be sad that his son is not with him, because the joy of the Garden of Eden and the joy of basking in the light of the Divine Presence [*Shekhina*] remove all sorrow and grief.[67]

In short, the medieval sources criticize parents who mourn the death of their children too much; yet they acknowledge that such mourning is not unusual and show understanding for their feelings. This is illustrated in *Sefer Ḥasidim*, where parents of young children are instructed not to actively display affection to their children in front of friends whose children have died.[68] This sensitivity shows the great awareness of death and its sorrows in medieval society. Most of the sources emphasize the limits society set on this sorrow, suggesting that overcoming the grief was the greatest difficulty faced by parents. An additional story in *Sefer Ḥasidim* illustrates this:

> Once there was a scholar who had a son who was a young man.[69] And his father taught him Torah, and the son died childless, and the father cried out in his sorrow: "Joseph, my son, come and study." And when it was time to eat, he cried: " Joseph, my son, come and eat." Once the father woke up early to study and he cried: "Joseph, my son, come and study," as he used to call him when he was alive, and a phantom in the image of his son came and stood next to him. Immediately, he understood that it was not his son but a phantom. He spit on him and said: "Go, go, impure one from here and run away." The phantom fled. Therefore one should not indulge in sorrow too much; rather, one should mourn as is customary.[70]

In another story a woman whose son died went insane after his death, and her sanity was restored by music for "one sings songs to a sorrowful soul" (Prov. 25:20).[71]

Contemporary Christian authors also discuss the sorrow parents felt and the mourning process they went through after the death of a child. They too scold parents for devoting too much attention to mourning for their children, while neglecting God and proper worship. For example, the thirteenth-century Dominican Thomas Cantimpratanus said that his grandmother had lost her eldest son and refused to be comforted until her son appeared to her in a dream. She saw him walking behind a joyful group of boys, and asked him why he walked alone and not in their company. Her son replied that he carried a jug with all of her tears and that the burden of that weight caused him to lag behind. The son instructed her to shed tears for God and to pour her heart out for the Holy Eucharist or in charity. Other similar examples can be found in Christian writings, describing parents who were immobilized with grief, until a local patron or saint came to their aid.[72]

These examples demonstrate the grief and sorrow felt after children's death, as well as the attempt made by scholars and advisors to turn the feelings of sorrow into productive ways of worshiping God. In these sources, it is hard to find any evidence of parents who treat the death of their children unemotionally and accept such deaths passively. The sources also document equal consternation over the death of girls and boys, and a number of texts specifically mention parents mourning the death of a son or a daughter. In addition, we have seen no distinction between the grief of mothers and that of fathers over the death of their children. Many of the sources examined above discussed the penances parents took upon themselves when their children died. These penances consisted mainly of fasting, and both mothers and fathers took fasts upon themselves. Such fasting was common practice and is mentioned in many sources, among them, the writings of Ḥasidei Ashkenaz. People fasted for a variety of reasons, often doing so on Mondays and Thursdays over a set period of time. In the context of family relationships, the sources mention fasting when children were ill or in danger or after the death of a child as a means of atonement.

There are, however, some distinctions in the discussions of grief over the death of children. The main distinction is related to the age of the deceased child. A number of sources suggest that parents, and especially fathers, mourn their elder children (those seven, eight, or even older) more than they mourn their infants and toddlers. For example, in the story quoted above in which the father continued to search for his dead son and attempted to call him back to the world of the living, the son was of marriageable age.[73]

The distinction between the grief felt at the death of an infant, as opposed to that felt for an older child, is not restricted to medieval times; it is also evident in ancient discussions of burial practices. Children who died as newborns, before they reached the age of thirty days were buried in private, while those who died after thirty days were buried in a more public ritual.[74] Massekhet Smaḥot also distinguishes between funerary procedures for children according to their ages.[75] The medieval sources, however, contain few discussions of these procedures and distinctions. In addition, Massekhet Smaḥot's distinctions revolve around the ages of five and seven,[76] the age at which boys joined the adult male world and began their schooling. These distinctions are reinforced and echoed in the medieval sources.

The differences between parental grief for the death of younger and older children correspond, to a certain extent, to the gender differentiations between the "natural" love of mothers and the more spiritual love of fathers. Just as the father's spiritual love was more valued, so too, an older child, who can be educated and is thus, a worthy recipient of spiritual love, is more valued. The passage quoted above, from R. Judah the Ḥasid's *Sefer Gematriyot*, conveys this idea:

> There are people of whom it is decreed that their children will die without successors, and they [the children] die at ten years of age and older. And why did they not die young, at age one, so that he [the parent] would not be so sad? Because it is known to the Creator of the world at what hour a person will experience great sorrow and be condemned to die, and the son dies so that the father or the mother will live. This is why the child lived until age ten, so that the father will be deeply sorrowful, and he will be atoned for [by the sorrow] and live.[77]

This source clearly describes the difference in reactions to the death of an infant and to that of a ten-year-old and emphasizes the greater investment fathers have in the older children. It also distinguishes between fathers' and mothers' responses to the death of their children.[78]

The Dark Side of Child Care: Abandonment and Infanticide

The issues discussed above — parental love and responses to children's deaths — were, as described in the introduction, the impetus for rich scholarly discussions on the darker side of medieval life, spurring investigation into a variety of topics, such as infanticide and abandonment. The proponents of this research were of two opposing viewpoints: While some wished to prove that medieval parents neglected and abandoned their children, others sought to prove the opposite.[79] Some Jewish scholars have argued that, whereas Christian parents did not love their children, Jewish parents did.[80] In the earlier parts of this chapter, I have argued that, in medieval Ashkenaz, Jews and Christians had similar values and understandings of human nature and of parent-child relationships. These similarities stem from a shared culture and from shared material and physical surroundings.

In this section, I will discuss several other aspects of medieval Christian society that were examined as part of the debate over Ariès's thesis. We have already seen that the medieval world recognized two different types of parental love: "natural" love, characteristic of mothers, and paternal love, which was supposed to be of a higher quality and of greater importance. This distinction highlights the competing values within medieval society, without which we cannot make sense of medieval life. This distinction can also help explain many of the issues that were often summoned as proofs that medieval parents did not value their children's lives. One such issue is the employment of wet nurses, which, some scholars argued, was, in and of itself, an indication of a lack of concern on the part of parents, and especially, mothers, since children fed by wet nurses died far more frequently. We have already seen that on this issue Jews were not much different from their neighbors, and that urban Jews, like urban Christians, employed wet nurses. Although Jewish sources voiced some concern over wet-nursing practices, these concerns were restricted to the employment of non-Jewish women, and, as we saw, even those concerns were not major ones.

Another issue that arose in Jewish sources is remarriage. The authorities were concerned that the new spouse might compete with the parents', and especially the mothers', affection and nurture. This is another issue in which cross-cultural comparison should help further our understandings of medieval family life, especially in light of different approaches to marriage and divorce. To this topic, we must add infanticide and abandonment of children, both of which have been studied extensively in the context of medieval Christian urban life. These issues will be examined in the following pages.

Remarriage

As we saw in the previous chapter, the suspicion of infanticide on the part of the mother was raised as a consideration in the talmudic discussions on the remarriage of women during the twenty-four-month nursing period. The Palestinian Talmud cited this suspicion as the reason for forbidding remarriage, whereas the Babylonian Talmud rejected this suggestion, although they both arrived at the same legal ruling. The medieval commentators mention both traditions, often raising this consideration before summarily dismissing it.

In the nonlegal sources, we find that infanticide is viewed as a possible and in some cases probable option practiced by some women seeking to remarry. *Sefer Ḥasidim* relates:

> A woman wanted to take a husband. The man said: "Because she has so many children, I do not want to marry her." She took the hands of her children and put them on the hands of those who had died, and they [the dead children] called after them [the live children] and they died.[81]

This story recounts a fascinating technique of causing death and provides insight into the medieval understanding of the relationship between the living and the dead. In this case, touching dead children's skin caused the dead children's souls to call the living children's souls and resulted in their eventual death. More interesting, however, for our discussion is the strong desire attributed to the woman. She wants to remarry so badly that she is willing to kill her children. This woman was probably not alone, since, as we saw in a case mentioned in the previous chapter, the widow from Krakow was also willing to go to great lengths in order to remarry (although her actions were not similar to the woman in this story from *Sefer Ḥasidim*). In addition, R. Tam's strict attitude, preventing widows and divorcees from remarrying during the nursing period, as well as the reinforcement of his opinion, indicate that the social norm was for these women to remarry quickly.

This phenomenon of quick remarriage, alluded to in the Jewish texts, is discussed in contemporary Christian sources as well. In the Christian case, remarriage shortly after the death of a spouse was not forbidden by law. In most places, however, local custom was to wait at least a year before remarrying. During this year, the widow could often find herself in a very difficult financial situation, if she was not a wealthy woman. In Christian society, the rights of wives to their husband's property after his death varied from place to place according to local laws and customs. In some places, women were allowed to take only their jewelry, personal possessions, and a small part of the husband's estate and were not allowed to remain in the family house. In other places, they had more rights. The specific economic and social circumstances surely influenced the decisions made by widows regarding remarriage.[82]

In Christian society, young widows who decided to remarry sometimes had to make difficult decisions. In certain cases, the deceased husband's family would refuse to give them any part of the deceased husband's estate and even take custody of any children from the previous marriage. Hence, many widows were in a no-win situation. If they were not wealthy enough to survive on their own, remarriage was a necessary choice. However, in some cases, the price of remarriage was the relinquishing of their children. Furthermore, in the case of young widows, society was often uncomfortable with these young unmarried women, as they feared that they would tempt other men and endanger the morals of society.[83] Even in cases in which these women returned to their father's homes after becoming widows, their families often urged them to remarry as quickly as possible, so as not to burden their families.[84]

Comparing the social circumstances of Christian society with the neighboring Jewish society is a complicated matter. First of all, we can assume there were proportionately more women who could potentially remarry in Jewish society than in Christian society: Mortality of spouses was probably similar in both societies, but the option of divorce, which existed in Jewish society, did not exist in Christian law. Second, no one has thoroughly investigated widowhood in medieval Ashkenaz. Cheryl Tallan, who has written a number of articles on the topic, has emphasized the advantages enjoyed by wealthy widows, but little work has focused on the less fortunate.[85] Jewish widows were supported by their husband's estate and lived in their husband's house until they decided to remarry. Alternatively, a widow could demand her ketubbah and terminate her financial connection to her deceased husband's family. There were, however, often complications in these procedures. Many responsa indicate that widows often had to contend with financial claims made by their deceased husband's family and his children.[86] Furthermore, the sources rarely enable us to distinguish between younger and older widows and between the pressures to remarry on women in either category. Based on the sources and the surrounding European culture, one can assume that Jewish widows, especially young ones, felt a need to remarry fairly quickly. The discussions of how quickly widows and divorcées could become engaged or get married after the dissolution of their previous marriage testify to this.[87]

In the case of remarriage, we see that despite the belief in the "natural love" of mothers for their children, under certain conditions, this love was not trusted as sufficient. If mothers were suspected of not cherishing their children when they were desperate to remarry, stepmothers were often portrayed as an outright danger to their stepchildren. *Sefer Ḥasidim* portrays good stepmothers as exceptions to the rule:

One man's wife died and he had children from her, and he married another woman and had children with her. And his second wife was good to the children of the first wife. And she [the second wife] died, and they wanted to give him another wife and money and he refused. They said to him: "Why don't you take a wife?" He said: "She is cruel and will be wicked to the children of my second wife, who was kind to the first wife's children, and I will not be ungrateful."[88]

The treatment of this subject displays clear-cut gender distinctions. Although, as we saw in the first part of the chapter, fathers also were understood as "naturally" feeling compassion for their children, there was no expectation whatsoever that stepfathers would be considerate of already existing stepchildren, and there are hardly any discussions of stepfathers' attitudes toward their wives' children.

Abandonment

The abandonment of infants in medieval Europe, a topic mentioned fairly often in the sources of the period, has been the subject of many modern studies as well. *Expositio* was a crime for which parents, and especially mothers, were blamed—the commonly portrayed situation being that of a woman who left her child on the church steps or at the entrance to the local monastery. Some modern scholars have argued that such acts were an almost certain death verdict for the abandoned children, since their chances of finding someone to care for them were minimal. Others, first and foremost, John Boswell, have argued that the "kindness of strangers" often saved these children's lives.[89] The phenomenon of abandonment is more heavily documented from the thirteenth century on, although there is evidence of the practice from ancient times. According to one legend, after frequently witnessing infants cast into the Tiber River by their mothers, Innocent III (1160–1216) established a home for foundlings. During the course of the thirteenth and fourteenth centuries, many foundling homes were established.[90] It is impossible to determine whether the practice of abandoning infants became more widespread or if the relative wealth of sources creates the impression of a new social concern. While some have claimed that the practice stemmed from the cruelty of parents, others have argued that children were abandoned only by those whose economic and social circumstances—extreme poverty, mothers of children born out of wedlock—did not permit them to keep them. Furthermore, the children were left in places where they believed that their child's chance of survival was greatest.[91]

Turning to Jewish society, we find few cases of abandonment in medieval Jewish society. The Talmud does include two categories of foundlings—*asufi* and *shetuki*. Both terms refer to children found in the marketplace. The distinction between them is that an asufi is found in the marketplace and taken in (*la'asof*—to gather), and the identity of his/her parents is unknown. In the case of a shetuki (from the verb *lishtok*—to be silent), the identity of his/her mother is known, but not that of the father. These children are mentioned in the context of forbidden marriages, since when these abandoned children grow up and wish to marry, their parentage is not known and certain legal problems come up.[92] There are few references to these categories in medieval literature, and, on the whole, these mainly repeat what was already said in the Talmud. For example, R. Jacob Ḥazan of London, who discussed the case of foundlings at length, summarizes Maimonides' resumé of the Talmud, without adding anything new to the discussion.[93]

Biblical interpretations of Exod. 2:6 demonstrate the medieval Jewish awareness of abandonment practices. The verse reads: "When she opened it, she saw that it was a child, a boy crying. She took pity on it and said: 'This must be a Hebrew child.'" A number of commentators explain that Pharaoh's daughter understood that Moses was not a foundling when she discovered his basket on the banks of the Nile. This explanation was based on the repetition in the verse "she saw that it was a child, a boy crying." According to R. Samuel b. Meir (Rashbam), when she opened the basket she expected to see a child, as foundlings were often abandoned in this way. When she saw, however, that Moses was a boy and circumcised no less, she understood that he was a Jewish child and not a foundling. On the other hand, had she been a girl, one could have assumed she was a foundling.[94] R. Judah Ḥasid explains the repetition in the verse to mean that not only was Moses by the Nile, but his brother Aaron was there too. Pharaoh's daughter saw the child in the basket and then she saw a boy crying; these were two different children—Moses and Aaron. According to R. Judah, she understood that Moses was not a foundling because he was accompanied by his brother.[95]

These interpretations show an awareness of the phenomenon of foundlings, as well as an inherent belief that Jewish children were not foundlings. I have found, however, one reference to the abandonment of a baby. An unpublished responsa from the collection of R. Meir b. Barukh's responsa reads as follows: "It happened that there was a baby abandoned in the street, and a rumor circulated about a single woman who had given birth to him, and it was an incessant rumor, and she became betrothed to a *cohen* [a person of priestly descent]."[96] According to this short report, there were rumors that a certain unmarried woman had given birth to a child and abandoned him. Unfortunately for us, the supplicant is more interested in determining the status of her subsequent marriage than in providing details about the abandonment of the child. Hence, we have no further details about the child's abandonment and we do not know what happened to the infant. In fact, had the woman not been subsequently betrothed to a cohen, we would have probably never heard about the matter.

This case certainly refutes any claims that Jews could not or would not abandon children for reasons of moral superiority. While I would agree that cases of abandonment were few and far between within the Jewish community, they were by no means unheard of.[97] In addition, this woman, who purportedly abandoned her baby, was, like many of the Christian women accused of the same crime, a single mother. Abandonment cases were probably fewer among Jews than among Christians for two reasons: First, the Jewish communities in Ashkenaz were small and tight-knit—hiding a pregnancy in such a community was probably very difficult, and abandoning a baby after attempting to hide a pregnancy—even harder. As the case above demonstrates, there were incessant rumors about the identity of the mother of the abandoned baby. A second reason Jewish mothers, even in dire circumstances, would have been more hesitant to abandon their infants than Christian women, is that Jews were a minority culture. According to Jewish law, an abandoned baby found in a Christian city was by definition not a Jew. Furthermore, if this infant were taken in by passersby, they could just as well be Christians as Jews. In other words, abandoning an infant probably meant abandoning him to Christianity.[98]

Infanticide

Boswell and others have indicated that abandonment on the church steps or in the marketplace was only one of the ways for parents to rid themselves of unwanted offspring. In addition, some infants were killed immediately after birth, often by their mothers and the women who attended her. Some of these children were born with handicaps and peculiarities and were killed out of dread of such physical impairments.[99] *Sefer Ḥasidim* discusses a case in which an infant was born with "teeth and a tail." Some people recommended that the infant be killed immediately, but eventually, following the advice of the sage, they cut off the teeth and the tail and allowed the child to live.[100] In this case, it was not the mother who wanted to kill her child but "some people." This fear of deformed infants, a fear that exists in modern times as well, does not illustrate medieval cruelty so much as the fear of deformity. In medieval times, malformed children were often considered bewitched or changelings, causing parents to fear them and at times even to expose or kill them.[101]

Despite this fear, and the fact that many of these infants died for natural and unnatural reasons, medieval Christian sources manifest the tremendous devotion of some mothers to their deformed children. They searched for remedies and went on pilgrimages to holy sites, praying for miracle cures.[102] Perhaps the case mentioned in *Sefer Ḥasidim*, in which the sage is asked for his advice, is a Jewish parallel to the quest for miraculous cures.

Other children killed at birth were those born to unwed mothers or the fruit of an adulterous relationship.[103] Two such cases are reported in *Sefer Ḥasidim*:

> In one city, there was a single woman who fornicated and became pregnant, and when she gave birth, her [female] relatives advised her to kill the child and she did so. And He who is Blessed delivered them into the hands of evil people and they [the evil people] took their money and tortured them until they fled the city.[104]

And:

> A woman became pregnant as a result of fornication, and she questioned another as to what to drink to abort her fetus. And one person [male] wanted to teach her, but they said to him: "Don't sin by assisting her to abort the infant." He responded: "She is better off aborting before the infant is born than killing it after it is born." They responded: "It is preferable that she sin without your help. Moreover, perhaps the child will rescued from her or she will die and the child will live."[105]

In the first case, the mother is a single woman and those supporting her at birth recommend killing the infant, the evidence of her illicit affair. In the second case, it is not clear if the woman is married or not. She turns to a woman who must have been known to provide assistance to women who wished to abort, and she somehow is referred to a man who can give her advice. The story raises some interesting issues. First, there is a surprising lack of secrecy surrounding the case, but perhaps this can be accounted for by the didactic genre of the book and the lesson the author wants to teach his readers. A second and more important point is that the man who had intended to advise her on the abortion is certain that if she does not abort the baby at this stage, she will kill it immediately after birth.

The same idea appears in a different story told by Caesarius of Heisterbach concerning a motif that appears throughout the centuries in anti-Jewish literature. Caesarius tells of a Jewish maiden who had an affair with a Christian priest and discovered she was pregnant. The girl feared that her father would kill her if he found out about the affair and the pregnancy, and together the young couple convinced her parents that she was about to give birth to the Messiah. When the infant was born and turned out to be a girl, one of the members of the Jewish community killed the baby.[106] Although I have not found other sources that distinctly mention killing unwanted infants, the circumstances mentioned here as those leading to infanticide — unknown or illegitimate paternity — accord with those outlined in contemporary Christian sources.

I would suggest that, in general, insofar as they were concerned with premarital and extramarital sexual relations and the handling of the unwanted results of such relations, Jews strongly resembled their Gentile neighbors.[107] We know that Jewish sources refer to the obligation of midwives to testify about the infant's parentage. The assumption was that if the infant was illegitimate, the parturient would disclose the father's name during labor.[108] The sources also discuss extramarital affairs, which were not uncommon, especially when husbands were traveling.[109] A quote from *Sefer Ḥasidim* summarizes the situation:

> Those scouting out the land to find a place to live should pay attention to the population in each city. What are the ways of the gentiles? For if they practice licentiousness, know that if Jews come to live in that city, their sons and daughters will also behave just as those gentiles do. For in each and every city the customs of the gentiles are, in most cases, those of the Jews who dwell with them.[110]

Crib Death

Another topic studied in the context of parental and especially maternal neglect is that of infants found lifeless in their parents' bed. In some of these cases, the deaths were probably crib death (SIDS).[111] Some scholars, however, have seen this as evidence of a method of infanticide—overlying, and have argued that these children (many of them girls) died because of neglect, indicating a lack of emotional attachment to children. This accusation of modern scholars echoes, at least to a certain extent, medieval attitudes toward parents who found their children dead in their beds. Canon law treated such cases as instances of murder, although the penalties and penances in such cases were relatively lenient.[112]

Jewish law, like canon law, treated these cases as a sin that required penance.[113] A number of medieval penances discuss overlaying:

> I found an answer about a woman who found her child dead in her bed. If she is not pregnant and is not nursing, and is also healthy, let her do penance for a year, but only if her husband wishes that she do so. And if she is young and is not used to fasting, let them [the woman and her husband] fast Mondays and Thursdays until they complete a year of fasting. And it is good if, to the greatest extent possible, they do not lay the children down in their beds, unless they see a need.[114]

Another response on the same topic is attributed to R. Meir b. Barukh:

> Maharam was asked about a woman who lay on her son and killed him, what her penance should be. And R. Meir instructed her to fast for a full year: not to eat meat or drink wine except for on the Sabbath and the holidays and New Moons, and Ḥanuka and Purim, when she should eat meat and drink wine. And in compensation for those holidays and new moons and Ḥanuka and Purim, on which she does not fast, she should fast on other days instead, until she has completed 365 days of fasting. And subsequently, she should fast every week—on Mondays and Thursdays, according to her strength. And she should eat meat and drink wine. Throughout all of her pregnancy and her days of nursing, she should not fast, and she should be careful not to let her son rest [in the same bed] with her.[115]

This response was well known in subsequent generations as well.[116] The legal authorities refer not only to the penance but also to the need to educate parents to lay their children down to sleep in cradles and not in their beds.[117] It is clear from the penances mentioned above, that the authors realize that at certain times, the children must be in their mother's bed. They encourage the mothers, however, to place the child back in his/her own bed after nursing.[118] While none of these penances voice the assumption that the child was overlaid on purpose, they all seem to assume that it is the mother, rather than her husband, who might be with the child in the same bed and who is responsible for the overlying.

Based on these penances from the thirteenth century, Urbach argued that the problem of overlaying arose in Ashkenaz at the end of the thirteenth century. He suggested that the reason was a deterioration in Jewish living quarters at this time. There is little evidence, however, that such a change took place at the end of the thirteenth century. Moreover, as Urbach himself noted, Christian penitential manuals discuss this problem from the sixth century onward. The Christian penance was to fast for a year, during which the penitent should eat only bread and drink only water and refrain from eating meat and drinking wine for two more years.[119] It is unlikely that Jews and Christians whose material surroundings were similar would have different overlying rates.

The Jewish sources that discuss overlying do not mention any details related to the physical surroundings of the home. In contrast, Christian sources are willing to condone overlying in poor homes much more readily than in affluent ones, although the punishment is still sometimes very harsh.[120] As Peter Abelard remarked:

> For look, some poverty-stricken woman has a little baby at the breast and doesn't have enough clothes to be able to meet the needs both of the little one in the crib and of herself. So, moved by pity for the little baby, she puts him by her side to warm him with her own rags. In the end, overwhelmed in her own feebleness by the force of nature, she is driven to smother the one she embraces with the greatest love. Augustine says: "Have charity and do whatever you want." Yet when she comes to the bishop for atonement, a heavy penalty is exacted from her, not for a fault she committed, but to make her or other women more careful about anticipating such dangers.[121]

Jewish sources do not distinguish between incidents of overlying in poor and in more affluent homes. It thus seems problematic to assume that a change in physical conditions in the thirteenth century gave rise to these penances. It seems more likely that as penances became more and more integral to mainstream Judaism, these penances became accepted for cases of overlying.

These different instances of children's deaths reveal the problems in generalizing about child care in the past. Within Jewish society, as within Christian society, there were instances of neglect and abuse due to individual nature or, more often, extenuating circumstances such as poverty and single motherhood. An examination of these cases of neglect, however, along with the norms outlined in the first part of the chapter reveals the value system of medieval Jews. We will examine one additional and rather extraordinary facet of this question — the killing of children during times of persecution in sanctification of the name of God.

A Different Mode of Abandonment

We have witnessed the competing interests that could obstruct parental love and devotion and at times endanger children. Because women gave birth and because care of young children was the mothers' responsibility, many of the instances discussed above had to do with neglect or lack of care on the mothers' part. These competing interests may be illuminated by examining another, very different category of actions.

Some scholars who have discussed maternal "cruelty" in medieval Christian society have not limited their study to infanticide practices, but also to the cases of mothers who wished to enter convents and abandoned their children, either to relatives or elsewhere. Some suggested that this willingness to leave children so the mothers could enter a holier way of life was additional proof that medieval parents did not care for their children.[122] In two studies on women and motherhood written during the last decade, Clarissa Atkinson and Barbara Newman have suggested a different way of looking at such cases. They have argued that mothers who left their children in order to enter a convent, or even expressed joy at the death of their children, did not do so out of cruelty. Rather, they saw their sacrifice as a way of advancing their spirituality. Martyrs such as St. Felicitas and St. Perpetua, who preferred martyrdom even when they were forced to abandon their nursing infants, served as role models and sources of encouragement. Three additional figures that were popular in medieval Germany were St. Julita, St. Felicitas, and St. Symphorosa (fig. 9). They are almost mythological figures, each of whom was killed with a number of infants.[123]

Biblical models were also called upon in this context. The Virgin Mary, who sacrificed her son, was one, as were biblical stories such as the sacrifice of Isaac, the dedication of Samuel to the Temple, and the story of Jepthe's daughter.[124] According to Newman and Atkinson, these role models enabled medieval women to express their grief over parting from their children, while arguing that they had sacrificed their most precious possessions — their children — to serve the Lord.[125] According to Newman's interpretation, Chaucer's Griselda serves as an example of such behavior and response. Griselda, who was told of the death of her children, responded without tears and with meekness. However, when she discovered that her children were alive, she wept like a mother.[126] Newman interprets her weeping "like a mother" as a description of expected motherly behavior, in contrast to her previous behavior that expressed, not cruelty, but her devotion to her husband and to God. In this light,

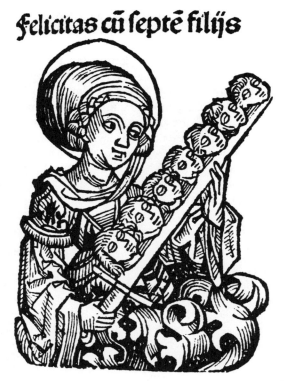

Figure 8. *"Felicitas cum septem filiis."* Schedel, Hartmann (1440–1514); Wolgemut Michael (1434–1519); Pleydenwurff Wilhem (d.1493), *Liber chronicarum — Nuremberg Chronicle* (A. Koberger, 1493). Photo courtesy of Archives and Research Collections, William Ready Division, McMaster University, Hamilton, Ontario, Canada.

we may consider those women who left their children in order to enter a convent as making a difficult choice in order to further their spirituality, rather than women whose maternal instincts and compassion were impaired.[127]

In Jewish society there was no equivalent to monastic life, and a spiritual life lived outside of the framework of the family was not a viable option for either women or men. As such, this case of Christian parental behavior has no clear parallel. Nevertheless, the study of women who chose monastic life can provide us with a better understanding of medieval Jewish society. The Jewish practice of sanctifying the name of God (*Kiddush haShem*), which included the killing of children in order to prevent their baptism, serves as a comparative case study. This practice became part of the Ashkenazic tradition in wake of the First Crusade, when a number of communities chose death over baptism. The chronicles that report these events, which were all written well after the Crusade, go to great lengths to describe the parents, and especially the mothers, who chose to take their children's lives rather than allow them to be captured by the Crusaders.[128]

Although I do not argue that the abandonment of a child in order to enter a convent and the killing of a child can be equated, Jews and Christians used the same models to justify their behavior. Jews during the First Crusade alluded to the sacrifice of Isaac as a model for their deeds,[129] and there are some hints at a tradition that extols the killing of the daughter of Jephte as well.[130] In addition, the story of the mother and her seven sons was an extremely popular one in medieval Jewish literature. The narratives of parents, many of them mothers, who chose to kill their children emphasize the tremendous sacrifice of the parents who insisted on their children's death.[131] The mother in *Sefer Yossipon*, the popular medieval account of the mother and her seven sons, calls upon what was understood as the essence of motherhood in order to encourage her son's death (figure 9). She says:

> My son, forsake all this! For I bore you in my belly for nine months and nursed you for three years. And after I nursed you . . . I sustained you with food until this very day and taught you the fear of the Lord. And now, my son, look up to the heavens and see the earth and the sea with your brothers. . . . Go, my son, and cleave onto your brothers, and may you enjoy the lot of their glory. And I shall come with you there and rejoice with you as on your wedding day and partake of the rewards of your righteousness with you.[132]

The medieval text introduces certain elements not present in the narrative in 2 and 4 Maccabees. In 2 Maccabees, the mother speaks "in the spirit of a man" and "in the language of the fathers." She claims that she "does not know how they entered her womb" and emphasizes her pregnancy, but these details emphasize her reversal of roles in this scene in which she acts with 'man-like courage.'"[133] In 4 Maccabees, the narrator emphasizes that were the mother to act like a mother, "if the woman had been weak in spirit—being, as she was, a mother—she would have complained and lamented 'in vain my sons did I endure those many travails for you.'"[134] In the medieval text, she claims her rights as a mother who bore the children in pain, fed them and nursed them, and with this power commands them to die rather than save themselves.

The shared models—both the biblical stories and the figure of the mother and her seven sons—were central to Christian and Jewish traditions in the Middle Ages. The expectation that women would devote themselves to their children is what made their decision to devote themselves to God and as a result sacrifice their children whether by abandonment or death all the more admirable.[135]

In light of this, one can see the choices made by Christian and Jewish parents as reflecting similar value systems, although those values were part of two traditions that were often in conflict.[136] Devotion to God was expressed by giv-

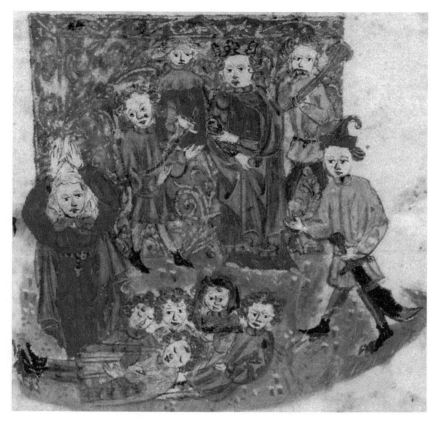

Figure 9. The Mother and Her Seven Sons. Cod. Heb. 37, fol. 79b, Germany, 1427. Photo courtesy of Hamburg Staats- und Universitätsbibliothek.

ing up an aspect of life that was particularly dear. An examination of the Jewish sources does not strengthen the claim that Jews, unlike Christians, valued their children's lives. Rather, it demonstrates that medieval Jews and Christians shared the same world.[137]

Jews who faced the choice of baptism or death preferred death for themselves and for their children. The idea that the death of a child is to be preferred over his baptism into Christianity appears in other sources as well, even those not dealing with times of duress, such as attacks on the community. R. Tam decrees that one should not mourn the death of a Jewish child who converted to Christianity. He discusses what one should do if such a child dies. When converted adult Jews died, they were not mourned by their families. The question concerns whether converted children should be mourned, as they did not consent to their conversions. Some felt that they should be mourned as if they were still part of the community. Although R. Tam disagreed,[138] the question in and of itself is evidence of the tremendous dilemma around this issue.

The Crusade chronicles also provide ample evidence for the dilemmas faced by parents forced to choose between their children's physical and spiritual welfare. This is evident in both the words attributed to parents who chose to kill their children and the words of those who did not. The narrative contrasts the parents' instinctive behavior toward their children with their actions, both when describing their actions and in the choice of biblical imagery. Thus, the women are called merciful and loving mothers, even as they choose to kill their own children. In addition, those parents who chose not to sacrifice their children do not receive the same attention. Entire communities, as in the cases of Metz and Regensburg, made this choice, and, as R. Solomon b. Samson explains, they did as the Crusaders instructed them in order to save their children.[139]

The case of R. Isaac b. David (of Mainz) who converted and then returned to the community demonstrates that the children were a central concern. He explains his decision to convert by stating: "I listened to the enemies only in order to save my children from these evil people."[140] When he decides to return to the community and be killed as a Jew together with his children, he chooses the spiritual over the physical. The story of the mother Marat Rachel illuminates these ideas as well. Marat Rachel, the wife of R. Judah and the daughter of R. Isaac b. Asher, kills her four children rather than allowing them to fall into the hands of Christians. She tells her friends:

> I have four children. On them as well have no mercy, lest these uncircumcised come and seize them and they remain in their erroneous faith. With them as well you must sanctify the Holy name.[141]

After killing three of her four children, she chases after her youngest, Aaron, vowing not to have mercy on him. Her husband then sees the four dead children and kills himself as well.[142]

In this story, which has been read and reread in recent years, it is Rachel, the daughter and wife of prominent rabbis, who does not act like a mother. Yet the narrative is constructed to highlight the difficulty of this ordeal, ending with the words *"Em al banim rutsha"* — when mother and babes were dashed to death together (Hos. 10:14) — that evoke the well-known opposing quotation "the mother of the children rejoices" (Ps. 113: 9).[143]

Several other cases are reported in the chronicles, in which mothers express their painful deliberations on the decision as to whether to allow their husbands to kill their children. Zipporah of Worms, who is described, like Sarah the Matriarch, as having waited years to have a child, begs her husband to kill her before he kills their child, so that she will not have to witness such horror.[144] Ultimately, maternal pity must give way before spiritual piety. Concern for the spiritual welfare of the child was to be favored over concern for his physical welfare.[145]

The response of Christian society to this behavior suggests that Christians saw and understood what these Jews were doing as a double insult to Christianity. Not only did they refuse to convert to Christianity, but by killing their children they expressed the ultimate contempt for the Christian religion. Scholars have described the tremendous anger with which Christians greeted the Jewish response to the Crusade. While this anger had many facets, the shared attitude toward children and the affront to this value that Christians perceived in the deeds of the Jews were certainly components of the Christian response.[146]

These actions of Jewish parents and especially of mothers were described as "unnatural" and as contrary to the order of society.[147] In Germany and northern France, parenthood was understood in similar cultural terms in Jewish and Christian society; both societies privileged the spiritual over what was understood as the physical and natural. Looking back at this society from a modern perspective, we must not judge this preference as evidence of the cruelty or lack of affection of parents for their children. Rather, attitudes toward children and childhood should be seen as a reflection of medieval society's principles and ideals. The understandings of women and the tasks they were allotted in child rearing also reflected their place in society and the gender hierarchies of their communities. Consequently, in order to attain a higher spiritual level, whether as martyrs or as *mulieres spirituales*, women were required to abandon the normative and physical attitudes toward children. This chapter has revealed the shared nature of Jewish and Christian medieval society, and the joint examination of Jewish and Christian parenting norms demonstrates how the tensions between the two religious groups were shaped by this shared framework. Jews and Christians used the same symbols and models, and their own particular and often polemical interpretations derived from a shared heritage and culture. This shared heritage and value system is expressed even in the extreme and drastic circumstances of martyrdom and *Kiddush haShem*, in which the two religions were embattled with each other and at a time when Jews and Christians were emphasizing the distinction between themselves and their surrounding cultures.

Conclusions

IN THESE PAGES, we have followed the lives of children in their early years, when they were sheltered by parental care. When the boys of medieval Ashkenaz reached the age of five, six, or seven, they took a step toward independence, as they began their schooling, accompanied by an elaborate ritual. The path followed by these boys from this point on is fairly well documented — either they chose to become scholars, or, in most cases, businessmen. The course pursued by the girls is not as well evidenced. They remained within the home with their mothers, preparing themselves for their roles as mothers, wives, and financial supporters of their future families. In many cases, they too were educated, although their education was notably different from that of their brothers, focusing on the practical laws of running a household and without the emphasis on textual knowledge that characterized boys' education.[1] These modes of education reflected both the values of medieval Jewish society and the future roles boys and girls were expected to assume.

The issues of parents and children in medieval Jewish society were examined within the context of the surrounding Christian world as one chapter of a wider social history of the Jews. By examining daily life alongside the theological and ideological debates recorded in the texts written by the medieval rabbis, we come to understand better the roles of women and children within their families. We may also situate family and community rituals and daily life within a wider social and cultural context. Despite the limitations of extant medieval Jewish sources, these texts provide significant information and reflections of the social reality of the Jewish families and communities as well as of the Christian society in which they lived. In this way, I have tried to supply the other side of the coin to the theological issues that have been so central in research to date.

This study has sought to further our knowledge of medieval Ashkenazic society in three ways. On a descriptive level, I have outlined the contours of family life and child care within the nuclear family. The nature of the sources and the information they provide has led me to organize my analysis around the stages of life and development of the children, rather than attempt to fully describe the material surroundings of the family. As such, this study is a first step toward the writing of a fuller history of family life. Secondly, examining the family and the ways in which mothers and fathers cared for their children has revealed some of the communal structures and hierarchies that shaped and were shaped by the family's every day needs. On a third level, the study illuminates the manifold social and intellectual relations between Jews and Christians and the cultural appropriations of practice and belief in medieval Jewish society.

CONCLUSIONS

In examining the nuclear family, I have detailed the daily praxis as well as the division of labor between men and women, fathers and mothers, in medieval Jewish society. While these divisions of labor were sometimes the result of religious beliefs and their interpretation, we also witnessed how medieval cultural understandings and concepts shaped common practice in ways different than those of previous generations. Many components of medieval family life remained constant throughout the Middle Ages and were a direct continuation of more ancient practices. This applies to attitudes as well as to expected behavior of children and their parents. The sources of the period attest both to concern and care for children, and to the awareness of childhood as a unique period of life. At the same time, we find different parenting practices that present variations of more ancient models, and we find competing medieval attitudes toward parenthood.

Despite the clear continuity of various traditions throughout the Middle Ages, we can also discern a number of changes in the lives of medieval parents and children. While at times these changes are small and almost inconsequential, in other cases they are more substantial. Together, they present a society that altered and reshaped itself over time. Many such examples have been discussed in the different chapters of his book and I will not repeat them here. Rather, I will point to number of such changes and link them to some of the more general conclusions that can be drawn from the evidence. Some of the variations derive from new social patterns that changed over time. For example, in the eleventh century, a divorced woman with a young infant could remarry fairly quickly, if she desired to do so. Her counterpart 150 years later would have faced nearly insurmountable barriers to such a remarriage and would have been required to wait longer. While it is easy to point to the legal precedent that instituted this change, I attempted to outline the social circumstances that were the impetus for the legal decision and the dilemmas such women faced as single mothers of young children. The relentless battles that the different rabbis waged against the marriage of women with children under age two demonstrated how pressing these issues were.

Examining the nuclear family and its daily and ritual life also offered us a new view of Jewish society and of some of the tensions that existed within it — both between families and along gender lines. Our ability to hear women's voices, voices one has to pry out of the male rabbinic narrative that characterizes most of the medieval Jewish sources, was greater when examining sites of tension. When discussing birth, we heard the midwives' voices mediated by their "colleagues," the circumcisers. It was not always possible to hear these voices, and in some cases we had to make do with a look at women's behavior and attempt to deduce their attitudes and stances from their described actions. For example, in the case of birth rituals, we hear of women's desires and actions most clearly when the male rabbinic authorities oppose them. Although in many cases my conclusions pointed to society's eventual acceptance of the ideas and behavior recommended by the male legal authorities, the exposure of the social negotiation processes within the halakhic and textual sources was the key to understanding the society's values.

The attempt to include Jewish women in the medieval historiographic tradition is a recent one. As such, the aspects of women's lives discussed in this book are a first step toward a fuller picture of women's lives. When looking for information relating to women, we found it easier to locate when examining topics such as motherhood and birth, which have inherent female aspects. Furthermore, since these women are presented as part of their communities and surroundings, the study of medieval women reveals many new aspects of their society. At the same time, we saw important male involvement in matters that have traditionally been considered of female concern, such as issues around the *Kindbetterin*, as well as constant contact between women and areas that have traditionally been considered male. For example, when studying midwives we learned about medical practice within the Jewish community, a practice that often refers to women only in passing. In a different case, when discussing attitudes toward overlying and the death of children, we found a richly documented practice of penances and ways of atonement that have until now been studied in almost exclusively male terms.

One can conclude that motherhood is not only an important topic of research in and of itself, but also a key to understanding other aspects of Jewish society. Women had many roles, and motherhood was a central one. By looking for mothers and information on women as mothers, we may learn much about other aspects of society that have little to do with being a mother, but, as they touch on the lives of women, they are discussed in similar contexts.

From a methodological point of view, studying women along with children and the wider community (rather than women alone) sheds light on various aspects of society and elucidates the complexities of medieval life. Limitations placed on female religious practice took on new meanings when such change affected children as well. While the Jewish society in question was a patriarchal one, our examination shows that the divisions between male and female realms were not always straightforward. One of the central conclusions of this book, as illustrated through observations on the changing ceremony of circumcision, was that women's place in religious ritual underwent substantive change during the thirteenth century and that these changes were part of broader social changes.

As other studies, first and foremost Ivan Marcus's *Rituals of Childhood*, have shown, and as was described briefly in the appendix to chapter 2, the participation of male children in religious rituals changed during the course of the thirteenth century. Whereas previously young boys were encouraged to perform a variety of commandments—such as wearing ẓiẓit and donning tefillin—in the thirteenth century, these obligations were postponed until after age thirteen. While age thirteen has always borne special significance within

Jewish society, the postponement of the observance of the commandments to this age reinforced and renewed the importance of age thirteen as the age of religious obligation. These developments demonstrate the social and religious changes taking place within Jewish society.[2] The thirteenth and fourteenth century were, however, also the period in which Jewish women were excluded from ritual practices in which they had participated previously. Thus, future research can combine an understanding of the changes in ceremonial practices of adolescent and preadolescent boys with those encompassing women and examine how the ideal Jewish participant had now become the adult male.

The examination of the larger family framework in which women and children were members demonstrates what may be gained from such a perspective. We come to see that the changing place of Jewish women and children in religious ritual was not primarily the result of a new attitude toward women or a changed understanding of childhood. The changes in Jewish ritual that have been outlined here and in other studies over recent years demonstrate changes in women's and children's places in religious ritual both public and private. By examining the changes as an ensemble, we may come to understand the function of these changes within the Jewish community at large.

One possible explanation for the changing place of women and children in religious ritual is connected to the Jewish community's self-image. Scholars have demonstrated that, as a result of the difficult events that communities endured during the late eleventh and twelfth century, the Ashkenazic Jewish communities came to see themselves as a holy community.[3] In the descriptions of these events, women and children are strikingly portrayed as active participants; some have suggested that this inclusion heightened the image of the entire community as a holy entity.[4] More recently, this self-image has been called into question, particularly in the work of Susan Einbinder, who has shown that the place of women in the depiction of the community and its events changed tremendously over the course of the twelfth and thirteenth centuries.[5] While a fuller explanation for the changing place of women and children in medieval Jewish society requires further research, some answers have been provided in this book. When discussing religious ritual we have witnessed the sacralization of the circumcision ritual, as well as a new trend describing circumcision as a sacrifice. We have seen a growing importance attributed to men's fulfillment of certain roles—that of circumciser and ba'al brit—as well as an increased need to define male and female spheres of action, as witnessed by R. Meir of Rothenburg's response concerning women who served as ba'alei brit.

If we now move from the focus on the processes within the Jewish community to an examination of Jews within their broader cultural context (as we have tried to do throughout this study), we find that the changes within Jewish society were to a great extent characteristic of the majority society within which Jews lived. Here we see that some of the conclusions of my study correspond with those of scholars of medieval Christian society. Recent research has shown a change in Christian women's and children's participation in religious ritual life as well. In the High Middle Ages, the age of confirmation was postponed and women's religiosity was sharply curtailed.[6] While these changes can be explained by internal developments within the church and Christian society, the close comparison of Jewish and Christian culture has helped us identify these trends as a part of more general, wider processes affecting members of both religious traditions.

Joint explanation does not exclude internal explanations of specific changes within each tradition, but expands our understanding of both internal community issues and more general matters. This approach recognizes the social reality in which Jews and Christians lived as close neighbors as well as their shared intellectual milieu. While it does not detract from the clear religious distinction between Jews and Christians that existed in medieval society, it enables a better understanding of the shared aspects of medieval life, some of which transcend presupposed differences and transgress boundaries.

Furthermore, our attempt to compare Jewish and Christian society in general, rather than in specific instances, allows for a systematic study of medieval Jewish society that examines the Jews as an integral part of their surroundings. This study has shown that not only were there many similarities between the way Jews and Christians chose to live their lives, but that the daily contacts between Jews and Christians were constant and numerous. The Jewish family, which some have portrayed as a haven in which Jews were isolated from their non-Jewish neighbors, was not an insular environment. Contact with Christians was part of everyday family life.

One aspect that has stood out in this study is the wealth of contact between Jewish and Christian women. Jewish and Christian women were medical colleagues and they met as neighbors. Christian women worked in Jewish homes, and Jewish children were cared for in Christian homes. The study of women, Jewish and Christian, is the result of the recent interest in women's and gender studies, areas of interest that have developed methodologies for uncovering the lives of women in the past and examining their lives in the context of the society within which they lived. These issues have only just begun to be addressed in medieval Jewish studies, and it is my hope that many more studies addressing the place of women and gender understandings and conceptions will be undertaken in the coming years.

We may ask whether the connections between Jewish and Christians women that were central to our discussion were the exception to the norm or typical of contacts between Jewish and Christian men as well. While the contacts between Jewish and Christian men were probably more frequent than research to date has demonstrated, I would argue that Jewish women were particularly immersed in the lives of their Christian neighbors, because so many of their daily contacts revolved around the home and child care, in which there was employment of, and frequent contact with, Christian women. As such,

Jewish and Christian women's interactions can be seen as a channel and a link between Jewish and Christian society.

While some instances demonstrated great similarity between Jewish and Christian society, in other cases we saw significant differences. Some of these differences resulted from an intentional effort to separate the two societies and religious identities, while in other cases I suggested that the difference was the result of the distinction between a minority and a majority society. In all these instances, we can only identify the nature of these differences and similarities by examining the Jewish communities within the wider cultural milieu. Christian practices that have previously been read in light of theological outlooks or religious motivations, such as churching or co-parenting, may be seen in a different light when compared with changes in Jewish practice. When examining Jewish practices, we have seen a great degree of similarity to Christian practices. These comparisons underline the fact that differences between Jewish and Christian society were not always organized around theological or religious motivations, and in some cases the same practices were upheld by Jews and Christians and supported by different explanations.

Our examination of the family as a unit, and of mothers in particular opens a new area of historical inquiry into medieval Jewish history and offers a richer understanding of Jewish life in the past. This study is a first step toward a more depthful social history of Jewish families in medieval Ashkenaz that will include other stages in family life as well as a fuller economic and cultural history. The focus on the close contacts between Jews and Christians and the world they shared opens new vistas for research and encourages historians of both Jewish and Christian society to search for and learn from these comparisons. By comparing and filling in the blanks when necessary, we can piece together a larger picture of the knowledge shared by Jews and Christians, men and women, in medieval society, and we can identify avenues along which Jews and Christians learned and appropriated ideas that were incorporated into both Jewish and Christian cultures. It is my hope that by examining the strategies medieval Jews used both consciously and unconsciously, while preserving their identity and introducing change and innovation into their daily and ritual lives, we have allowed voices that had not yet been heard be sounded. We can learn from this inquiry that isolation is not necessarily the only way for a minority group to maintain distinct national and religious identities and to survive as a minority.

NOTES

NOTES TO INTRODUCTION

1. Abelard explains that he is quoting Héloise herself. Recently, Gadi Algazi has suggested that this passage describes Héloise's circumstances and not Abelard's: "Abelard, Héloise and Astralabe," in *Women, Children and the Elderly: Essays in Honour of Shulamith Shaḥar*, eds. Miriam Eliav-Feldon and Yitzhak Hen (Jerusalem, 2001), 85–98.

2. Peter Abelard, *The Letters of Abelard and Héloise*, trans. Betty Radice (Hammondsworth, 1974), 71.

3. The separation of boys from the female sphere is described in Ivan Marcus, *Rituals of Childhood: Jewish Acculturation in Medieval Europe* (New Haven and London, 1996), 75–78.

4. For example: Clarissa Atkinson, *The Oldest Vocation: Christian Motherhood in the Middle Ages* (Ithaca, N.Y. and London, 1991), 6–7.

5. Examples are multiple, and this is true not just of remarks in passing but also in studies focusing on the Jewish family. For example: Solomon Schechter, "The Child in Jewish Literature," *Studies in Judaism* (Philadelphia, 1896), 1:282–312; William Moses Feldman, *The Jewish Child: Its History, Folklore, Biology and Sociology* (London, 1917); Franz Kobler, *Her Children Call Her Blessed: A Portrait of the Jewish Mother* (New York, 1955); Rachel Monika Herweg, *Die jüdische Mutter. Das verborgene Matriarchat* (Darmstadt, 1994).

6. (Paris, 1960).

7. Barbara Hanawalt, "Medievalists and the Study of Childhood." *Speculum* 77(2002):440–60.

8. For example: Lawrence Stone, *The Family, Sex and Marriage in England 1500–1800* (New York, 1977); Lloyd de Mause, "The Evolution of Childhood," *The History of Childhood* (New York, 1974), 1–73.

9. Shulamith Shaḥar, *Childhood in the Middle Ages* (London and New York, 1990); Barbara Hanawalt, *The Ties That Bound: Peasant Families in Medieval England* (New York, 1986); Danièle Alexandre-Bidon et Monique Closson, *L'enfant à l'ombre des cathédrales* (Lyon and Paris, 1985); Pierre Riché et Danièle Alexandre-Bidon, *L'Enfance au Moyen Age* (Paris, 1994); Didier Lett, *L'enfant des miracles. Enfance et société au Moyen Age (XIIe–XIIIe siècle)* (Paris, 1997); James Schultz, *The Knowledge of Childhood in the German Middle Ages, 1100–1350* (Philadelphia, 1995); Nicholas Orme, *Medieval Children* (New Haven, 2001) and for modern times: Linda A. Pollock, *Forgotten Children: Parent-Child Relations 1500–1900* (Cambridge and New York, 1983).

10. Elisabeth Badinter, *L'Amour en plus: L'histoire de l'amour maternel (XVIIe–XXe siècle)* (Paris, 1980).

11. For a survey of the early research: Etienne van de Walle, "Recent Approaches to Past Childhoods," in *The Family in History: Interdisciplinary Essays*, eds. Theodore K. Rabb and Robert I. Rothberg (New York, Hagerstown, San Francisco, and London, 1973), 171–78, and more recently the articles in the volume: Cathy Jorgenson Itnyre (ed.), *Medieval Family Roles: A Book of Essays* (New York, 1996).

12. Clarissa Atkinson, *The Oldest Vocation*; Mary Dockray-Miller, *Motherhood and Mothering in Anglo-Saxon England* (London, 2000); and the collections of essays: Anneke B. Mulder-Bakker (ed.), *Sanctity and Motherhood: Essays on Holy Mothers in the Middle Ages* (New York, 1995); John Carmi Parsons and Bonnie Wheeler (eds.), *Medieval Mothering* (New York and London, 1996).

13. Joan Scott, *Gender and the Politics of History* (New York, 1988), 43–44 virtually ignores motherhood; Marianne Hirsch, "Feminism and the Maternal Divide: A Diary," in *The Politics of*

Motherhood: Activist Voices from Left to Right, eds. Alexis Jetter, Annelise Orleck and Dianna Taylor (Hanover, N.H. and London, 1997), 352–68; Sara Ruddick, "Rethinking 'Maternal' Politics," ibid, 369–81.

14. Yvonne Knibiehler, *Les Pères aussi ont une histoire* (Paris, 1987); Jean Delumeau et Daniêl Roche (eds.), *Histoire des pères et de la paternité* (Paris, 1990) and for early modern Europe: Steven Ozment, *When Fathers Ruled: Family Life in Reformation Europe* (Cambridge, Mass., 1983).

15. Christiane Klapisch-Zuber, "Including Women," trans. Arthur Goldhammer, *History of Women in the West*, ed. Christiane Klapisch-Zuber (London and Cambridge, Mass., 1992), 2:7–10.

16. A recent study has demonstrated how much can be learned from such an analysis of the medieval author's gender and identity. See the articles in Catherine M. Mooney (ed.), *Gendered Voices: Medieval Saints and Their Interpreters* (Philadelphia, 1999); and for earlier discussions of these issues: Gabrielle M. Spiegel, "History, Historicism and the Social Logic of the Text in the Middle Ages." *Speculum* 65(1990): 59–86.

17. Scott, *Gender*, 28–50; Gisela Bock, "Challenging Dichotomies: Perspectives on Women's History," in *Writing Women's History. International Perspectives*, eds. Karen Offen, Ruth Roach Pierson and Jane Rendall (Bloomington and Indianapolis, 1991), 1–24.

18. I emphasize the word *relatively* because there are far more sources for the ninth and tenth centuries in Christian society than for Jewish sources for that time period.

19. Doris Desclais Berkvam, *Enfance et maternité dans la littérature française des XIIe et XIIIe siècles* (Paris, 1981); Schultz, *The Idea of Childhood*; Lett, *L'enfant des miracles*.

20. For example: Pierre Toubert, "The Carolingian Moment," in *A History of the Family*, eds. André Burguière et al., trans. Sarah Hanbury Tension et al. (Cambridge, Mass., 1996), 1:379–406; Janet Nelson, "Parents, Children and the Church," in *The Church and Childhood*, ed. Diana Wood (*Studies in Church History*, 31) (Oxford, 1994), 81–115.

21. For example: Beatrice Gottlieb, *The Family in the Western World from the Black Death to the Industrial Revolution* (New York, 1993).

22. Mordechai Breuer, "The "Black Death" and Antisemitism," in *Antisemitism Through the Ages. A Collection of Essays*, ed. Shmuel Almog (Jerusalem, 1980), 139–52 [in Hebrew]; Zefira Entin Rokéaḥ, "The State, the Church and the Jews in Medieval England," ibid., 99–126; William Chester Jordan, *The French Monarchy and the Jews: From Philip Augustus to the Last Capetians* (Philadelphia, 1989), 214–38.

23. Michael Toch, *Die Juden im mittelalterlichen Reich* (*Enzyklopädie deutscher Geschichte*, 44) (München, 1998), 55–67; Franz-Josef Ziwes, *Studien zur Geschichte der Juden im mittleren Rheingebiet während des hohen und späten Mittelalters* (Hanover 1995), 220–66.

24. This issue has been discussed at length by various scholars over the past years. While some have argued for complete distinction between the areas, others have demonstrated the advantage of studying both areas together. For a discussion of this issue: Israel Ta-Shma, *Early Franco-German Ritual and Custom* (Jerusalem, 1992), 14–16; 22–27 [in Hebrew]. See further discussion of this in note 30.

25. Many documents related to the formation of the communities were published by Julius Aronius, *Regesten zur Geschichte der Juden im fränkischen und deutschen Reiche bis zum Jahre 1273* (Berlin, 1902, repr. Hildesheim and New York, 1970), 25–92.

26. For settlement of Jews in Germany: Avraham Grossman, *The Early Sages of Ashkenaz: Their Lives, Leadership and Works* (900–1096) (Jerusalem, 2001[3]), 9–18 [in Hebrew]; Ziwes, *Studien zur Geschichte der Juden*; Michael Toch, "The Formation of a Diaspora. The Settlement of the Jews in the Medieval German Reich," *Aschkenas* 7 (1997), 55–78; Alexander Pinthus, *Die Judensiedlungen der deutsche Städte. Eine stadtbiologische Studie* (Berlin, 1931), 13–47; and most recently: Markus J. Wenninger, "Zur Topographie der Judenviertel in den mittelalterlichen deutschen Städten anhand österreichischer Beispiele," in *Juden in der Stadt*, eds. Fritz Mayrhofer und Ferdinand Opll (Linz, 1999), 81–117. The last two studies focus on the layout of the cities. I thank Professor Israel J. Yuval who referred me to Pinthus's and Wenninger's work.

NOTES TO INTRODUCTION 193

27. For settlement in France: Avraham Grossman, *The Early Sages of France: Their Lives, Leadership and Works* (Jerusalem, 2001³), 13–21 [in Hebrew].

28. Grossman, *Sages of Ashkenaz*, 27–28.

29. An additional geographic area that could have been part of our frame of reference is that of Poland, to which many German Jews emigrated during the high and late Middle Ages. However, the state of research about Poland during this period does not allow for a close examination.

30. Although Grossman distinguished between Germany and France when writing his histories of the Sages' lives, he treats them as one area when examining women: *Pious and Rebellious: Jewish Women in Europe in the Middle Ages* (Jerusalem, 2001) [in Hebrew]. Others have argued for greater differentiation: Eric Zimmer, *Society and Its Customs: Studies in the History and Metamorphosis of Jewish Customs* (Jerusalem 1996) [in Hebrew] as well as the review of this book: Haym Soloveitchik, "Review Essay of *Olam Ke-Minhago Noheg*," *AJS Review* 23(1998): 223–25 and most recently: "Piety, Pietism and German Pietism: 'Sefer Ḥasidim I' and the Influence of 'Ḥasidei Ashkenaz.' " *JQR* 92(2002): 455–93. For a discussion of this issue in broader terms: Carlrichard Brühl, *Deutschland-Frankreich: Die Geburt zweier Völker* (Köln and Vienna, 1990).

31. As noted above, n. 24.

32. For example: Shaḥar, *Childhood*; Eadem, *The Fourth Estate: A History of Women in the Middle Ages*, trans. Chaya Galai (London and New York, 1983); Mary Martin McLaughlin, "Survivors and Surrogates: Children and Parents from the Ninth to the Thirteenth Centuries," in *The History of Childhood*, ed. Lloyd de Mause (New York, 1974), 101–81; Hugh Cunningham, *Children and Childhood in Western Society since 1500* (London and New York, 1995); Gottlieb, *The Family in the Western World*; Alexander-Bidon and Closson, *L'enfance à l'ombre des cathédrales*; Luke DeMaitre, "The Idea of Childhood and Childcare in Medical Writings of the Middle Ages," *Journal of Psychohistory* 4(1976/77): 461–90; John Boswell, *The Kindness of Strangers: The Abandonment of Children in Western Europe from Late Antiquity to the Renaissance* (New York, 1988). James Casey, in his *The History of the Family* (Oxford and New York, 1989) protests the exclusion of Spain from these discussions.

33. For example: Berkvam, *Enfance et maternité*, who focuses on France; Schultz, *Knowledge of Childhood*, focuses on Germany; and Nicholas Orme, "The Culture of Childhood in Medieval England"; *Past and Present* 148(1994): 48–88; idem, *Medieval Children*, discusses medieval England. See also: Linda Paterson, "L'enfant dans la littérature occitane avant 1230"; *Cahiers de civilization médièvale Xe-XIIe siècle* 32(1989): 233–45; Jenny Swanson, "Childhood and Child Rearing in *ad status* Sermons by Later Thirteenth Century Friars"; *Journal of Medieval History* 16(1990): 309–30; Kathryn Ann Taglia, "The Cultural Construction of Childhood: Baptism, Communion and Confirmation," in *Women, Marriage and Family in Medieval Christendom. Essays in Memory of Michael M. Sheehan*, eds. Constance M. Rousseau and Joel T. Rosenthal (Kalamazoo, MI, 1998), 255–88.

34. This issue is discussed at length in chapter 1. See also: Joseph Shatzmiller, *Jews, Medicine and Medieval Society* (Berkeley, Los Angeles, and London, 1994).

35. In this statement I include the scholars whose Hebrew writings have reached us. Although they wrote in Hebrew, this was not the language in which they conducted most of their business and family lives.

36. For example: Marcus, *Rituals of Childhood*, 74–101.

37. Esther Cohen and Elliott Horowitz, "In Search of the Sacred: Jews, Christians and Rituals of Marriage in the Later Middle Ages," *Journal of Medieval and Renaissance Studies* 20(1990): 225–27.

38. Jacob Katz, *The "Shabbes Goy": A Study in Halakhic Flexibility*, trans. Yoel Lerner (Philadelphia, 1989), 49–68.

39. Only in Speyer were the Jews originally settled in a separate area, over the river: "Speyer," *Germania Judaica*, 1:328.

40. A wonderful example of this familiarity can be found in a response concerning a widow

from the twelfth century: "Once a certain widow lit the Sabbath candles in her home and went to the synagogue. She left her house sealed, closing the door so that the wind would not blow out the candle. When she returned from the synagogue she found that the candles had fallen to the ground. And a gentile woman came over to light the candles because she [the gentile woman] was extremely knowledgeable of Jewish law." MS Paris héb. 326, fol. 19a. The same story appears in MS Oxford Bodl., Hunt. 404, (794), 796b–80a. Other examples of such familiarity appear in the halakhic literature, for example: R. Meir b. Barukh, *Teshuvot Psakim uMinhagim*, (Responsa, rulings and Customs), collected, annotated and arranged by Isaac Ze'ev Cahana (Jerusalem, 1960) 2: responsa no. 36.

41. William Chester Jordan, *Women and Credit in Pre-Industrial and Developing Societies* (Philadelphia, 1993), 35–39; Idem, "Jews on Top: Women and the Availability of Consumption Loans in Northern France in the Mid–Thirteenth Century." *Journal of Jewish Studies* 29 (1978): 39–56.

42. Cohen and Horowitz, "In Search of the Sacred," 225.

43. See chapter 1, pp. 48–49.

44. For example: Leopold Löw, *Die Lebensalter in der jüdischen Literatur: von physiologischem, rechts-, sitten-, und religionsgeschichtlichem Standpunkte betrachtet* (Szegedin, 1875, repr. Jerusalem, 1969), 77–80.

45. Marcus, *Rituals of Childhood*, 8–13; Robert Bonfil, *Jewish Life in Renaissance Italy*, trans. Anthony Oldcorn (Berkeley, Los Angeles, and London, 1994), 101–104, 114–16, and in greater detail in his "Cultura ebraica e cultura cristiana in Italia meridionale," *Tra due mondi. Cultura ebraica e cultura cristiana nel Medioevo* (Napoli, 1996), 3–11.

46. This method has been used and adopted in different ways by many medieval scholars. For example: Israel J. Yuval, *"Two Nations in Your Womb": Perceptions of Jews and Christians* (Tel Aviv, 2000) [in Hebrew]; Jeremy Cohen, "Between Martyrdom and Apostasy: Doubt and Self-Definition in Twelfth-Century Ashkenaz." *Journal of Medieval and Early Modern Studies* 29(1999): 431–71.

47. Nils Roemer, "Turning Defeat into Victory: *Wissenschaft des Judentums* and the Martyrs of 1096," *Jewish History* 13(1999): 65–80.

48. His magnum opus, *A Social and Religious History of the Jews*, 18 vols. (Philadelphia, 1952–1983), contains fifteen volumes that are devoted to aspects of the Middle Ages, yet within this tremendous corpus there is not a single chapter devoted to women or family.

49. Jacob Katz, *Tradition and Crisis: Jewish Society at the End of the Middle Ages*, trans. Bernard Dov Cooperman (New York, 1993), 113–31, and criticism of his thesis: Chava Weissler, "The Missing Half and the Other Half: A Feminist and Anthropological Response"; *Jewish Social Studies* 2:(1996), 98–105, 108–15; Elisheva Carlebach, "Early Modern Ashkenaz in the Writings of Jacob Katz," in *Pride of Jacob. Essays on Jacob Katz and his Work*, ed. Jay M. Harris (Cambridge, Mass., 2002), 65–83.

50. For example: Löw, *Lebensalter*; Adolf Berliner, *Aus dem inneren Leben der deutschen Juden im Mittelalter nach gedruckten und ungedruckten Quellen. Zugleich ein Beitrag für deutsche Kultur-geschichte* (Berlin, 1871); Israel Abrahams, *Jewish Life in the Middle Ages* (Philadelphia, 1896); Moshe Güdemann, *Sefer haTorah veHeḤayim beArzot Ashkenaz beYemei haBenayim*. 3 vols. (Warsaw, 1897).

51. For example, Abrahams, ibid., states: "The Jewish home was a haven of rest from the storms that raged around the very gates of the ghettos, nay a fairy palace in which the bespattered objects of the mobs' derision threw off their garb of shame and resumed the royal attire of freemen," 129.

52. This has changed only over the past decade and a half. I have indicated only a partial list of the research that has flourished during the past fifteen years. On the family and women: Steven M. Cohen and Paula Hyman (eds.), *The Jewish Family: Myths and Reality* (New York, 1986); Judith R. Baskin (ed.), *Jewish Women in Historical Perspective* (Detroit, 1998^2); Lynn Davidman and Shelley Tennenbaum (eds.), *Feminist Perspectives on Jewish Studies* (New Haven, 1994); Miriam Peskowitz and Laura Levitt (eds.), *Judaism since Gender* (New York, 1997). In Hebrew, such re-

search has flourished only during the past seven or eight years: Yael Azmon (ed.), *A View into the Lives of Women in Jewish Societies* (Jerusalem, 1995), [in Hebrew]; Reneé Levine-Melammed, ed., *"Lift up Your Voice": Women's Voices and Feminist Interpretation in Jewish Studies* (Tel Aviv, 2001) [in Hebrew]; Israel Bartal and Isaiah Gafni, eds., *Sexuality and the Family in History: Collected Essays* (Jerusalem, 1999) [in Hebrew]; and most recently Grossman, *Pious and Rebellious*. In addition see a number of articles: Ivan G. Marcus, "Mothers, Martyrs and Moneymakers: Some Jewish Women in Medieval Europe"; *Conservative Judaism* 38(1986): 34–45; Judith R. Baskin, "From Separation to Displacement: The Problem of Women in *Sefer Ḥasidim*"; *AJS Review* 19 (1994):1–18; Eadem, "Silent Partners: Women As Wives in Rabbinic Literature," in *Active Voices: Women in Jewish Culture*, ed. Maurie Sacks (Urbana and Chicago, 1995), 19–37. On childhood: Simḥa Goldin, "Jewish Children and Christian Missionizing," *Sexuality and the Family in History. Collected Essays*, ed. Israel Bartal and Isiah Gafni (Jerusalem, 1999), 97–118 [in Hebrew]; Idem, "Die Beziehung der jüdischen Familie im Mittelalter zu Kind und Kindheit," *Jahrbuch der Kindheit* 6(1989): 211–56; Ephraim Kanarfogel, "Attitudes toward Childhood and Children in Medieval Jewish Society"; *Approaches to Judaism in Medieval Times* 2(1985): 1–35; idem, *Jewish Education and Society in the High Middle Ages* (Detroit, 1992), 33–41; Israel Ta-Shma, "Children in Medieval Germanic Jewry: A Perspective on Ariès from Jewish Sources"; *Studies in Medieval and Renaissance History* 12(1991): 263–81; William C. Jordan, "A travers le regard des enfants," *Provence Historique* 37(1987): 531–43.

53. In general, as Judith M. Bennett ("Medievalism and Feminism," in *Studying Medieval Women. Sex, Gender and Feminism*, ed. Nancy Partner (Cambridge, Mass., 1991, 7–29) has argued, gender studies reached the area of medieval studies rather late. In the case of medieval Jewish studies, gender perspectives were made part of research even later.

54. Ephraim E. Urbach, *The Tosaphists: Their History, Writings and Methods*; (Jerusalem, 1980[4] [in Hebrew]; Grossman, *Sages of Ashkenaz*; Idem, *Sages of France*; Robert Bonfil, *Rabbis and Jewish Communities in Renaissance Italy*; trans. Jonathan Chipman (London-Washington, 1993); Yedidya Alter Dinari, *The Rabbis of Germany and Austria at the Close of the Middle Ages: Their Conceptions and Halacha-Writings* (Jerusalem, 1984) [in Hebrew]; Israel Jacob Yuval, *Scholars in Their Time: The Religious Leadership of German Jewry in the Late Middle Ages* (Jerusalem, 1988) [in Hebrew].

55. One of the early and most important studies was that of Jacob Katz, *Exclusiveness and Tolerance: Studies in Jewish-Gentile Relations in Medieval and Modern Times* (London, 1961); and more recently: Gavin I. Langmuir, *History, Religion and Antisemitism* (Berkeley, 1990).

56. This assumption stands out in much of the literature that examines the lives of the Rabbis. For example: Grossman, *Sages of Ashkenaz*, 23: "The sources for the history of the early Ashkenazic sages are mainly internal." Urbach, *The Tosaphists*, 20, notes the contacts between Torah scholars and local Christian scholars but warns his readers: "One should not forget the intimate connection of the Tosafists to the world of Talmud and halakha." In contrast, others have pointed to the necessity of examining Ashkenazic Jewry in its broader cultural context: Marcus, *Rituals of Childhood*; Jeremy Cohen, *"Be Fertile and Increase: Fill the Earth and Master It": The Ancient and Medieval Career of a Biblical Text* (Ithaca and London, 1989); Eleazar Tuitto, "Shitato haParshanit shel Rashbam al Reka haMeẓut haHistorit shel Zemano," in *Studies in Rabbinic Literature, Bible and Jewish History*, ed. Yizḥak D. Gilat, Chaim Levine and Ẓvi Meir Rabinowitz (Ramat Gan, 1982), 48–74 [in Hebrew].

57. For example: Yom Tov Assis, *The Golden Age of Aragonese Jewry* (London-Portland Or., 1997), in his introduction, begins with the "profound impact that Gentile society made on the Jews," 1; David Nirenberg, *Communities of Violence: Persecution of Minorities in the Middle Ages* (Princeton, 1996), 8–9.

58. For example: Grossman, *Sages of Ashkenaz*, by index; Urbach, *The Tosaphists*, by index.

59. The contrast of these two approaches can be seen in the works of Yuval, *Two Nations*, and Elḥanan Reiner, "From Joshua to Jesus: The Transformation of a Biblical Story to a Local Myth:

A Chapter in the Religious History of The Galilean Jews," in *Sharing the Sacred. Religious Contacts and Conflicts in the Holy Land, First to Fifteenth Centuries CE*, eds. Arieh Kofsky and Guy Stroumsa (Jerusalem, 1998), 223–71.

60. Grossman has published a number of studies over the years and they have recently been synthesized in his *Pious and Rebellious*. Grossman is not the first to examine these topics. Many studies concerning marriage have been written over the past decades: Abraham Ḥaim Freimann, *Seder Kiddushin veNissuin Aharei Ḥatimat haTalmud. Meḥkar Histori Dogmati beDinei Yisrael*; (Jerusalem, 1945); Ze'ev Falk, *Jewish Matrimonial Law in the Middle Ages* (Oxford, 1966); Cohen and Horowitz, "In Search of the Sacred," 225–50; Roni Weinstein, *Jewish Marriage in Italy during the Early Modern Era: A Chapter in Social History and History of Mentality*. Ph.D. Diss., Hebrew University (Jerusalem, 1995) [in Hebrew].

61. Joshua Trachtenberg, *The Devil and the Jews: The Medieval Conception of the Jew and Its Relation to Modern Antisemitism* (New Haven, 1943) and more recently: Miri Rubin, *Gentile Tales: The Narrative Assault on Late Medieval Jews* (New Haven, 1999).

62. Different scholars have discussed these modes of living together that existed in the Middle Ages: Alfred Haverkamp, "'Concivilitas' von Christen und Juden in Aschkenas im Mittelalter," in *Judische Gemeinden und Organisationsformen von der Antike bis zur Gegenwart*, eds. Robert Jütte und Abraham P. Kustermann (Vienna-Köln and Weiman, 1996), 103–36; Nirenberg, *Communities of Violence*, 8–10.

63. Bonfil, *Tra due mondi*, 4–9.

64. Shlomo Dov Goitein, *A Mediterranean Society: The Jewish Communities of the Arab World As Portrayed in the Documents of the Cairo Geniza*; 6 vols. (Berkeley, Los Angeles, and London, 1967–1983); Joseph Shatzmiller, *Recherches sur la communauté juive de Manosque au Moyen Age, 1241–1329* (Paris, 1973); Assis, *The Golden Age of Aragonese Jewry*; Bonfil, *Jewish Life in Renaissance Italy*.

65. Louise A. Tilly, "Women's History and Family History: A Fruitful Collaboration or Missed Connection."

66. Supra. n. 51.

67. Kanarfogel, *Jewish Education and Society*, 39–51.

68. Goldin, "Die Beziehung der jüdischen Familie," 230–31. This idea is expanded in his monograph: *Uniqueness and Togetherness: The Enigma of the Survival of the Jews in the Middle Ages* (Tel Aviv, 1997), 42–66 [in Hebrew].

69. Ta-Shma, "Children in Medieval Germanic Jewry," 264–66: "We can safely accept the basic assumption as to the substantially different treatment accorded small children in Jewish and gentile families" (p. 266).

70. Abrahams, *Jewish Life*, 113, 127, 131, 137, 140, 156.

71. For a partial list of such publications in recent years, supra. n. 52.

72. For example: Baskin, "Problem of Women"; Eadem, "Male Piety, Female Bodies: Men, Women and Ritual Immersion in Medieval Ashkenaz," (forthcoming); Eadem, "Reading Women into the Sources: Reassessing Jewish Women in Medieval Ashkenaz," (forthcoming). I thank the author for allowing me to read her articles prior to their publication.

73. Martin King Whyte, *The Status of Women in Preindustrial Societies* (Princeton, 1978).

74. There are many examples of such comparison. One such was recently discussed by Maria Diemling, *"Christliche Ethnographien" über Juden und Judentum in der Frühen Neuzeit: Die Konvertiten Victor von Carben und Anthonius Margaritha und ihre Darstellung jüdischen Lebens und jüdischer Religion*, Dissertation zur Erlangung des Doktorgrades der Philosophie eingericht an der Geisteswissenschaftlichen Fakultät der Universität Wien (Vienna, 1999), 168–69.

75. This is true for any discussion that relates past and present: Judith M. Bennett, "Medieval Women, Modern Women: Across the Great Divide," in *Culture and History 1350–1600. Essays on English Communities, Identities and Writing*, ed. David Aers, (Detroit, 1992), 147–75.

76. Catherine Bell, *Ritual Theory, Ritual Practice* (New York, 1992), 171–81; Pierre Bourdieu,

"Rites As Acts of Institution," *Honor and Grace in Anthropology*, eds. John G. Peristiany and Julian Pitt-Rivers (Cambridge, 1992), 81–88.

77. For example: Natalie Z. Davis, "The Reasons of Misrule," in *Society and Culture in Early Modern France* (Stanford, 1975), 97–123; Robert Darnton, "A Bourgeois Puts His World in Order: The City As a Text," in *The Great Cat Massacre and other Episodes in French Cultural History* (New York, 1985), 116–24; Susan C. Karant-Nunn, *A Reformation of Ritual: An Interpretation of Early Modern Germany* (London and New York, 1997); Edward Muir, *Ritual in Early Modern Europe* (Cambridge and New York, 1997).

78. Marcus, *Rituals of Childhood*; Weinstein, *Jewish Marriage*; Lawrence A. Hoffman, *Covenant of Blood: Circumcision and Gender in Rabbinic Judaism* (Chicago and London, 1997); Nissan Rubin, *The Beginning of Life: Rites of Birth, Circumcision and Redemption of the Firstborn in the Talmud and Midrash* (Tel Aviv, 1995) [in Hebrew]. For a general overview: Harvey E. Goldberg, "Coming of Ages of Jewish Studies, or Anthropology Is Counted in the Minyan," *Jewish Social Studies* n.s. 4(1997): 29–63.

79. Marcus, *Rituals of Childhood*.

80. For example: Hoffman's analysis of the circumcision ceremony is not historical. Rather he discusses the circumcision ritual as an anthropologist, often ignoring historical developments pertaining to the ritual. See: Nissan Rubin, "Review of L. A. Hoffman, *Covenant of Blood: Circumcision and Gender in Rabbinic Judaism*," *Zion* 63(1998): 225–30, esp. 230.

81. For a summary of these approaches, see: Ivan G. Marcus, *The Religious and Social Ideas of the Jewish Pietists in Medieval Germany: Collected Essays* (Jerusalem, 1986), 11–24 [in Hebrew].

82. This approach has been adopted by others who have studied family life, for example: Grossman, *Pious and Rebellious*. Grossman does not discuss this issue in his book, however his broad use of sources from *Sefer Ḥasidim* throughout the book, illustrates the approach I am describing.

83. For example: David Herlihy and Christiane Klapisch-Zuber, *Tuscans and Their Families: A Study of the Florentine Catasto of 1427* (New Haven, 1985).

84. For example: Caroline Walker Bynum, *Holy Feast and Holy Fast: The Religious Significance of Food to Medieval Women* (Berkeley, 1987); Barbara Newman, *From Virile Woman to WomanChrist: Studies in Medieval Religion and Literature* (Philadelphia, 1995).

85. For example: R. Eleazar b. Judah, *Sefer Rokeaḥ haGadol* (Jerusalem, 1960), no. 296.

86. Men, women, and children frequented the synagogue. Evidence concerning women's attendance has not yet been studied systematically. See: Löw, *Der Synagogale Ritus* (Krotoschin, 1884), ch. 5; *SHP*, no. 464–65, no. 468. Medieval Jews contributed large amounts of money to beautify their synagogues: Richard Krautheimer, *Batei Knesset beYemei haBenayim*, trans. Amos Goren (Jerusalem, 1994), 47–56; Sigmund Salfeld, *Martyrologium des Nürnberger Memorbuches* (Berlin, 1898), 87–94. The fact that many medieval synagogues were turned into churches after the Jews were expelled from their cities is evidence of their splendor. See Mary Minty, "'Judengasse' into Christian Quarter: The Phenomenon of the Converted Synagogue in the Late Medieval and Early Modern Holy Roman Empire," in *Popular Religion in Germany and Central Europe 1400–1800*, eds. Bob Scribner and Trevor Johnson (Basingstoke, 1996), 58–86.

87. Supra., n. 23.

88. Pinthus was interested in understanding the changes in the relationship between the Jewish quarter and other parts of the city, and only a very small part of his book (43–47) deals with the living conditions of families. Alexander Pinthus, *Die Judensiedlungen*, 13–47. Recently Markus Wenninger has taken up some of these issues: "Zur Topographie der Judenviertel," 81–117.

89. For comparative work regarding Christian society: Jack Goody, *Production and Reproduction: A Comparative Study of the Domestic Domain* (Cambridge, 1976); Michael Mitterauer, *Historisch-Anthropologische Familienforschung. Fragestellungen und Zugangsweisen* (Vienna, 1990), 26–31, 35–37, 87–100; Pierre Toubert, "The Carolingian Moment," 383–88.

90. Martha Howell, *The Marriage Exchange: Property, Social Place and Gender in Cities of the*

Low Countries, 1300–1550 (Chicago and London, 1998), 98–100; Henri Bresc, "Europe: Town and Country," in *History of the Family*, eds. André Burguière, Christiane Klapisch-Zuber, Martine Segalen, and Françoise Zonabend (Cambridge, Mass., 1996), 461–66. Bresc's comparison of Jewish and Christian societies is problematic because he compares Geniza society in Egypt and medieval European cities.

91. Grossman, *Pious and Rebellious*, 63–87; idem, "Background to Family Ordinances—R. Gershom Me'or haGolah," in *Jewish History. Essays in Honor of Chimen Abramsky*, eds. Ada Rappaport-Albert and Steven J. Zipperstein (London, 1988), 3–23; Zeev Falk, *Jewish Matrimonial Law*, 86–112.

92. Grossman discusses the importance of lineage at length in his *Sages of Ashkenaz*, 400–411, but he only hints at family sizes, 8, n. 32.

93. Kenneth R. Stow, "The Jewish Family in the Rhineland in the High Middle Ages: Form and Function." *American Historical Review* 92(1987): 1085–1090.

94. There is a need for further research concerning these networks. Irving A. Agus, *Urban Civilization in Pre-Crusade Europe: A Study of Organized Town-Life in Northwestern Europe during the Tenth and Eleventh Centuries based on the Responsa Literature* (New York, 1965), 256–309; idem, *The Heroic Age of Franco-German Jewry* (New York, 1969), 101–44 is one of the few scholars to discuss these issues to date.

95. Grossman, *Sages of Ashkenaz*, 400–412.

96. A comparison with the data Goitein collected about Jewish society in medieval Fustat reveals that although families often lived in shared courtyards, each conjugal unit was independent financially: Goitein, *A Mediterranean Society* (Berkeley, 1978), 2:188; 3;130; 231; 291.

Notes to Chapter 1

1. A Mishnaic term for a miscarriage. For example: Niddah, 3:4.

2. For example, the summary of previous research in Cohen, *"Be Fertile."* Cohen surveys the intellectual history of the biblical commandment "Be fruitful and multiply," but does not examine its social contexts. For further discussion of Cohen's book, see p. 25.

3. Ibid., and Ron Barkai, *A History of Jewish Gynecological Texts in the Middle Ages* (Leiden, Boston, and Köln, 1998) have described at length the place of birth in intellectual traditions. Although much has been written on the social aspects of birth in Christian society, nothing has been written on these aspects in medieval Jewish society.

4. I am borrowing this formulation from Gail McMurray Gibson, "Scene and Obscene: Seeing and Performing Late Medieval Childbirth," *Journal of Medieval and Early Modern Studies* 29(1999): 7–24, esp. 9–11.

5. Sherry Ortner, "Is Female to Male Like Nature Is to Culture?" in *Making Gender* (Princeton, 1996), 21–42; Helen Callaway, "The Most Essentially Female Function of All: Giving Birth," in *Defining Females. The Nature of Women in Society*, ed. Shirley Ardener (Oxford and Providence, 1993), 146–67.

6. Shaḥar, *The Fourth Estate*, 98–106. Silvana Vecchio, "The Good Wife," in *A History of Women in the West*, ed. Christiane Klapisch-Zuber (London and Cambridge, Mass., 1992), 2:106–107; Berkvam, *Enfance et maternité*, 77. Although men also became fathers and were expected to marry, they were primarily educated to study Torah and acquire a profession. We should note the difference between being educated to be a wife and being educated to be a mother. The extent to which the distinctions discerned by Vecchio apply to contemporaneous Jewish culture have only recently been examined. See Grossman, *Pious and Rebellious*, 216–29.

7. MS Oxford Bodl., Opp. 170, (1205), fol. 104 b–c. This manuscript contains a commentary on *piyutim* mentioning many thirteenth-century scholars from northern France.

8. Ibid., fol. 105 c–d. For the *piyut*, see: *Maḥzor le-Vamim nora'im*, ed. Daniel Goldschmidt

(Jerusalem, 1970), Rosh haShana, 69–71. For this *piyut*, see Davidson, *Thesaurus of Medieval Hebrew Poetry*, (New York, 1970), 1: 314.

9. I deviate from the JPS translation, "Sarah's lifetime [sing.]," as his comment is based on the plural form of the Hebrew.

10. Judah b. Samuel Ḥasid, *Perushei haTorah leRabbi Yehuda heḤasid*, ed. Isaac Samson Lange (Jerusalem, 1973), 28, *Ḥayei Sarah*, 23:1.

11. BT Nedarim 64a.

12. *SHP*, nos. 367, 1170.

13. *SHP*, no. 1155.

14. For example: Jacob Katz, "Marriage and Sexual Life among the Jews at the Close of the Middle Ages," *Zion* 10(1945): 22–23, 40 [in Hebrew].

15. Cohen and Horowitz, "In Search of the Sacred," 225–50; Stow, "The Jewish Family," 1103–1104.

16. In a broader context, we should note that differences of opinion with respect to procreation were common in polemics between different religious groups. In antiquity, a variety of groups besides Christians and their opponents, argued for celibacy or procreation — David Herlihy, *Medieval Households* (Cambridge, Mass., and London, 1985), 23–26.

17. The process for women is described in detail in Jane Tibbets Schulenburg, *Forgetful of Their Sex: Female Sanctity and Society, ca. 500–1100* (Chicago, 1998), 127–75. See also: John A. Nichols and Lillian Thomas Shanks, *Distant Echoes: Medieval Religious Women* (Kalamazoo, Mich., 1984); Penelope Johnson, *Equal in Monastic Profession: Religious Women in Medieval France* (Chicago and London, 1991), 133–65, 229–47. Kirsten Hastrup discusses these ideas outside the medieval context in her article: "The Semantics of Biology: Virginity," in *Defining Females. The Nature of Women in Society*, ed. Shirley Ardener (Oxford and Providence, 1993), 34–50, and esp. 40–44. Even when women lived as celibate virgins, the expectations of them were different from those of men. See Barbara Newman, "Hildegard and Her Hagiographers: The Remaking of Female Sainthood," in *Gendered Voices*, ed. Catherine Mooney (Philadelphia, 1999), 16–34.

18. Caroline W. Bynum, "And Woman His Humanity: Female Imagery in the Religious Writing of the Later Middle Ages," in *Fragmentation and Redemption: Essays on Gender and the Human Body in Medieval Religion* (New York, 1991), 151–79; Atkinson, *The Oldest Vocation*, 64–100.

19. Cohen, "*Be Fertile*"; 231.

20. For example, according to R. Eleazar b. Judah, *Sefer Rokeaḥ*, no. 353, wheat was thrown on the bride and groom, and they were told "be fertile and multiply."

21. Dyan Elliot, *Spiritual Marriage: Sexual Abstinence in Medieval Wedlock* (Princeton, 1993), 137–38; Jean Gaudemet, *Le mariage en Occident* (Paris, 1987), 181–88; Christopher Brooke, *The Medieval Idea of Marriage* (Oxford, 1989), 273–80.

22. Ton Brandenberg, "Saint Anne: A Holy Grandmother and Her Children," in *Sanctity and Motherhood. Essays on Holy Mothers in the Middle Ages*, ed. Anneke B. Mulder-Bakker (New York-London, 1995), 31–65; Kathleen Ashley and Pamela Sheingorn (eds.), *Interpreting Cultural Symbols. Saint Anne in Late Medieval Society* (Athens, Ga., 1990).

23. It should be noted that these conclusions do not shed light on attitudes toward family or children in the Early Middle Ages in Jewish or Christian society. These issues warrant a separate study.

24. Jeremy Cohen, "Conjugal Sex in RaABaD," *Jewish History* 6 (1992): 65–78, esp. 71–74.

25. Dalia Ḥoshen, *The Fire Symbol in Talmuddic-Aggadic Exegesis*, Diss. submitted for Ph.D. Phil. (Bar Ilan University, 1989), 132–57, and esp. 142–45 [in Hebrew]; Eadem, "Sexual Relations between Husband and Wife," *S'vara* 3 (1993): 39–45 [in Hebrew].

26. MS Oxford Bodl. Mich. 84 (784), fol. 148b. This story does not appear in the printed editions of *Sefer Ḥasidim*.

27. *SHP*, no. 984, 989. This attitude has been emphasized in the work of Baskin, "Problem of Women," 1–18.

28. This was suggested many years ago by Yitzhak Baer in his article: "The Religious-Social Ten-

dency of *Sepher Hasidim*," *Zion* 3(1938): 1–50 [in Hebrew], but subsequently rejected. Recently, Talya Fishman has revived this idea: "The Penitential System of Ḥasidei Ashkenaz and the Problem of Cultural Boundaries," *Journal of Jewish Thought and Philosophy* 8 (1999): 201–30.

29. David Berger, *The Jewish-Christian Debate in the High Middle Ages* (Philadelphia, 1979), section 205, 209. Comments on the same topic also appear in sections 42, 69–70.

30. Ibid., 70; Bernhard Blumenkranz, *Les auteurs chrétiens latin du moyen âge sur les juifs et la judäisme* (*Etudes juives*, 4), (Paris, 1963), 98.

31. Sylvie Laurent, *Nâitre au moyen âge: De la Conception à la naissance, la grossesse et l'accouchement XIIe–Xve siècle* (Paris, 1989); Jacques Gélis, *L'Arbre et le fruit: La naissance dans l'occident moderne* (Paris, 1984).

32. Rashi, Eruvin 27a, s.v. *"P'riyah ureviyah"*; Rashi, Kiddushin 34a, s.v. *"UP'riyah ureviyah."*

33. For example in connection with *tefillin* (phylacteries), women are excluded from performing this *mitzva* because of requirements of *guf naki* — a clean body. See R. Samson b. Zadok, *Sefer haTashbez* (Warsaw, 1901), no. 270.

34. John W. Baldwin, *The Language of Sex: Five Voices from Northern France around 1200* (Chicago and London, 1994), 206–10.

35. For example: Catherine M. Mooney, "Claire of Assisi and Her Interpreters," in *Gendered Voices*, 69–70.

36. This idea comes across in the word used in *Midrash Yezirat haValad Ozar Midrashion*, ed. Judah David Eisenstein (New York, 1915), 1: 244, where the woman's body is referred to as a *k'li*, or receptacle.

37. Ron Barkai, "Greek Medical Traditions and Their Impact on Conceptions of Women in the Gynaecological Writings in the Middle Ages," *A View into the Lives of Women in Jewish Societies. Collected Essays*, ed. Yael Azmon (Jerusalem, 1995), 124–26 [in Hebrew]; Joan Cadden, *Meanings of Sex Difference in the Middle Ages: Medicine, Science and Culture* (Cambridge, 1991).

38. This is outlined in the versions of *Midrash Yezirat haValad*, 1:244–45.

39. *SHP*, no. 1188, and see a fuller discussion of this source (ch. 4, n. 14).

40. These laws appear in Tractate *S'machot* (7:15) and are repeated throughout the Middle Ages. See for example: *Sefer Or Zaru'a*, Hilkhot Evel (Laws of Mourning), no. 448.

41. In some cases, special magical chants and prayers were said to help ensure the birth of a son, especially in cases where a man had already fathered several daughters. Some of these formulas appear in MS Oxford Bodl., Mich. 9, (1531), fols. 175a–186a.

42. For example: Rashi, Shabbat, s.v. *"Ga'aguin — bremors* . . . and this cure does not pertain to females since the father does not love them as much from the start." For this preference in Christian society, see Gélis, *L'arbre*, 163.

43. In an excerpt from a thirteenth-century commentary on Genesis from northern France, the author writes: "And she was named Dinah": It is not explained why she was named thus, for it is not necessary to explain except in the case of males, for they are the *ikar* — the core (cf. MS Vatican 123, fol. 8b); *Sefer Tosafot haShalem*, Gen. 30: 21, no. 10 "and named her Dinah": One does not give thanks for the birth of a daughter like for a son."

44. Gélis, *L'arbre*, 160–64.

45. On child brides: Grossman, *Pious and Rebellious*, 63–87. Some girls were sexually active even before reaching sexual maturity. For example: *SHP*, no. 1155; MS Paris héb. 1120, fol. 66b, discusses difficulties during birth. One of the difficulties mentioned is: "And if for internal reasons, the girl conceives before she brought signs [of sexual maturity] and her straits are narrow." For the history of this text, see: Ron Barkai, "A Medieval Treatise on Obstetrics," *Medical History* 33(1988): 96–119. This passage describes the difficulties of young girls giving birth. Another fifteenth-century source voices concern over girls sexually active from a young age and recommends that doctors instruct these girls on how to prevent conception. See MS Paris héb. 1122, 46a, on pregnancy and birth control: "And you should know that the doctor must give these medicines to a woman so that she does not conceive when she is young and has not yet reached her time." It seems

that fourteen was considered the age at which women commonly gave birth. See *Sefer Tosafot haShalem*, Gen. 25:26, no. 9. Eleven was seen as the age at which girls were deemed able to give birth: Rashi, Ketubbot 39a, s.v. *"Pahot mikan"* and s.v. *"Veyeter al ken."*

46. Karen E. Paige and Jeffrey M. Paige, *The Politics of Reproductive Ritual* (Berkeley, Los Angeles, and London, 1981); Whyte, *The Status of Women*, 53–54, 80.

47. This idea comes across in the medieval marriage and inheritance laws as well. Israel J. Yuval, "HaHesderim haKaspiyim shel haNissuin beAshkenaz beYemei haBenayim," in *Religion and Economy: Connections and Interactions. Collected Essays*, ed. Menahem Ben Sasson (Jerusalem, 1995), 191–207, esp. 193–96, 199–205.

48. Vern Bullough noted this paradox in his path-breaking article written almost thirty years ago: "Medieval Medical and Scientific Views of Women," *Viator* 4(1973): 497.

49. See pp. 35–36.

50. Jacqueline Murray, "On the Origins and the Role of 'Wise Women' in Cases for Annulment on the Grounds of Male Impotence," *Journal of Medieval History* 16(1990): 241–45. For an illustration of these examinations, see: Laurent, *Nâitre au moyen âge*, illustration 16. For an example in the Jewish sources: *Sefer Or Zaru'a*, 1: no. 652.

51. *SHP*, no. 380.

52. See, for example, in the *Sefer Assaf*, published by Zusman Muntner, *Korot* 5(1970): 58, no. 682.

53. Supra, n. 50.

54. It is not clear who would have performed the examination. *Sefer Or Zaru'a*, 1: no. 653.

55. For examples of women bewitching in cases of fertility as well as in other cases, see Joseph Dan, "Sippurim demonologim mi-kitvei R. Judah he-Hasid," in *The Religious and Social Ideas of the Jewish Pietists in Medieval Germany*, ed. Ivan G. Marcus (Jerusalem, 1987), 288, no. 29 [in Hebrew]. Witches are often called by their German name, *"streya,"* for example *SHP*, no. 1465–67, as well as Dan, ibid., 278, no. 2; 280, no. 5.

56. Lett, *L'Enfant des miracles*, 242–44.

57. See, for example, R. Gershom Me'or HaGolah's discussion of a woman who does not menstruate but shows no exterior signs of physical difference. R. Gershom b. Judah, *Teshuvot Ragmah*, ed. Shlomo Eidelberg (New York, 1956), no. 84, and parallel source: Mordekhai, *Yevamot*, no. 113.

58. MS Oxford Bodl., Opp. Add. 14 (1101), fol. 187a–b. This experiment was omitted from the printed version of the *Lekah Tov*.

59. Laurent, *Nâitre au moyen âge*, 48. The *Trotula* texts have been thoroughly examined over the past years by Monica Green. See her articles "The Development of the *Trotula*," *Revue d'histoire des textes* 16(1996): 119–203; and "A Handlist of Latin and Vernacular Manuscripts of the So-called *Trotula* Texts." *Scriptorum* 50(1996): 137–75; 51(1997): 81–103. See Green's translation of the text: *The Trotula: An English Translation of the Medieval Compendium of Women's Medicine* (Philadelphia, 2002).

60. These cures appear in a manuscript of the book *Sefer Zori haGuf* by Nathan b. Joel Falquera, MS Paris héb. 1122, fol. 4b, 45a. On the author, see David Margalith, "Falquera, Nathan b. Joel," *EJ* 6: 1140, and the passing references to him in Barkai, *Jewish Gynecological Texts*, 88; Joseph Shatzmiller, *Jews, Medicine and Medieval Society*, 53–54.

61. For example: "Sefer Assaf"; *Korot* 4(1968): 531 no. 325.

62. James Brundage, *Law, Sex and Christian Society in Medieval Europe* (Chicago-London, 1987), 39, 115, 143–45.

63. Murray, "Role of Wise Women," 235–50.

64. These statutes are documented in Louis Finkelstein, *Jewish Self-Government in the Middle Ages* (New York, 1964), 20–30, 139–47. For the different opinions on the dating of the manuscripts and evidence, see: Grossman, *Pious and Rebellious*, 122–33. Recently, this topic has been discussed by Elimelech Westreich, *Transitions in the Legal Status of the Wife in Jewish Law* (Jerusalem, 2002), 62–96 [in Hebrew].

65. It should be noted that this is a unique Ashkenazi approach. In Spain, during the Middle Ages, polygamy was allowed. Grossman, ibid.; Yom Tov Assis, "The 'Ordinance of Rabbeni Gershom' and Polygamous Marriages in Spain," *Zion* 46:(1981), 251–77.

66. Elimelech Westreich, "Polygamy and Compulsory Divorce of the Wife in the Decisions of the Rabbis of Ashkenaz in the Eleventh and Twelfth Centuries," *Bar Ilan Law Studies* 6(1988): 118–64, esp. 143–63 [in Hebrew].

67. BT Ketubbot 64a; BT Yevamot 65a.

68. BT Yevamot 65a.

69. R. Solomon b. Isaac, *Responsa Rashi*, ed. Israel Elfenbein (New York, 1943), no. 207.

70. Grossman, *Pious and Rebellious*, 415–23.

71. Nedarim 11: 12; BT Nedarim 91a–b.

72. *Sefer Or Zaru'a*, 1: no. 653; *Teshuvot Maimoniyot*, no. 6. On this response, see Urbach, *The Tosaphists*, 1:262–63.

73. Avraham Grossman, "The Origins and Essence of the Custom of "Stopping the Service," *Milet* 1(1983): 199–219 [in Hebrew].

74. *Sefer Or Zaru'a*, 1: no. 652.

75. Grossman, *Pious and Rebellious*, 415–23. For a different approach to this responsum, see: Ephraim Shoham-Steiner, *Social Attitudes Towards Marginal Individuals in Medieval European Society*, Ph.D. Diss., Hebrew University (Jerusalem, 2002), 299–302 [in Hebrew].

76. R. Meir b. Barukh, *Shut Maharam* (Prague), no. 947.

77. Mordekhai, *Yevamot*, no. 113.

78. Grossman's book, *Pious and Rebellious*, 415–24, discusses infertility. Although Grossman discussed many of the same sources examined in this chapter, his interpretation differs from that offered here because of the geographic provenance of his sources and the general thrust of his argument. While I agree with Grossman that claims of impotence became one of the channels for women demanding divorce, especially after other options were no longer accessible because of the growing restriction legal authorities put on such claims, I do not read these sources as evidence of the strength of women's position in society. The question of what divorce records may teach us about the place of women in society requires a broader theoretical and empirical basis. For example, does a higher frequency of divorce indicate stronger or weaker male status?

79. Ortner, *Making Gender*, 38.

80. Zeev W. Falk, *Marriage and Divorce: Reforms in the Family Law of German-French Jewry* (Jerusalem, 1961), 20–25 [in Hebrew], discusses the possibility of Christian influence on the Jewish rabbis. For Regino of Prum, see J. Laudage, "Regino," *LdM* 7: 579–80. For Burchard of Worms and his decrees, see: Brundage, *Law, Sex and Christian Society*, 172, 200–203; Laurent, *Naître au moyen âge*, 13–14.

81. R. Solomon b. Isaac, *Responsa Rashi*, no. 207.

82. Grossman cites many sources from Spain in discussing this issue. See *Pious and Rebellious*, 422–24.

83. MS Parma Palatina 2757, fol. 73a, no. 263.

84. Mc Murray Gibson, "Scene and Obscene."

85. For recent literature on birth in medieval and early modern society, see Ya'ara Bar-On, *The Crowded Delivery Room: Gender and Public Opinion in Early Modern Gynecology* (Haifa, 2000) [in Hebrew]; Hilary Marland (ed.), *The Art of Midwifery: Early Modern Midwives in Europe* (London-New York, 1993); Michel Salvat, "L'accouchement dans la littérature scientifique médiévale," *L'enfant au moyen âge. Littérature et civilisation* 9(1980): 87–106.

86. This literature is listed and reviewed extensively in chapter 3.

87. Barkai, *Jewish Gynecological Texts*; idem, *Les infortunes de Dinah: Le livre de la generation, la gynecologie juive au moyen âge* (Paris, 1991).

88. Amanda Carson Banks, *Birthchairs, Midwives and Medicine* (Jackson, MS, 1999), 1–32.

89. For example, in *SHP*, nos. 1046–1047.

90. MS Oxford, Bodl., Opp. 170 (1205), fol. 131b–c.

91. David Herlihy and Christiane Klapisch-Zuber (*Tuscans and Their Families*), have estimated that approximately one fifth of all women there died in childbirth.

92. According to Jewish law, when one bakes bread, a small portion of the dough must be set aside and burned.

93. Shabbat 2:6.

94. *Midrash Tanḥuma*, trans. into English with Introduction, Indices and Brief Notes (S. Buber recension), by John T. Townsend (Hoboken, N.J., 1989), Gen. Parasha II: 31–32.

95. *SHP*, no. 1046.

96. MS Cambridge Add. 3127, fol. 32b: "To bless a woman: 'He who blessed Sarah, Rebecca, and Rachel and Hannah.' And if he bless a woman about to give birth, he shall say: 'Sarah, Rebecca, Rachel and the greatest of righteous women; He who cured the King of Judah from his illness and the prophetess Miriam from her leprosy; He who sweetened the Waters of Marah through Moses and who cured the waters of Jericho through Elisha, may He bless and cure *Marat Ploni* daughter of *Ploni* in recompense for what *ploni* or *plonit* has vowed to give in charity. May the Omnipresent send her His good word and heal her and grant life to her offspring.' And if he blesses a woman, he should say, 'And bring her labor pangs to a successful end and lengthen her days and years and send her a speedy recovery in body and flesh and in all of her limbs, along with all the sick of Israel, quickly and in good time, amen.' " This manuscript is also from the late fourteenth century (1399).

97. The biblical text does, however, distinguish between pain and death. Eve's curse only included pain: Newman, *From Virile Woman to WomanChrist*, 82.

98. BT Sotah 12a.

99. Ulrike Rublack, "Pregnancy, Childbirth and the Female Body in Early Modern Germany," *Past and Present* 150(1996): 90–93.

100. See for example: Elisheva Baumgarten, "'Thus Sayeth the Wise Midwives': Midwives and Midwifery in Thirteenth-Century Germany," *Zion* (60)2000: 68; Weissler, *Voices of the Matriarchs: Listening to the Prayers of Early Modern Jewish Women* (Boston, 1998), 66–75.

101. This Midrash appears in a number of printed and manuscript sources: *Midrash Tanḥuma*, ed. Shlomo Buber (New York, 1946); P'kudei, 3:131–33; *Ozar Midrashim*, 1: 243–45 and in manuscript: MS Parma 563/40, fols. 136b–138a; Ms Oxford Bodl., Heb. d. 11 (2797/2), fols. 11a–14a; MS Vatican ebr. 44/11, fols. 323a–24b; Darmstadt, 25/11, fols. 28d–29b.

102. *Midrash Yezirat haValad*, 243–45.

103. I am intentionally using male pronouns in my translation, as the entire Midrash seems completely divorced from women.

104. For an outline of Aristotelian views, see: Cadden, *Meanings of Sex Difference*, supra, n. 37.

105. Lev. 12.

106. BT Berakhot 60a.

107. There was a belief that in exceptional, miraculous cases, the gender of the baby could be changed even after forty or eighty days. In their discussions of the birth of Dinah, the daughter of Jacob, some medieval commentators suggest that Dinah was actually supposed to have been a boy. She was changed into a girl because, had she been a boy, she would have become Leah's seventh son. Consequently, Rachel would have been deprived of her allotted number of sons (as Jacob had been allotted a total of twelve sons). Thus, Dinah was turned into a female after she had already been created as a male. *Sefer Tosafot haShalem*, Gen. 30:21, no. 3 (as well as MS Vatican ebr. 123, fol. 48b "and she bore a daughter."

108. The idea appears in BT Niddah 31a, and many commentators repeat it. For example, *Sefer Tosafot haShalem*, Gen. 29:16 no. 3; Rashi, Gen. 46:15, s.v. "these are the sons of Leah"; *Moshav Zekenim on the Torah*, ed. Shlomo David Sasson (London, 1959), Lev. 12:2; *SHP*, no. 509. This idea, originating in classical medical sources, was widely accepted in Christian society as well. See Michel Salvat, "L'accouchement"; Claude Thomasset, "Quelques principes de l'embryologie médiévale," *L'enfant au moyen âge. Littérature et civilisation* 9(1980): 107–21.

109. BT Shabbat 129a.

110. *SHP*, nos. 109, 264, 517, 565. Pious women would prepare hot water before the Sabbath

so as to avoid heating water on the Sabbath. Although this act was permitted when a woman was about to give birth, they preferred not to violate the Sabbath. *SHP*, no. 515 as well as R. Moses Parnas, *Sefer haParnas* (Vilna, 1895), nos. 283–84; R. Eleazar b. Judah, *Perush haRokeaḥ al ha-Torah* (New York, 1978), Yitro 20: 12.

111. *Sefer Tosafot haShalem*, Gen. 38:5, no. 5; 27, no. 2.

112. Rashi, Berakhot 3a, s.v. "*Shilya*," and see Arsène Darmsteter and David S. Blondheim, *Les Glosses françaises dans les commentaries talmudiques de Raschi* (Paris, 1926), 146 no. 1058.

113. For example, his commentary on Hos. 6:11; 13:13.

114. R. Isaac b. Nathan, *Perush Rivan leMassekhet Yevamot*, ed. Efraim Kupfer (Jerusalem 1977), 42a, 193.

115. Marianne Elsakkers, "In Pain You Shall Bear Children: Medieval Prayers for a Safe Delivery," in *Women and Miracle Stories. A Multidisciplinary Explanation*, ed. Anne Marie Korte (Leiden, Köln, and Boston, 2001), 179–210.

116. Rashi, Bava Kama 59a, s.v. "*Nekhi ḥaya*." Compare: Ann Giardina Hess, "Midwifery Practice among the Quakers in Southern Rural England in the Late Seventeenth Century," in *The Art of Midwifery. Early Modern Midwives in Europe*, ed. Hilary Marland (London and New York, 1993), 56–57.

117. Klaus Bergdolt, "Schwangerschaft und Geburt," *LdM*, 7: 1612–16.

118. Gerhard Baader, "Der Hebammenkatechismus des Muscio—ein Zeugnis frühmittelalterlichen Geburtshilfe," in *Frauen in Spätantike und Frühmittelalter*, ed. Werner Affeldt (Sigmaringen, 1990), 115.

119. R. Ḥayim b. Isaac, *Sefer She'elot uTeshuvot Maharaḥ Or Zaru'a*, no. 8 s.v. "*Yelamdenu al otah isha*"; *and see also* R. Joseph b. Moses, *Sefer Leket Yosher*, 2: 20, for another example of the wise women's expertise.

120. R. Asher b. Yeḥiel, *Shut haRosh*, no. 33.

121. Baumgarten, "Midwives," 73, and in R. Gershom *haGozer, Sefer Zikhron Brit*, ed. Jacob Glassberg (Berlin, 1892), 142. This supports the suggestion made by Monica Green almost a decade ago (Monica Green, "Women's Medical Practice and Health Care in Medieval Europe," *Signs* 14(1989): 434–73, esp. 438–46), in which she suggested that women served as medical practitioners of many different kinds and were not restricted to gynecology. Thus, the distinction sometimes made in modern literature between doctors and midwives is irrelevant. The women referred to as wise women in the Jewish texts should be included in any account of medical professionals.

122. See, for example, *SHP*, no. 68 where a midwife is listed as the only female professional not obliged to fast when a city is under siege.

123. Theodore Kwasman, "Die mittelalterlichen jüdischen Grabsteine in Rothenburg o.d. Tauber," in *Zur Geschichte der mittelalterlichen judischen Gemeinde in Rothenburg ob der Tauber; Rabbi Meir ben Baruch von Rothenburg zum Gedenken an seinen 700 Todestag*, ed. Hilde Merz (Rothenburg o.d. Tauber, 1993), tombstones nos. 40, 154. The practice of recording midwifery as a female profession on gravestones is known from antiquity. See, for example, Nancy Demand, *Birth, Death and Motherhood in Classical Greece* (Baltimore and London, 1994), 152.

124. She is mentioned in Salfeld, *Martyrologium*, 90.

125. Thus in the lists of the dead from Rothenburg in 1298 we hear of Marat Yuta haMeyaledet who was killed with her great grandson Avraham (ibid., 43). Marat Beila, the midwife of Würzburg, was killed in 1298 with her daughter and three of her great-grandchildren (ibid., 57). Marat Berla, the midwife of Winheim, was killed with her sons, daughters, and four of her grandchildren (ibid., 56). In a list from Nürnberg (1298) we hear of Marat Zarlieb haZekana (the old) haMeyaledet and Marat Miriam haMeyaledet (ibid., 36). In 1349 in Worms the midwife Marat Minna was killed with her son and his wife together with the midwife Marat Ogia who was killed with her daughter (ibid., 75–76).

126. Zvi Avineri, "Nürnberg"; *Germania Judaica* II 2: 598–604 as well as Moritz Stern, "Verze-

ichnis der Judenbürger zu Nürnberg, 1338," *Die Israelitische Bevölkerung der deutschen Städte* 3 (1893/4):9–14.

127. As they were widows, they were listed as individual taxpayers. There might well have been additional midwives in the community who were not widows and, consequently, were not listed.

128. This seems to be a general feature of midwives in the Christian sources.

129. The literature on this period has grown tremendously over the past years. See, for example: Merry E. Wiesner, *Working Women in Renaissance Germany* (New Brunswick, 1986), 55–73; Hess, "Midwifery Practice," 67.

130. Weisner, *Working Women*, 56–60.

131. One of the abilities often attributed to midwives in fifteenth- and sixteenth-century Europe is their literacy. However we do not know if medieval midwives, Jewish or Christian, could read. See Weisner, ibid., 55–73. Already in ancient times, doctors recommended that midwives know how to read. For example: *Souranus' Gynecology*, ed. Oswei Temkin (Baltimore, 1956), 5–7. The question of the literacy of Jewish women demands further investigation. See: Judith Baskin, "Some Parallels in the Education of Medieval Jewish and Christian Women; *Jewish History* 5(1991): 41–52 and more recently Grossman, *Pious and Rebellious*, 277–82, 293–99.

132. Vivian Nutton, "Medicine in Medieval Western Europe 1000–1500," in *The Western Medical Tradition 800 B.C. to A.D. 1800*, eds. Lawrence Conrad et al. (Cambridge, 1995), 153–59. He explains that some medieval medical treatises were purely theoretical with no base in experience.

133. Barkai has described these texts and translated some of them in his work, *Jewish Gynecological Texts*; n. 62.

134. This book was published by Zusman Muntner in several volumes of the journal *Korot*, 1966–71.

135. Joseph Shatzmiller, " 'Doctors and Medical Practices in Germany around the Year 1200': The Evidence of *Sefer Asaph*," *PAAJR* 50(1983): 149–64.

136. See, for example, *Korot* 3: 422, 532–5; 4: nos. 321–44, (pp.) 531–33; no. 1182, 618; nos. 1311–13, 644; 5: no. 650, 49; no. 696, 61; nos. 755, 166; nos. 914, 319; nos. 997, 444; nos. 1018, 447.

137. For example: MS Parma Palatina 2342, fol. 262b–286b; MS Oxford Bodl., Opp. Add. 14 (1101), fol. 187a–b; Ms Oxford Bodl., Mich 9, (1531), fol. 121b.

138. This manual was published at the end of the nineteenth century, supra n. 121. It was one part of a new genre of practical manuals produced in Ashkenaz from the thirteenth century onward. On this genre, see Israel Ta-Shma, "HaSifrut haHilkhatit haMikzo'it beAshkenaz," in *Ritual, Custom and Reality in Franco Germany, 1000–1350* (Jerusalem, 1996), 96.

139. For a different opinion on the dating of the chapter, see Grossman, *Pious and Rebellious*, 203, n. 61.

140. A detailed analysis of these issues can be found in Baumgarten, "Midwives."

141. Lyndal Roper, *Oedipus and the Devil: Witchcraft, Sexuality and Religion in Early Modern Europe* (London-New York, 1994), 199–225.

142. *SHP*, no. 380. It seems that it was the midwives who attended women using the mikve. Little is known about medieval mikves and this subject certainly requires further inquiry. For preliminary comments, see Shaye J. D. Cohen, "Purity, Piety and Polemic: Medieval Rabbinic Denunciation of 'Incorrect' Purification Practices," in *Women and Water: Menstruation in Jewish Life and Law*, ed. Rahel R. Wasserfall (Hanover N.H. and London, 1999), 82–100.

143. Rashi, Sotah 22b, s.v. *"Kegon Yoḥani bat Retavi."*

144. MS Oxford, Bodl. Opp. 540 (1567), published by Dan, "Sippurim Demonologim," 282 no. 13. Yoḥani bat Retavi is mentioned in other medieval sources as well: R. Nathan b. Yeḥiel, *Sefer Arukh haShalem*, ed. Alexander Kohut (Vienna, 1926), "Yoḥani," 4: 117–18; R. Nissim b. Jacob of Kirouan, *Ḥibbur haYafe min haYeshu'a*, trans. and introduction by Ḥaim Z. Hirshberg (Jerusalem, 1954), 35–36.

145. For example: Barbara Newman, *Sister of Wisdom: St. Hildegard's Theology of the Feminine* (Berkeley and Los Angeles, 1987), 144.
146. Baumgarten, "Midwives," 68.
147. Barkai, *Infortunes de Dinah*, 234.
148. For example: *SHP*, no. 1186, *SHB*, no. 172. This is also discussed in halakhic deliberations concerning the case of a woman who is hungry on Yom Kippur.
149. BT Shabbat 66b.
150. Michelle Klein, *A Time to Be Born: Customs and Folklore of Jewish Birth* (Philadelphia, 1998), 93.
151. Baumgarten, "Midwives," 70. Carol Rawcliffe, *Medicine and Society in Later Medieval England* (Gloucester, 1995), 194–97.
152. Hildegardis Bigiensis, *Liber subtilitateum diversarum naturam creaturarum*, eds. Charles Daremberg and F. A. Reuss, *PL* 197 (Paris, 1855), 1255 "De Sardio."
153. Avodah Zara, 2:2.
154. Shlomo Simonsohn, *The Apostolic See and the Jews* (Toronto, 1988), 1: no. 23 (Canterbury, before 1179); no. 56 (Provence, 1267); Solomon Grayzel, *The Church and the Jews in the Thirteenth Century* (New York, 1966), 1: 306 (Paris, 1213): "Statuimus . . . ne Christiane obstetrices intersint puerperio Judeorum."
155. See chapter 4, p. 136.
156. See chapter 4, p. 89 for a detailed list of the decrees regarding Christian wet nurses.
157. R. Elḥanan b. Isaac, *Tosfot al Massekhet Avodah Zara*, ed. David Fränkel (Husiatyn, 1901), 56 s.v. "*Aval lo beino leveinah*."
158. *Sefer Or Zaru'a*, 1: *Piskei Avodah Zarah*, nos. 146–47.
159. Joseph Shatzmiller, "Doctors and Medical Practices in Germany around the Year 1200: The Evidence of *Sefer Hasidim*," *Journal of Jewish Studies* 33(1982): 583–93.
160. R. Gershom, *Zikhron Brit*, 143.
161. Ibid.
162. Hess, "Midwifery Practice," 60.
163. Frederic C. Tubach, *Index Exemplorum* (Helsinki, 1969), 221, no. 2806; *Das Viaticum narrationem des Heunmannus Boniensis*, ed. A. Hilka (Berlin, 1935), 59, no. 39; Michel Tarayre, *La Vièrge et le miracle. Le 'Speculum historiale' de Vincent de Beauvais* (Paris, 1999), 91–94.
164. Charles Caspers, "Leviticus 12, Mary and Wax: Purification and Churching in Late Medieval Christianity," in *Purity and Holiness. The Heritage of Leviticus*, eds. M.J.H.M. Poorthuis and Joshua Schwartz (Leiden, Boston, and Köln, 2000), 307, n. 58; C.G.N. de Vooys, *Middelnederlandse Marialegenden* (Leiden, 1903), 1; 357–59.
165. Merry E. Wiesner, "The Midwives of South Germany and the Public/Private Dichotomy," *The Art of Midwifery. Early Modern Midwives in Europe*, ed. Hilary Marland (London and New York, 1993), 86–88.
166. *SHP*, nos. 1917–18.
167. Frederick M. Powicke and Christopher R. Cheney (eds.), *Councils and Synods with Other Documents Relating to the English Church* (Oxford, 1964), 2: 35.
168. *SHP*, no. 1352.
169. This practice is the subject of a rabbinic discussion. Since swaddling sometimes changed the shape of infants' bodies, questions arose as to the permissibility of swaddling on the Sabbath. Rashi and Rabbenu Tam hold differing opinions on the matter (Rashi, *Sotah* 12a, s.v., *Meshaper*). The infants remained swaddled for the first years of their lives. See Alexandre-Bidon and Closson, *L'enfant à l'ombre des cathèdrales*, 94–99.
170. As the Rashba stated: "Men do not birth women" (R. Solomon b. Aderet, *Teshuvot ha-Rashba* (Benei Berak, 1957), 2: no. 182).
171. Rashi, Bava Kama 59a, s.v. "Nekhi ḥaya."
172. Baumgarten, "Midwives," 74.

173. I assume this is based on what women desire in other traditional societies today, where the wish for sons is often predominant.
174. For example: *Sefer Tosafot haShalem*, Gen. 38:28, no. 5.
175. R. Gershom, *Zikhron Brit*, 139–40.

Notes to Chapter 2

Wolfram von Eschenbach, *Willelham*, ed. Albert Letzmann (Tübingen, 1961), 307, lines 23–24: "der juden touf hât sundersite: den begênt mit einem snite."

1. For a detailed description of reproductive rituals, see: Paige and Paige, *Reproductive Ritual*.
2. For a discussion of the importance of circumcision in antiquity, see: Sacha Stern, *Jewish Identity in Early Rabbinic Writings* (Leiden, 1995), 63–68.
3. Rubin, *Beginning of Life*. See also Lewis M. Barth (ed.), *Berit Mila in the Reform Context* (New York, 1990).
4. Hoffman, *Covenant of Blood*. Hoffman's analysis relies heavily on a book written over one hundred years ago that is still extremely relevant: Löw, *Lebensalter*, 81–92.
5. Paige and Paige, *Reproductive Ritual*, 4–14; John W. M. Whiting, "Adolescent Rituals and Identity Conflicts," in *Cultural Psychology*, eds. James W. Stigler, Richard A. Schweder, and Gilbert Herdt (Cambridge and New York, 1990), 357–65; Gilbert Herdt, "Sambia Nosebleeding Rites and Male Proximity to Women," *ibid.*, 366–400.
6. Howard Eilberg-Schwartz, *The Savage in Judaism: An Anthropology of the Israelite Religion and Ancient Judaism* (Bloomington and Indianapolis, 1990), 141–76; Rubin, *Beginning of Life*, 75–86.
7. For example, he discusses the role of women in the circumcision ceremony in the Middle Ages in light of his findings concerning an earlier time period, rather than in its historical context: *Covenant of Blood*, 190.
8. For a survey of approaches to ritual, see: Bell, *Ritual Theory*, 197–218. For a critical assessment of some of these approaches, see: Bourdieu, "Rites As Acts of Institution," 81–88, as well as Paige and Paige, *Reproductive Ritual*, 43–53. In our context, I will argue that despite the seemingly marginal role of women in this male ritual, the place of women in the ritual elucidates the place of women in society at large. For an analysis of rituals as defining social hierarchies, see: Stephen Lukes, "Political Ritual and Social Integration," *Sociology* 9(1975): 289–91; 300.
9. Tosefta Kiddushin, ed. Saul Lieberman (New York, 1973), 1:11; Mishna, Kiddushin, 1:7.
10. Hoffman assumes that the prayers for the circumcision ceremony, like many other prayers, were shaped during the time of the compilation of the Mishna (*Covenant of Blood*, 54–63). Hoffman supports this point, citing the detailed account of John's circumcision ceremony. However, no blessings are mentioned there.
11. Tosefta Berakhot, ed. Saul Lieberman (New York, 1955), 6;12; PT Berakhot, 9c; BT Shabbat 137b.
12. *Siddur R. Sa'adjah Gaon*, eds. Israel Davidson, Simha Assaf, and Issachar Joel (Jerusalem, 1941), 98–100; *Seder R. Amram Gaon*, ed. Daniel Goldschmidt (Jerusalem, 1932), 179–81. For the differences between the ritual in these two books see Lawrence A. Hoffman, *The Canonization of the Synagogue Service* (Notre Dame and London, 1979), 136–39. For the dating of the books, see Robert Brody, "The Enigma of *Seder Rav 'Amram*,'" in *Knesset Ezra. Literature and Life in the Synagogue: Studies Presented to Ezra Fleischer*, eds. Shulamith Elizur et al. (Jerusalem, 1994), 21–34. Ginzberg argued that the blessing for the mother was a later addition and did not appear in the Gaonic sources: Louis Ginzberg, *The Geonim and Their Halakic Writings* (New York, 1909), 1:143. In circumcision ceremonies conducted in the East, only the blessing for the child appears (*Siddur R. Shlomo b. R. Nathan haSigilmasi*, ed. Shmuel Haggai, (Jerusalem, 1995), 142).

13. Daniel Lasker, "Transubstantiation, Elijah's Chair, Plato and the Jewish-Christian Debate," *REJ* 143 (1984): 31–58.

14. Richard Schenk, "Covenant Initiation: Thomas Aquinas and Robert Kilwardy on the Sacrament of Circumcision," in *Ordo Sapientis et Amoris. Hommage au Professeur Jean-Pierre Torrell*, ed. Carlos-Josaphat Pinto de Oliveira (Fribourg, 1993), 555–93.

15. Baptism usually took place at the time of the Easter celebrations. For a survey of the changes in the ritual, see Joachim Jeremias, *Die Kindertaufe in den ersten vier Jahrhunderten* (Göttingen, 1958²); Victor Saxer, *Les rites de l'initiation chrétienne du IIe au Vie siècle. Esquisse historique et signification d'après leurs principaux témoins* (Spoleto, 1988); John D. C. Fisher, *Christian Initiation: Baptism in the Medieval West: A Research in the Disintegration of the Primitive Rite of Initiation* (Alcuin Club Collection 47), (London, 1965); Peter Cramer, *Baptism and Change in the Early Middle Ages, c. 200–c. 1150* (Cambridge, 1993). I thank Professor Evelyn Patlegean for referring me to Saxer's book.

16. The medieval authors themselves were very much aware of this distinction. R. Joseph Bekhor Shor explains that in lieu of circumcision, Jewish women observe the laws of menstrual purity (*Perush al haTorah*, ed. Yehoshafat Nevo (Jerusalem, 1994), Gen. 17:11). Professor Shaye Cohen of Harvard University has undertaken a study of this difference and has published one part of his study to date. See Shaye J. D. Cohen, "Why Aren't Jewish Women Circumcised?" *Gender and History* 9(1997): 560–78.

17. Cramer, *Baptism and Change*, 221–66, argues strongly that baptism lost some of its importance in the later Middle Ages. Other scholars have suggested baptism became less important as early as the ninth century: Jaroslav Pelikan, *The Growth of Medieval Theology 600–1300. The Christian Tradition: A History of the Development of Doctrine* (Chicago and London, 1978), 3:29–32.

18. Powicke and Cheney (eds.), *Councils and Synods* (Oxford, 1962), 2:35.

19. Bernhard Jussen, "La parrainage à la fin du Moyen Age: Savoir publique attentes théologique et usages sociaux," *Annales E.S.C.* 47(1992): 483.

20. Cramer, *Baptism and Change*, 130–78; Joseph Lynch, *Godparenthood and Kinship in Early Medieval Europe* (Princeton, 1986), 285–332; Arnold Angenendt, "Taufe und Politik im frühen Mittelalter," *Frühmittelalterliche Studien* 7(1973): 143–68; Bernhard Jussen, *Patenschaft und Adoption im frühen Mittelalter: Künstliche Verwandtschaft als soziale Praxis* (Göttingen, 1991), 271–98.

21. For baptism in the Byzantine Empire: Evelyn Patlegean, "Christianisation et parents rituelles: Le domaine de Byzance," *Annales E.S.C.* 33(1978): 625–36; Ruth Macrides, "The Byzantine Godfather," *Byzantine and Modern Greek Studies* 11(1987): 139–62. For baptism during the Carolingian reform: Jean-Paul Bouhot, "Explications du rituel baptismal à l'époque carolingienne," *Revue des études Augustiniennes* 24(1978): 278–301; Marie Magdalene van Molle, "Les fonctions du parrainage des enfants en Occident: Leur apogée et leur degradation (du VIe au Xe siecle)," *Paroisse et Liturgie* 46(1964): 121–46; Cyrille Vogel, *Medieval Liturgy: An Introduction to the Sources*, trans. and revised by William Storey and Niels Rasmussen (Washington, D.C., 1986), 164–66; Lynch, *Godparenthood*, 285–89.

22. Lynch, *Godparenthood*, 125–26; 170; van Molle, "Fonctions du parrainage," 122.

23. Christiane Klapisch-Zuber, "Les femmes dans les rituels de l'alliance et de la naissance à Florence," in *Riti e rituali nelle società medievali*, eds. Jacques Chiffoleau et al. (Spoleto, 1994), 3–22; Eadem, "Au péril des commères: L'alliance spirituelle par les femmes à Florence," in *Femmes, mariages, lignages, XII-XIV siècles, Melanges offerts à George Duby*, eds. Pierre Toubert, et al. (Brussels, 1992), 215–32; compare this with Lynch, *Godparenthood*, 205–206.

24. Joseph H. Lynch, "*Spiritale Vinculum*: The Vocabulary of Spiritual Kinship in Early Medieval Europe," in *Religion, Culture, and Society in the Early Middle Ages: Studies in Honor of Robert E. Sullivan*, eds. Thomas F. X. Noble and John J. Contreni (Kalamazoo, Mich., 1987), 181–204; John Bossy, "Blood and Baptism: Kinship, Community and Christianity in Western Eu-

rope from the Fourteenth to the Seventeenth Centuries," in *Sanctity and Secularity: The Church and the World*, ed. Derek Baker (*Studies in Church History*, 10), (Oxford, 1973), 129–43; idem, "Godparenthood: The Fortunes of a Social Institution in Early Modern Christianity," in *Religion and Society in Early Modern Europe 1500–1800*, ed. Kaspar von Greyerz (London, Boston, and Sydney, 1984), 194–201.

25. Sidney W. Mintz and Eric R. Wolf, "An Analysis of Ritual Co-Parenthood (Compadrazgo)," *Southwestern Journal of Anthropology* 6(1950): 341–68; Sidney W. Mintz, "Culture: An Anthropological View"; *The Yale Review* (1982): 506–08; see p. 82 for a discussion of their work.

26. Berger, *The Jewish-Christian Debate*, English section, 172, no. 157.

27. Supra, unnumbered note.

28. Sara Lipton, *Images of Intolerance: The Representation of Jews and Judaism in the Bible moralisée* (Berkeley, 1999), 18.

29. For example: *Siddur R. Solomon b. Samson of Worms*, ed. Moshe Hershler (Jerusalem, 1972), 246–47; 282–90; *Perushei Siddur haTefila laRokeah*, eds. Moshe Hershler and Judah Alter Hershler (Jerusalem, 1992), 2:722–32, and in manuscript: MS Verona Seminar 34, fol. 177a–b; see also the mahzor (prayer book) from 1470 where a blessing for the baby in Hebrew appears: MS Parma 403/2, fol. 87a. For a discussion of the omission of these blessings in Ashkenaz, see *Sefer Or Zaru'a*, 2: no. 107; R. Jacob b. Gershom, *Zikhron Brit*, 60.

30. The main Talmudic sources on circumcision are Mishna Shabbat, 19:2–6; BT Shabbat 134–35.

31. For example, Luke 1:59; PT Hagiga 2:1 fol. 9b.

32. *Sefer Sha'arei Tzedek* (Jerusalem, 1966), 3, section 5, 51, no. 11: "Whether to circumcise an infant on sand or water or to bring the infant to the synagogue — it does not matter. As it is not forbidden either way, we will not instruct you to change your custom."

33. For early modern Europe, see: Bonfil, *Jewish Life in Renaissance Italy*, 192; Richard I. Cohen, *Jewish Icons: Art and Society in Modern Europe* (Berkeley and London, 1998), 34–52; Elliot Horowitz, " 'A Different Mode of Civility': Lancelot Addison on the Jews of Barbary," in *Christianity and Judaism*, ed. Diana Wood (*Studies in Church History*, 29), (Oxford, 1992), 322.

34. This becomes clear through the comparison of a newborn to a groom. See, for example, p. 189, as well as sources from the Cairo Geniza: Goitein, *A Mediterranean Society*, 3:230–31. I have not been able to establish where the circumcision ceremony took place in medieval Geniza society.

35. Lynch, *Godparenthood*, 290–304.

36. Bourdieu, "Rites of Institution."

37. Bell has noted that even if a ritual is performed with no alterations or changes, there is great importance to this continuity (*Ritual Theory*, 204–23). For an opposing view, see: Jack Goody, "Against Ritual: Loosely Structured Thoughts on a Loosely Defined Topic," in *Secular Ritual*, eds. Sally F. Moore and Barbara G. Myerhoff (Assen, 1977), 34.

38. For the compiling and editing of this book as well as for the genre of mahzorim that existed in medieval France in the late eleventh and early twelfth centuries, see Grossman, *Sages of France*, 395–403; Israel M. Ta-Shma, "*Al Kama Inyanei Mahzor Vitry*," '*Alei Sefer* 11 (1984): 81–89; Simha Emanuel, "*Lehnyano shel Mahzor Vitry*," '*Alei Sefer* 12 (1986):129–30; Israel Ta-Shma, "Response to Simha Emanuel," '*Alei Sefer* 12 (1986):132. For manuscripts of the Mahzor in which the laws of circumcision appear: MS Oxford Bodl., Opp. 59, (1100), fol. 224a–229b; JTS mic. 8092, fol. 161a–164e dated to 1203; MS Parma 403, fol. 228a–229b; MS Moscow Günzburg 481, fol. 225a–229d; MS Paris héb. 1408, fol. 140a–141b. The printed version is based on MS London British museum 655 with the exception of the first few pages, which are based on the Oxford 1100 manuscript. I have used this edition unless otherwise noted.

39. In some manuscripts the blessing is "So may he enter mizvot." See, for example, MS Oxford Bodl., Opp. 59, fol. 229a and MS JTS mic. 8092, fol. 164b.

40. *Mahzor Vitry*, nos. 506–507. A slightly more detailed version is MS JTS mic. 8092. These details will be discussed later in this chapter, pp. 65, 70.

41. See p. 67.
42. Exod. 13:48; Pesaḥim, 5:3. I thank Gidon Rothstein with whom I discussed this issue.
43. R. Jacob b. Gershom, *Zikhron Brit*, 94–95. This source seems to allude to another name given the child before the circumcision ceremony. I will return to this point in chapter 3.
44. Rashi, Kiddushin, 74a, s.v. *"Kol shiv'a."*
45. R. Jacob b. Moses Mulin, *Sefer Maharil. Minhagim*, ed. Shlomo J. Spitzer (Jerusalem, 1989), Hilkhot Mila, no. 19.
46. Taglia, "Cultural Construction of Childhood," 258–65.
47. The idea that uncircumcised babies need help reaching heaven appears in the Midrash, and this fact is recounted many times in medieval literature. *Midrash Bereshit Rabbah* 19 [in Hebrew]. The Midrash is dated to the fifth century in Palestine. This Midrash is repeated time and again in medieval Ashkenaz: for example, R. Jacob b. Gershom, *Zikhron Brit*, 91–92; R. Eleazar b. Judah, *Perushei Siddur* 2:727. For a Christian comparison, see Caroline Bynum, *Fragmentation and Redemption*, 239–97.
48. When the father did perform the circumcision himself, a special blessing was recited. See Benjamin Shlomo Hamburger, *Shorshei Minhag Ashkenaz* (Jerusalem, 1995), 357–82.
49. For example, see Goitin, *Mediterranean Society*, 3:230–31.
50. *Maḥzor Vitry*, no. 506.
51. For example, see MS Darmstadt Cod. Or. 25, fol. 76d: "And as for someone who has a son to circumcise, do not take a circumciser because of the love of the person; [choose] rather an expert." In this text, the same stipulation applies to midwives. This too seems to indicate a professional connection between midwives and circumcisers.
52. For example: R. Moses Parnas, *Sefer he Parnas* (Vilna, 1897), no. 138.
53. BT Shabbat 134a.
54. 1 Macc. 1:60, 2 Macc. 6:10.
55. Charlotte Elisheva Fonrobert, *Menstrual Purity: Rabbinic and Christian Reconstructions of Biblical Gender* (Stanford, 2000), 128–59.
56. BT Avodah Zara 27a.
57. Yaacov S. Spiegel, "Woman As Ritual Circumciser—the Halakhah and Its Development," *Sidra* 5(1989): 150–54 [in Hebrew].
58. See, for example: R. Jacob b. Gershom, *Zikhron Brit*, 52–53, who says a woman can circumcise if no man can do the job as well.
59. Compare my analysis to that of Grossman: *Pious and Rebellious*, 332. While Grossman also summarizes Spiegel's article, he does not cite Spiegel's entire argument. He merely states that until the thirteenth century, many Ashkenazic rabbis allowed women to circumcise and that this opinion was restricted somewhat during the course of the thirteenth century. He terminates his discussion without stating that subsequently women were forbidden to circumcise. He also states that the permission for women to circumcise is an indication of their high status. This line of argument seems unproductive. Since, prior to the Middle Ages, women were allowed to circumcise, the main focus should be on the limitation of women's roles.
60. See p. 62.
61. *Maḥzor Vitry*, no. 507. This meal will be discussed in greater detail in chapter 3.
62. MS Oxford Bodl., Opp. Add. 34 (641), fol. 93b: "On the day before the circumcision ceremony, the father and the *ba'al brit* bathe in order to beautify the commandment (*hidur hamizva*), and the community also bathes with them out of respect for circumcision." R. Jacob the circumciser reports the same practice (*Zikhron Brit*, 63–64). A fourteenth-century manuscript of Sefer haTashbez reports on immersion in the mikve (MS Paris héb. 643, fol. 34a).
63. For example: *Sefer Maharil*, Hilkhot Mila, no. 14; ibid., no. 1. Compare: *Zikhron Brit*, 64–66; *Sefer Or Zaru'a*, 2: no. 107; R. Eleazar b. Judah, *Sefer haRokeaḥ*, no. 113.
64. *Sefer Tashbez*, no. 398 and parallels: R. Meir b. Barukh of Rothenburg, *Teshuvot Psakim uMinhagim*, 2: Psakim uMinhagim no. 204; Mordekhai, *Shabbat*, nos. 472, 473; R. Asher b.

Yehiel, *Shut haRosh*, no. 12, n. 3. The accepted halakhic ruling that the honor should be given to the first person it was promised to is attributed to Rabbenu Tam: MS Oxford Bodl., Opp. Add. 34 (641), fol. 95b. "It happened in the days of Rabbenu Tam that a man had a son."

65. *Sefer Tashbez*, no. 398 and parallels: R. Zidkiya b. Abraham, *Sefer Shibolei haLeket haShalem*, ed. Shlomo Buber (Vilna, 1887), 196; Mordekhai, *Hullin*, no. 655.

66. R. Moses of Zurich, *Sefer haSamak miZurich*, ed. Isaac Har Shoshanim (Bnei Brak, 1973), 2: commandment 154, no. 77.

67. For later sources that use the term sandek, see Joseph b. Moses, *Sefer Leket Yosher*, 2:52.

68. *Midrash Tehillim haMekhune Shoher Tov*, ed. Shlomo Buber (Vilna, 1891), chapter 35. The manuscript in which this passage appears, MS Cambridge Or. 786, dated 1282, is called manuscript 6 (Vav) by Buber. On fol. 91c, it states "With my thighs I become a *sandikanos* for children who are circumcised on my knees." Note the difference between this and the printed version (thighs vs. knees).

69. For the dating of the Midrash, see: Leopold Zunz, *Die gottesdienstlichen Vorträge der Juden historisch entwickelt: ein Beitrag zur Alterthumskunde und biblischen Kritik, zur Literatur- und Religionsgeschichte* (Frankfurt, 1892), 278–80.

70. *Midrash Tehillim*, 248, n. 8.

71. R. Nathan b. Yehiel, *Arukh haShalem*, 6:83–84, "*sandikus*."

72. I follow the suggestion of Leopold Zunz, *Der Ritus des synagogalen Gottesdienstes, geschichtlich entwickelt* (Berlin, 1919^2), 4 n.a. For a contrasting view, see Israel M. Ta-Shma, "The Earliest Literary Sources for the Bar Mitzva Ritual and Festivity," *Tarbiz*, 68 (1999), 595–96 [in Hebrew]. Ta-Shma suggests that the role of *sandek* is an ancient one. See also Moshe Goshen-Gottstein, "Likrat Heker haShekiin shel Masorot haTirgumim haArami'im," in *Studies in Rabbinic Literature, Bible and Jewish History, Ezra Zion Melammed Festschrift*, eds. Isaac D. Gilat, Hayim Y. Levine and Tzvi M. Rabinowitz (Ramat Gan, 1982), 43–47.

73. Löw, *Lebensalter*, 83–84.

74. R. Yehiel b. Yekutiel haRofeh, *Sefer Tanya Rabbati* (Vilna, 1899), no. 96.

75. *Ozar HaGaonim: (Thesaurus of the Gaonic Responsa and Commentaries) Shabbat*, ed. Benjamin M. Lewin (Jerusalem, 1930), 139, no. 425.

76. *Sefer Or Zaru'a*, 2: no. 107. A similar quotation, explaining the chair prepared for Elijah, can be found in the Italian *Sefer haTanya*, there without mention of the ba'al brit, stating simply that the chair is for Elijah (*Sefer haTanya*, no. 96). This comment is similar to the wording of R. Isaac's quotation of R. Sherira, but omits mentioning the ba'al brit.

77. Elijah is, according to tradition, the angel of circumcision. See *Pirkei deRabbi Eliezer*, ed. Hayim M. Horowitz (Jerusalem, 1973), end of chapter 29.

78. JTS mic. 8092, fol. 164b.

79. *SHP*, no. 1287, and parallel: *SHB*, no. 407. There are differences between these versions as well as between the version as it appears in the Parma manuscript (*Sefer Hasidim according to MS Parma H3280*, introduction by Ivan G. Marcus (Jerusalem, 1985), no. 1287), and the printed version *SHP*, no. 1287. I have reconstructed the passage using all three sources.

80. Efraim Kupfer, *Teshuvot uPsakim* (Jerusalem, 1973), no. 71.

81. Published and referred to as *Zikhron Brit*; see chapter 1, n. 21.

82. *Zikhron Brit*, 64.

83. The wording is "as God had spoken to him" (*dibber*) and not commanded (*zivah*), as the text reports.

84. I have translated *mekho'ar* as ugly, because of the explicit sexual connotations the word has.

85. *Sefer Tashbez*, no. 397.

86. Kupfer explains that many of the responsa in this manuscript are from the twelfth and thirteenth century. In any case, the manuscript was copied by 1315–16.

87. The Verduner altar in Klosterneuburg, Austria, was designed by Nicholas of Verdun in 1184. Three circumcision scenes are depicted on it: that of Isaac, Samson, and Jesus. In all three scenes a woman is holding the infant.

88. R. Jacob Mulin, *Sefer Maharil*, Hilkhot Mila, no. 22, comment no. 3, "for it is the way of women to help their husbands to bring him [the infant] to the synagogue and then her husband takes from her."

89. It is hard to determine whether the Maharam's instructions became common practice before the fifteenth century. While some sources from the fourteenth century refer to the ba'alat brit consistently as the wife of the ba'al brit, they do not provide many details as to her tasks. See, for example, R. Moses Parnas, *Sefer he Parnas*, no. 237.

90. *Sefer Leket Yosher*, 2:52.

91. Compare: Grossman, *Pious and Religious*, 321–24.

92. See. p. 68.

93. Some scholars have suggested that the ba'alat brit mentioned in these sources was the mother (see, for example, Hoffman, *Covenant of Blood*, 196–97). I think, however, that the sources clearly show that the ba'alat brit, like the ba'al brit, was not the infant's parent.

94. R. Jacob Mulin, *Sefer Maharil*, Hilkhot Mila, no. 22, comment 3.

95. See pp. 101–5.

96. *Seder R. Amram Gaon*, 180.

97. For example: *Maḥzor Vitry*, no. 506; *Sefer Or Zaru'a*, 2: no. 107.

98. Ibid.

99. *Zikhron Brit*, 111.

100. It is possible that Maharil is simply quoting the Or Zaru'a, even if this was not the custom at his time. Other custom books from the period do not mention sending the cup of wine to the mother.

101. Israel M. Ta-Shma, "Birkhot haMila al haKos beTish'a beAv," *Early Franco-German Ritual and Custom*, 327–35; Daniel Sperber, "Al Hashka't haYayin biVrit Hamila"; *Milet*, 1(1983), 221–7; Idem, *Minhagei Yisrael* (Jerusalem, 1989), 1;60–66.

102. Bonfil, *Jewish Life in Renaissance Italy*, 252, discusses the circumcision when it took place at home. He writes that the wine was sent to another room for the mother. It is difficult, however, to know how this worked when the ceremony took place in the synagogue.

103. *Maḥzor Vitry*, no. 499. For recent research on this point, see Jeffrey Robert Woolf, "Medieval Models of Purity and Sanctity: Ashkenazic Women in the synagogue," in *Purity and Holiness: The Heritage of Leviticus*, eds. M.J.H.M. Poorthuis and Joshua Schwartz (Leiden, Boston, and Köln, 2000), 263–80, as well as Israel M. Ta-Shma, "Synagogal Sanctity — Symbolism and Reality," in *Knesset Ezra. Literature and Life in the Synagogue. Studies Presented to Ezra Fleischer*, eds. Shulamith Elizur et al. (Jerusalem, 1994), 351–64 [in Hebrew].

104. *Maḥzor Vitry*, 612.

105. The reasons for this change are discussed in greater detail in chapter 3.

106. This is clear in discussions on when women should wash themselves after birth. See Baumgarten, "Midwives," 69, as well as Barkai, *Les infortunes de Dinah*, 236.

107. R. Moses of Zurich, *Semak of Zurich*, 2: commandment 154, no. 77.

108. R. Joseph b. Moses, *Sefer Leket Yosher*, 2:52. The term *kvatter* takes on a new explanation in the fifteenth century when R. Jacob Mulin explains that the kvatter is called by this name because of a play on the words kvatter and k'toret (incense). He compares the kvatter to someone burning incense before God (*Sefer Maharil*, Hilkhot Mila, no. 1). The term kvatter is, however, the German *gevatter*.

109. Hermann von der Hardt, in discussing the circumcision ceremony, calls the ba'alei brit co-parents (*Juris Judaeorum canonici prodromus, de circumcisione* (Helmstadt, 1700), 79–84).

110. Lynch, "*Spiritale Vinculum*," 181–204.

111. Supra. n. 25.

112. van Molle, "Fonctions du parrainage," 12; Lynch, *Godparenthood*, 305–22.

113. *Sefer Or Zaru'a*, 2: no. 107.

114. The instruction not to honor the same person as ba'al brit more than once is made by *SHB*,

Zava'at Rabbenu Yehuda heHasid, no. 35. In reality, this custom might have been accepted by only a few.

115. For a summary of these incest restrictions, see Brundage, *Law, Sex and Christian Society*, 355–57.

116. This topic has not been addressed in the medieval context and is worthy of further investigation. For antiquity: Michael Satlow, *Jewish Marriage in Antiquity* (Princeton, 2001), and recently for the seventeenth and eighteenth centuries: David Warren Sabean, "Kinship and Prohibited Marriages in Baroque Germany: Divergent Strategies among Jewish and Christian Populations," *Leo Baeck Institute Year Book* 47(2002): 91–103.

117. For both of Bossy's articles on this topic, see supra, n. 4.

118. As described by Bell, *Ritual Theory*, 171.

119. Supra, n. 19 and n. 20, and most recently in his new book: *Spiritual Kinship As Social Practice: Godparenthood and Adoption in the Early Middle Ages*; translated by Pamela Selwyn (Newark and London, 2000), 29.

120. Supra, n. 111.

121. Jacob Katz, "Marriage and Sexual Life," 21–54; Grossman, *Pious and Rebellious*, 98–106. Much has been written about Christian marriage in the Middle Ages. See, for example: Gaudemet, *Le mariage en Occident*; Brooke, *The Medieval Idea of Marriage*; Georges Duby, *Medieval Marriage: Two Models from Twelfth Century France*; trans. Elborg Foster (Baltimore and London, 1978); Jean-Louis Flandrin, *Familles: parenté, maison, sexualité dans l'ancienne société* (Paris, 1976); Alan MacFarlane, *Marriage and Love in England: Modes of Reproduction 300–1840* (Oxford, 1986).

122. For discussion of some of these changes in the medieval period as well as a comparison with the Christian marriage ritual, see Abrahams, *Jewish Life*, 202–28; Cohen and Horowitz, "In Search of the Sacred," 225–50; Roni Weinstein, *Jewish Marriage*.

123. Bava Batra, 10:7–9; Sanhedrin, 3:5; Tosefta, Berakhot, ed. Saul Lieberman, 2:10; Pe'ah, 4:16; Shevi'it, 7:9; Shabbat, 17:4; BT Berakhot 61a; BT Eruvin, 18b; BT Succah 25b; BT Ketubbot, 6b, 77b; BT Gittin, 57a; BT Bava Batra, 144b–145a; BT Sanhedrin 27a. Only in BT Kiddushin 61a does shushvin appear in the female form, *shushvintae*. Stories about the shushvinim (pl.) can be found in a variety of Midraishim. In many of these stories, he appears along with a king and the king's daughter or wife. In such cases, the shushvin usually defends the woman's right to whatever was the issue in question. See, for example, Exodus Rabbah, 31:10; 41:6; 42:8; 43:7; 44:4; 46:1; 47:2; Leviticus Rabbah, 20:10; Numbers Rabbah 1:5; 2:15; 2:25; 18:12; 21:2; Deuteronomy Rabbah 1:2; 3:16; Midrash Tanhuma (Buber ed.), Ki Tisa 12:17, Ahrei Mot 8; Bamidbar 5; Korah 22; Tosefet leKorah 2; Pinhas 2; Vaethanan 2; Midrash Tanhuma (Vilna) Ki Tisa 24; Ekev 10, 1; Eikha Rabba 1:1.

124. For a review of some of the information concerning the shushvin, see Naftali Tur-Sinai, "Shushvin": in *Sefer Assaf. Kovetz Ma'amarei Mehkar*, eds. M. D. Cassuto, Joseph Klausner, and Joshua Guttman (Jerusalem, 1954), 316–22.

125. For example, R. Meir b. Barukh, *Shut Maharam* (Prague), no. 17; R. Hayim b. Isaac, *Shut Maharakh Or Zaru'a*, nos. 92, 125, 194; R. Jacob b. Meir, *Sefer haYashar leRabbenu Tam, She'elot uTeshuvot*, ed. Shraga Rosenthal (Berlin, 1895), no. 92.

126. Weinstein, *Jewish Marriage*, 242, describes the intense involvement of the shushvinim in the ritual. He shows that they were in some ways like additional grooms — they spoke, recited special prayers, and wore their *talitot* (ritual shawls) under the wedding canopy.

127. *SHP*, no. 587.

128. In his study of marriage rituals among the Jews of Italy in the Renaissance, Roni Weinstein has argued that the institution of the shushvin was very similar to that of the co-parent (224–58). While I agree that both are honor systems by which others are included in the ritual, I suggest that Weinstein's comparison reveals the strength of the co-parent-ba'al brit comparison suggested here. Indeed, both the shushvinim and the ba'alei brit, like the co-parents, expressed and forged bonds

between members of the community. Unlike the co-parents, however, and like the ba'alei brit, there were no female shushvins. This becomes evident in a comment of Rashi's when he explains the Talmud term *shushvinteh* — a female shushvin — as "the ba'alat brit" (BT Kiddushin 61 a s.v. "*Shushvintae*"). Had there been female shushvinim, Rashi would undoubtedly not have explained the word as he did.

129. For a description of this process and change, see Yuval, "*HaHesderim haKaspiyim*," 193–96, 199–205.

130. Ibid., 201–206.

131. For a more thorough, though still preliminary treatment of the subject, see the pioneering comparative study of Cohen and Horowitz, "In Search of the Sacred."

132. Paige and Paige, *Reproductive Rituals*, 53–67; 46: "Legitimate rights to a child in preindustrial societies are established by informal agreements and social consensus, but agreements may be broken and social consensus may vanish. The birth of a child tests agreements and threatens consensus because it immediately transfers the questions of legitimate rights from the hypothetical to the actual."

133. These two topics — marriage and the place of women in society — are certainly deeply related. The different theoretical issues behind them will not be properly addressed here but will be the subject of future research.

134. See pp. 68, 70–71.

135. Paige and Paige, *Reproductive Ritual*, 54–67.

136. Bourdieu, "Rites of Institution," 187–88.

137. Mary Douglas, *Purity and Danger: An Analysis of the Concepts of Pollution and Taboo* (London, 1989), 159–79, esp. 167–68. See also Goody, "Against Ritual," 34.

138. For recent research on purity and the synagogue, see the discussion above, p. 78.

139. See pp. 71–72.

140. The phrase appears in BT Menahot 30a, in which the Talmud discusses taking a Torah scroll from the market. The issue in this case is how honorable the deed of taking the Torah scroll is. However, the phrase "*Lahtof mizvah*" does not have a negative meaning. The phrase also appears in Leviticus Rabbah, 2:34:2. See also R. Meir (of Rothenburg) b. Barukh, *Shut Maharam* (Prague), no. 925.

141. For a detailed description of this process, see Talya Fishman, "A Kabbalistic Perspective on Gender-Specific Commandments: On the Interplay of symbols and Society," *AJS Review* 17(1992): 199–245.

142. For research on this topic, see Israel M. Ta-Shma, "Ma'amad hanashim hamitnadvot," *Ritual, Custom and Reality*, 262–79.

143. For example: *Sefer Or Zaru'a*, 2: no. 166.

144. For example: R. Samson b. Zadok, *Sefer Tashbez*, no. 270; R. Jacob Mulin, *Shut Maharil haHadashot*, ed. Yitzchok Satz (Jerusalem, 1977), no. 7; R. Jacob Barukh b. Judah Landa, *Sefer heAgur haShalem*, ed. Moses Hershler (Jerusalem, 1960), Hilkhot ZIzit, no. 27.

145. See for example: Brenda Bolton, "Mulieres Sanctae," in *Sanctity and Secularity: The Church and the World*. ed. Derek Baker (*Studies in Church History*, 10), (Oxford, 1973), 77–95; Nichols and Shank (eds.), *Distant Echoes; Medieval Religious Women*, vol. 1 (Kalamazoo, 1984); Bynum, *Holy Feast and Holy Fast*, 21–23.

146. Marcus, *Rituals of Childhood*, 83–101; Kanarfogel, *Jewish Education*, 40–41; Goldin, and Ta-Shma's objections to Marcus, "The Earliest Literary Sources," 591–96.

147. Tosafot, BT Eruvin, 96b, s.v. "*La salka da'atakh*"; Rashi, BT Brakhot 20b, s.v. "*UMin hatefillin*."

148. R. Samson b. Tzadok, *Sefer Tashbez*, no. 273.

149. R. Jacob Mulin, *Sefer maharil*, Hilkhot Tefillin, no. 10.

150. R. Meir b. Barukh, *Shut Maharam* (Prague), no. 529.

151. Taglia, "The Cultural Construction of Childhood," 258–65.

152. Orme, "Children and Church," 572–76.

153. Talya Fishman describes this process in her article, "Kabbalistic Perspective on Gender-Specific Commandments," 199–245.

Notes to Chapter 3

1. R. Moses b. Isaac Mintz, *She'elot uTeshuvot Rabbenu Moshe Mintz (Maharam Mintz)*, ed. Jonathan Shraga Domb, 2 vols. (Jerusalem, 1991), mentions this custom a number of times, nos. 19, 37, and 64, as does R. Jacob Weil, *She'elot uTeshuvot Mahari Weil*, ed. Yitzchok Satz (Jerusalem, 1988), no. 120. Earlier sources distinguish between Hebrew names (*shem kodesh*) and nicknames (*kinui*). For example: R. Barukh b. Isaac, *Sefer haTeruma*, (Warsaw, 1897), nos. 121, 128.

2. The only extensive treatment of this ritual to date is Hamburger, *Shorshei Minhag Ashkenaz*, 415–55, esp. 428–31. For a description of later developments of this custom, see Eli Katz, "Zeman Netinat Shem leBen uleBat," *Zefunot* 6(1990): 41–45.

3. These verses are generally recited as part of the Saturday night prayer service.

4. *Mahzor Vitry*, no. 507. This custom does not appear in the earlier manuscripts of the *Mahzor*. See Israel Ta-Shma, "Al Kama meInyanei *Mahzor Vitry*," 82.

5. Oskar Rühle, "Bibel," *HdA*, 1:1212–14. This was also the recommended way to help a child who cried incessantly at night, in cases in which the crying was believed to be the result of a spell cast by a demon. Similar beliefs concerning crying can be found in *SHP*, no. 172.

6. *SHB*, no. 1140.

7. *Sefer Huqqei haTorah* also reports a similar custom: "And on the eighth day, after he has been circumcised, they sit the child on a bed of sheets, with the Pentateuch on his head. And the elders of the community or the head of the Yeshiva will bless him, saying: 'May God give you of the dew of heaven' until 'Blessed they who bless you' (Gen. 27:28–29). And the head of the Yeshiva will put his hand on the Pentateuch and will say: 'This one shall learn what is written in this' three times, and then he will say: 'He shall fulfill what is written in this' three times. 'The teaching of the Lord may be in your mouth' (Exod. 13:9). 'Let not this Book of the Teaching cease from your lips etc.' (Josh. 1:8). And the father will host a feast of drinking and joy for the circumcision and for the dedication as it says in the case of Hannah: 'For as long as he [Samuel] lives, he is lent to the Lord' (1 Sam. 1:28)." Simha Assaf, *Mekorot le-Toldot haHinukh* (Tel Aviv, 1924), 1:13. This text discusses the customs of a select group that recommended dedicating a son to spend all of his days studying Torah. Historians have argued over the place of origin of this text. Although most recent research has pointed to Ashkenaz, as there remains some uncertainty, I have not included it in my discussion. For a discussion of the text and its history, see Kanarfogel, *Jewish Education*, 101–105, 195–97.

8. I have translated the word *hol* as "not holy," since the modern "secular" is not an accurate translation.

9. Supra no. 2. See also: Ernst N. Z. Roth, "Al haHollekreisch," *Yeda Am*, 7 [52] (1962), 86–88.

10. Florence Guggenheim, "Houlekraasch," *Israelitisches Wochenblatt Zürich*, 24(1958), 32.

11. Rashi, BT Shabbat 58b, s.v. "*Vela'Arisa*"; Rashi, Ta'anit 22a, s.v. "*'Arisa*"; Rashi, Sanhedrin 20b, s.v. "*Ha'Arisa*." Darmsteter and Blondheim, *Le Glosses françaises*, no. 143 a, b, c.

12. R. Moses Mintz, *She'elot uTeshuvot*, no. 19.

13. Isaac Satz, "Hagahat haGaon R. Israel b. haGaon Shalom Shakhna miLublin beInyan Zurat haOtiyot," *Moriah* 11 [7–8] (1982): 4.

14. R. Joseph Juspa Hahn Neurlingen, *Sefer Yosef Omez* (Frankfurt a.M., 1928), 362.

15. Güdemann, *Sefer haTorah vehaHayim*, 3:104–106; Joseph Perles, "Die Berner Handschrift des kleinen Aruch," *Jubelschrift zum siebzigsten Geburtstage des Prof. H. Graetz* (Breslau, 1887), 24–31; this suggestion was adopted by other scholars at the turn of the century. For example: Löw, *Lebensalter*, 105; Joshua Trachtenberg, *Jewish Magic and Superstition: A Study in Folk*

Religion (New York, 1939), 41–42. See, more recently, Herman Pollack, *Jewish Folkways in Germanic Lands (1648–1806): Studies in Aspects of Daily Life* (Cambridge Mass., 1971), 27–28; Dov Sedan, *Shay Olamot: Three Hundred and Ten Worlds: Twelve Folkloristic Studies*, ed. Dov Noy (Jerusalem, 1990), 7–24 [in Hebrew]. I thank Aaron Cohen for referring me to Sedan's article.

16. Hamburger, *Shorshei Minhag Ashkenaz*, 413, prefers to see the custom as strange and mysterious. The subtitle of his chapter is "a rare and inexplicable custom."

17. Viktor Waschnitius, *Perht, Holda und verwandte Gestalten* (Vienna, 1913), 4–179; Lotte Motz, "The Winter Goddesses: Percht, Holda and Related Figures," *Folklore* 116 (1984): 151–66; Bernhard Kummer, "Frau Holle," *HdA*, 2: 1772; Jacob Grimm, *Deutsche Mythologie*, ed. Elard Hugo Meyer (Tübingen, 1953), 1:207–62, esp. 212–13; 220–34; Bernhard Kummer, "Freyja," *HdA*, 3: 79–82; Grimm, *Deutsche Mythologie*, 2: 79; F. L. W. Schwarz, "Stampa," *HdA*, 8: 354–7; idem, "Frau Rose," *HdA*, 7: 781; idem, "Perhta," *HdA*, 6: 1478–93; Hans Naumann, "Befania," *HdA*, 1: 974–75. Motz, "Winter Goddesses," 151, points to a connection between these figures and Scandinavian figures. Frau Holle and Hulda were related to Scandinavian earth and winter goddesses. See Rudolph Simek, "Huldana" and "Hulda," *Dictionary of Northern Mythology*, 153–54, 165. I thank Dr. Oren Falk for his help on this point.

18. Will-Erich Peuckert, *Deutscher Volksglaube des Spätmittelalters* (Stuttgart, 1942), 97–112, devotes his chapter to Frau Holle. See also Karl Beth, "Brandopfer," *HdA*, 1: 1492–93, who discusses the burning of the first woven product each year as a sacrifice to Frau Holle; Lutz Mackensen, "Altweibersommer," *HdA*, 1: 354; Grimm, *Deutsche Mythologie*, 1:356, 495.

19. Supra, n. 17; Paul Sartori, "Advent," *HdA*, 1: 200; idem, "Fastnacht," *HdA*, 2: 1252; F. Ranke, "Kinderschreck," *HdA*, 4: 1369; Paul Sartori, "Lucia," *HdA*, 5: 1442–46; Karl Meuli, "Maske, Maskereien," *HdA*, 5: 1784; Ludwig Herold, "Schaf," *HdA*, 7: 974; Carl Mengis, "Seelenüberfahrt," *HdA*, 7: 1570; Grimm, *Deutsche Mythologie*, 1:280; F. Eckstein, "Backen," *HdA*, 1: 758, idem, "Brei," *HdA*, 1: 1604; idem, "Essen," *HdA*, 2: 1026; idem, "Gebildbrot," *HdA*, 3: 394–6; idem, "Kuchen," *HdA*, 5: 651; idem, "Neujahrs und Dreikonigsbäcke," *HdA*, 6; 1051; idem, "Pfefferkuchen," *HdA*, 6: 1572; idem, "Pfannekuchen," *HdA*, 6: 1552–65.

20. Motz, "Winter Goddesses," 155; Waschnitius, *Perht, Holda*, 55.

21. Burchardi Wormaciensis Episcopi, *Decretorum*, Liber 19, *PL* 140, 962, "Credidisti ut aliqua femina sit quae hoc facere possit quod quaedam, a diabolo deceptae, se affirmant necessario et ex praecepto facere debere, id est cum daemonum turba in similtudinem mulierum transformatum, quam vulgaris stutitia holdam vocat, certis noctibus equitare debere super quasdam bestias, et in eorum se consortio annumeratam esse? Si particeps fuisti illius incredulitatis, annum unum per legitimas ferias poenitere debes," trans. John T. Mc Neill and Helena M. Gamer, *Medieval Handbooks of Penance: A Translation of the Principal Libri Poenitentiales* (New York, 1990), 331; Heidi Dienst, "Zur Rolle der Frau in magischen Vorstellungen," in *Frauen in Spätantike und Frühmittelalter. Lebensbedingungen-Lebensnormen-Lebensformen*, eds. Werner Affeldt et al. (Sigmaringen, 1990), 178–79.

22. Waschnitius, *Perht, Holda*, 60, 321 quotes: Tractatus de septem vitiis: "Hodie pueri non ministrant Domino, sed diabolo, prius vadunt ad choream, quam ad ecclesiam, ante sciunt cantare de domina Perchta quam dicere Ave Maria."

23. Idem, 18–20; 52–55; 152. Norman Cohn, *Europe's Inner Demons: The Demonization of Christians in Medieval Christendom* (London, 1993), 166–71.

24. *SHP*, nos. 171–72; 1565–67. *Sefer Ḥasidim* also provides means of defense against them. See, for example, *SHP nos*. 1465–67.

25. *Sefer Or Zaru'a*, 1:362; Perles, "Die Berner Handschrift," 26; Trachtenberg, *Jewish Magic*, 41; Grimm, *Deutsches Mythologie*, 1:384.

26. Popular culture linked the Virgin Mary and Frau Holle. See Waschnitius, *Perht, Holda*, 20, 36, 128, 178; A. Wrede, "Maria," *HdA*, 5: 1650; Grimm, *Deutsche Mythologie*, 2:735.

27. This is what the sources seem to suggest. However, it is possible that the custom was more widespread.

28. See p. 113.

29. This custom has been treated in passing. See Perles, "Die Berner Handschrift," 23–24 and, more extensively, Elliott Horowitz, "The Eve of Circumcision: A Chapter in the History of Jewish Nightlife," *Journal of Social History* 13 (1989/90): 45–46.

30. See n. 39 for explanations of these terms.

31. *Mahzor Vitry*, no. 502.

32. Ibid., no. 506.

33. This ancient event is mentioned in later sources together with *shavu'a habat*, a celebration for a girl. Rubin rejects this idea, *Beginning of Life*, 117–19; 188, n. 226.

34. For example: Tosafot, Baba Kama 80a, s.v. "*LeBeit yeshu'a haben*"; Rashi, ibid., s.v. "*Shavu'a haben*"; Rashi, Sanhedrin 32b, s.v. "*Or haner beBrorhayil*"; Tosafot, ibid., s.v. "*Kol rehayim beBurani*"; "*Or haner deBrorhayil*," *Midrash Shoher Tov*, chap. 112, 468.

35. For the development of the custom, see Elliot Horowitz, "The Eve of Circumcision," 45–69; idem, "Coffee, Coffeehouses and Nocturnal Rituals," *AJS Review*, 14(1990): 39.

36. Jacques Brill, *Lilith ou la mère obscure* (Paris, 1981) compares Lilith and demons in different traditions. Siegmund Hurwitz, *Lilith die erste Eva. Eine Studie über dunkle Aspekte des Weiblichen* (Zurich, 1980), 112–14; Trachtenberg, *Jewish Magic*, 42, suggests that the Wachnacht ceremony was directed against Lilith.

37. Horowitz, "Eve of Circumcision," 61, n. 9; Güdemann, *Sefer haTorah veheHayim*, 3:103–104; Trachtenberg, *Jewish Magic*, 171–72. For Spain and Provence, see *Sefer haZohar*, 93:1–2; Aaron b. Jacob haCohen of Lunelle. *Sefer Orhot Hayim*, ed. Moses Schlesinger (Berlin, 1912), 2: nos. 1, 14.

38. Saxer, *Rites de l'initiation*, 144–48.

39. These foods are mentioned in other medieval sources as well: *Siddur Rashi*, ed. Jacob Freimann and Shlomo Buber (Berlin, 1911), no. 126; Rashi, BT Berakhot 42a, s.v. "*Lahmaniyot*: oublies" and in thirteenth century French sources such as *Sefer haMizvot leR. Abraham b. Ephraim*, MS Paris héb 392, fol. 60a, no. 381; MS Paris héb. 393, fol. 42b; 46b; MS Parma 813, fol. 118a. For the meaning of the old French words, see Darmsteter and Blondheim, *Le Glosses françaises*, no. 745. See also Buber's comments in his introduction to Siddur Rashi, LXII, no. 11.

40. For these items in Christian daily life, see Urban T. Holmes, *Daily Living in the Twelfth Century* (Madison, 1952), 80: "The citizens of Paris were very fond of bread and pastry. They loved *gaufres* [waffles], *nieules* [light pastry], *canestel* [little cakes], and *oublies* [wafers]." My thanks to Professor Haym Soloveitchik for referring me to this book.

41. Tosafot, Hullin 64a, s.v. "*Simanin*"; MS Paris héb 393, 46b.

42. Supra n. 1.

43. *Lebensalter*, 77–80. Löw was especially interested in showing how the ritual stemmed from the Jewish tradition. I am less interested in this aspect of the discussion than in the development of the medieval ritual. Hamburger (supra. n. 2) also discusses this custom, focusing on the blessings recited in the synagogue by the parturient; he devotes no attention, however, to the social context of the custom.

44. R. Jousep (Juspa) Schammes (1604–1678), *Minhagim deKehilat Kodesh Wormeisa (Wormser Minhagbuch)* (Jerusalem, 1988), no. 288; See appendix at the end of this chapter.

45. Compare: Roper, *Oedipus and the Devil*, 199–225.

46. As discussed in the previous chapter, these candles were part of every circumcision ritual, p. 62. Already in medieval times, there is discussion of women's role as candle makers. For example, Dulce, the wife of R. Eleazar b. Judah (Rokeah), is said to have made candles. See Haberman, *Gezerot Ashkenaz veZarfat* (Jerusalem, 1946), 167.

47. Jousep (Juspa) Schammes, *Wormser Minhagbuch*, no. 237.

48. This custom may have originated from motives similar to those of the custom of hiding the bride's head under a veil at wedding ceremonies.

49. R. Juda Kirchheim, *Minhagot Wormeisa* (Customs of Worms Jewry), ed. Isaac Mordechai Peles (Jerusalem, 1987), 317 [in Hebrew]. Hamburger, *Shorshei Minhag Ashkenaz*, 400, indicates that this custom varied and that in some communities, no synagogue ritual was held for the mother if her baby had died.

50. MS Nürnberg 7058, fols. 43v–44r, dated 1589, published by Roth, "Al haHollekreisch," 67–68.

51. Hamburger, *Shorshei Minhag Ashkenaz*, 398–400.

52. Glückel bas Judah, *Memoirs*, trans. Marvin Lowenthal (New York, 1977), 88.

53. Tracy Guren Klirs (ed.), *The Merit of Our Mothers: A Bilingual Anthology of Jewish Women's Prayers* (Cincinnati, 1992), 130–31.

54. This reasoning seems distinctly Jewish, in light of Christian attitudes toward sexuality.

55. Lev. 12:1–8.

56. Most sources that deal with this problem seem to suggest that some women first attended the mikve more than eighty days following birth. See Zimmer, *Society and Its Customs* (Jerusalem, 1996), 231–39 [in Hebrew].

57. Hamburger, *Shorshei Minhag Ashkenaz*, 398–400, 410–11 documents the geographic areas in which this custom was observed.

58. Leon Modena, *Historia de Riti Hebraici* (Venice, 1678), 102–103.

59. Most of the recent research concerning this ritual deals with the period after the Reformation. Two books written in the early nineteenth century contain much valuable information that served as the basis for modern research: Peter Browe S. J., *Beiträge zur Sexualethik des Mittelalters* (Breslau, 1932), 15–35; Adolf Franz, *Die kirchlichen Benediktionen im Mittelalter* (Freiburg, 1909), 2:186–240. Franz's book provides a detailed description of the liturgy of the ritual and its development, esp. 2:209, 223–27. Many books on medieval women mention the ritual in passing. For example: Hanawalt, *The Ties That Bound*, 217; Alexandre-Bidon et Closson, *L'enfant à l'ombre des cathédrales*, 67–71; Beatrice Gottlieb, *The Family in the Western World*, 125–29; Clarissa Atkinson, *The Oldest Vocation*, 184; Sylvie Laurent, *Naître au moyen âge*, 213–35; Henrietta Leyser, *Medieval Women*, 130. Two recent doctoral dissertations have addressed medieval churching: Paula Marie Rieder, *Between the Pure and the Polluted: The Churching of Women in Medieval Northern France 1100–1500*, Ph.D. Diss., University of Illinois (Urbana-Champaigne, 2000); Becky Rose Lee, *"Women ben purifyid of her childeryn": The Purification of Women after Childbirth in Medieval England*, Ph.D. Diss., University of Toronto (Toronto, 1998). For studies of churching in early modern Europe, see David Cressy, "Purification, Thanksgiving and the Churching of Women in Post Reformation England," *Past and Present* 141(1993): 106–46; idem, *Birth, Marriage and Death: Ritual, Religion and the Life-Cycle in Tudor and Stuart England* (New York, 1997), 197–228; Adrian Wilson, "The Ceremony of Childbirth and Its Interpretation," in *Women As Mothers in Pre-Industrial England, Essays in Memory of Dorothy McLaren*, ed. Valerie Fildes (London and New York, 1990), 68–107; William Coster, "Purity, Profanity and Puritanism: The Churching of Women, 1500–1700," in *Women in the Church*, eds. W. J. Sheilds and Diana Wood (*Studies in Church History*, 27), (Oxford, 1990), 377–87; Susan Karant-Nunn, *Reformation of Ritual* (London and New York, 1997), 74–78. My deep thanks to Professor Karant-Nunn for her help.

60. Rieder, *Churching of Women*, 1–46.

61. Caspers, "Leviticus 12, Mary and Wax," 295–309.

62. Luke 2:22–32.

63. On *imitatio Mariae*, see: Richard Kieckhefer, "Major Currents in Late Medieval Devotion," in *Christian Spirituality: High Middle Ages and Reformation*, ed. Jill Raitt (London and New York, 1987), 2: 89–93; Elizabeth A. Johnson, "Marian Devotion in the Western Church," in *High Middle Ages and Reformation*, ed. Jill Raitt (London and New York, 1987), 2: 392–414. For medieval adoration of Mary, see Marina Warner, *Alone of All Her Sex: The Myth and the Cult of the Virgin Mary* (New York, 1976), 255–69. Warner emphasizes Mary's connection to fertility and discusses the purification in passing, 67, 106; Stephan Beissel, *Geschichte der Verehrung Marias im 16 und 17 Jahrhundert: Ein Beitrag zur Religionswissenschaft und Kunstgeschichte* (Freiburg, 1909), 320–21.

64. Gail McMurray Gibson, "Blessing from Sun and Moon: Churching As Women's Theater," in *Bodies and Disciplines: Intersections of Literature and History in Fifteenth-Century England*, eds. Barbara A. Hanawalt and David Wallace (Minneapolis and London, 1996), 139–57. Recently, Rieder, *Churching of Women*, 45, has questioned the link between the biblical command and the medieval practices. She has argued for a more complex evolvement of the churching ritual and its relationship to the Feast of Purification and for greater involvement of women in the creation of the ritual. Nevertheless, the biblical practice is at the basis of the medieval practice and is a central shared component of the Jewish and Christian rites.

65. Franz, *Kirchlichen Benediktionen*, 1:442–60; Jacobus de Voragine, *Legenda Aurea*, recensuit par Theodor Graesse (Dresden and Leipzig, 1845), 158–67: "consuevit autem illud festum tribus nominibus appellari, scilicet purificatio, hypopanti et candelaria."

66. *Sefer Nizahon Vetus* discusses the purification of Mary as part of its polemic against Christianity. It asks why Mary had to be purified if, indeed, she was indeed a virgin giving birth to a holy son. See Berger, *Jewish-Christian Debate*, 44, section 6.

67. Gibson, "Sun and Moon," 141–44.

68. *Legenda Aurea*, 163: "Et quoniam difficile est consueta relinquere, christiani de gentibus ad fidem conversi difficile poterant relinquere huiusmodi consuetudines paganorum, ideoque Sergius papa hanc consuetudinem in melius commutavit et scilicet christiani ad honorem sancte matris domini omni anno in hac die totum mundum cum accensis candelis et benedictis cereis illustraren, ut solemnitas quidem staret sed alia intentione fieret." The Candlemass also had social significance, since it marked the period when new servants were hired and old ones let go. See Roger E. Reynolds, "Churching of Women," *Dictionary of the Middle Ages*, ed. Joseph Strayer, 3:382; Frederick G. Holweck, "Candlemass," *The New Catholic Encyclopedia*, 3:245–46.

69. Rieder, *Churching of Women*, 18–25, 42; Wilson, "Ceremony of Childbirth," 75–76, mentions a period that varied depending on the financial abilities of the family, usually between four and six weeks. Karant-Nunn, *Reformation of Ritual*, talks of a period of six weeks, 74–78.

70. See above, pp. 97–99.

71. My description is based on Wilson's and Rieder's descriptions, supra, n. 59.

72. Gibson, "Sun and Moon," 141–51.

73. This problem was addressed by Jews as well, as we remarked above, n. 66.

74. See for example: Hildegardis Bigensis, *Scivias*, ed. Adelgundis Führkötter O.S.B. collaborante Angela Carlevaris O.S.B. (*CCCM* 43) (Turnholt, 1978), 28, Visio secunda, pars prima, 21 (525–47): "Quare mulier post partum vel a viro corrupta I occulto maneat et ab ingressu templi abstineat. Sed et mulier cum prolem peperit fractis occultis membris suis templum meum nonnisi secundum legem per me sibi datam ingrediatur . . . quia Filium meum purissima Virgo genuit, quae integra absque ullo uulnere peccati fuit. Locus enim, qui in honorem eiusdem Vinigeniti mei consecratus est, integri ab omni corruptione liuoris ac uulneris esse debet; quoniam idem Vinigenitus meus integritatem uirginei partus in se nouit. Vnde et mulier quae integritatem uirginitatis suae cum uiro corrumpit, in liuore plagae suae qua corrupta est ab ingressu templi mei se contineat usque dum plaga uulneris ipsius sanetur secundum quod ecclesiastica disciplina ipsi de eadem causa certissime demonstrat." See: Browe, *Beiträge zur Sexualethik*, 27; Shaḥar, *Childhood*, 51, n. 106.

75. Rieder summarizes this point: *Churching of Women*, 268–69.

76. Browe, *Beiträge zur Sexualethik*, 18; Rieder, *Churching of Women*, 18; Gregorius, *MGH*, epist II, 3, 338: "Nam si hora eadem qua genuerit actura gratias intrat ecclesiam, nullo peccati pondere gravatur; voluptas enim carnis, non dolor in culpa est."

77. Browe, *Beiträge zur Sexualethik*, 25–33. Browe also discusses some of the same issues concerning menstruation, 5–14. Franz, *Kirchlichen Benediktionen*, 2:215–20, also discusses this issue. See Rieder, *Churching of Women*, 155–202.

78. Franz, *Kirchlichen Benediktionen*, 2:224–25. For example: versio 1, no. 3: "ut, sicut unigentus filius tuus cum nostre carnis substantia in templo est presentatus, ita facias hanc famulam

tuam purificatis tibi mentibus presentari." This sentence is taken from the purification ritual. See this prayer 1:143; 2:229.

79. Rieder, *Churching of Women*, 93–97.

80. Caspers, "Leviticus 12, Mary and Wax," 295–309.

81. Karant-Nunn, *Reformation of Ritual*, 76.

82. For churching customs related to the chasing away of demons and evil spirits, see: Marianne Beth, "Aussegnung," *HdA*, 1: 645–47; Gustav Jungbauer, "Freitag," *HdA*, 3: 56; Karl Beth, "Kathartik," *HdA*, 4: 1091; Hugo Hepding, "Knien," *HdA*, 4: 1580; Bernhard Kummer, "Wöchnerin," *HdA*, 9: 692–716.

83. Karant-Nunn, *Reformation of Ritual*, 78; Browe, *Beiträge zur Sexualethik*, 20–21.

84. For discussions of these developments in England and post–Reformation Germany, see Wilson, "Ceremony of Childbirth," 91–93.

85. It is possible that these differences are not all that significant, since we find similar distinctions between Jews and Christians in other instances. Jews lacked priests and the husband and cantor seem to be filling in for them in this case.

86. Keith Thomas, *Religion and the Decline of Magic: Studies in Popular Beliefs in Sixteenth- and Seventeenth-Century England* (London, 1971), 42–43.

87. This view of the process was suggested by Wilson, "Ceremony of Childbirth," 83–85, who argues that one cannot separate the churching ritual from the entire process the woman underwent after birth.

88. Ibid., 85–88.

89. Davis, *Society and Culture*, 124–51.

90. Wilson, "Ceremony of Childbirth," 88–93.

91. Ibid., 93–97.

92. Gibson, "Sun and Moon," esp. 142–44.

93. Rieder, *Churching of Women*, 233–74.

94. Chapter 2, p. 76.

95. R. Joseph Juspa Hahn Neurlingen, *Sefer Yosef Omez*, 343–44.

96. Moses Henochs Altschul-Jeruschalmi, *Brantspiegel*, ed. Sigrid Riedel (Frankfurt a.M., 1992), chap. 35.

97. R. Joseph Juspa Kashman, *Noheg kaZon Yosef* (Tel Aviv, 1969), 95, no. 4. It is interesting to note that Kashman emphasizes the fact that until four weeks have passed, in other words, until the parturient is ready to go to the synagogue, she should not perform ritual activities. He even suggests that she should bathe (but not immerse!) before doing so.

98. See introduction, p. 9.

99. William Chester Jordan, "Marian Devotion and the Talmud Trial of 1240," in *Religionsgespräche im Mittelalter*, eds. Bernard Lewis and Friedrich Niewöhner (Weisbaden, 1992), 61–76; Denis L. Despres, "Immaculate Flesh and the Social Body: Mary and the Jews," in *Jewish History* 12(1998): 47–70.

100. Mary Minty, " 'Judengasse' into Christian Quarter," in *Popular Religion in Germany and Central Europe 1400–1800*, eds. Bob Scribner and Trevor Johnson (Basingstoke, 1996), 58–86; Hedwig Röckelein, "Marienverehrung und Judenfeindlichkeit in Mittelalter und früher Neuzeit," in *Maria in der Welt. Marienverehrung im Kontext der Sozialgeschichte 10.–18. Jahrhundert*, eds. Claudia Opitz, Hedwig Röckelein, Gisela Signori and Guy P. Marchal (Zürich, 1993), 279–307.

101. Supra, n. 66. Jews' awareness of Mary was the result of theological debates and more mundane contacts. For example, in some parts of Germany, Lichtmess was the date on which new servants were employed and old ones let go. In addition, Hedwig Röcklein has noted that in some cases this was also a day on which Christians attacked their local Jewish communities. See Hedwig Röcklein, "Vom Umgang der Christen mit Synagogen und jüdischen Friedhöfen, Ashkenaz, Zeitschrift für Geschichte und Kultur der Juden 5(1995): 11–45, esp. 34–38 and note 134, chapter 1, pp. 49–52.

102. Quoted: Caspers, "Leviticus 12, Mary and Wax," 307.

103. This conclusion does not necessarily contradict arguments that churching was far more than just a rite of purification (for example Rieder, *Churching of Women*, 269–74). It could have served many purposes, including purification.

104. Karant-Nunn, *Reformation of Ritual*, 78–79.

105. These three angels are mentioned many times in the medieval literature and are known as angels who can protect the parturient and the baby from Lilith, R. Juspa Schammes, *Wormser Minhagbuch*, no. 288, n. 3.

106. The *windel* or *wimpel* is the cloth diaper used at the circumcision ceremony. It was made into a Torah binder: Joseph Gutmann, *The Jewish Life Cycle* (Leiden, 1987), 6–8; Barbara Kirshenblatt-Gimblett, "The Cut That Binds: The Western Ashkenazic Torah Binder As Nexus between Torah and Circumcision," in *Celebration: Studies in Festivity and Ritual*, ed. Victor Turner (Washington D.C., 1982), 136–45. The most detailed study of wimpels to date is Naomi Feuchtwanger-Sarig, *Torah Binders from Denmark*. Ph.D. Diss., Hebrew University (Jerusalem, 1999). Some scholars have suggested this custom originated at the time of Maharil (R. Jacob Mulin): Patricia Hidiroglou, *Les rites de naissance dans le Judaïsme* (Paris, 1997), 146.

107. I have followed the explanations of the editor of the *Wormser Minhagbuch* (see n. 44). The meaning here is not entirely clear, but the author is describing the drawing of the circle around the parturient's bed until the correct amount of time has passed, as he continues in the lines that follow.

108. On this custom: Güdemann, *Sefer haTorah veheHayin*, 1:204, n. 4.

109. *Kindbett* appears in many sources as a general term for this period spent in bed. For example: R. Juda Löw Kirchheim (d. 1632), *Minhagot Wormeisa*, 315; Eliyahu b. Moses Luntz, *Sefer Toldot Adam* (Koenigsburg, 1860, repr. Jerusalem, 1988), no. 37, 115–23, 135–40, 159–62. I thank Yemima Ḥovav who referred me to this book.

110. The *Sturz* and *Schleier* were both head coverings. The *Sturz* was less fancy and in this case worn over the fancier head covering, the *Schleier*. See *Wormser Minhagbuch* (n. 44), 2:159, nn. 25 and 26 as well as 1: no. 120, n. 1.

111. The *Röckli* (lit. little skirt) was the name for shrouds in Ashkenaz. In this case, the parturient is wearing shrouds over her clothing.

112. There were a number of different customs concerning when to bring the *wimpel* to the synagogue. See Hidiroglou, *Les rites de naissance*, 3; and Gutman, *The Jewish Life Cycle*, 9. This section is followed by a description of the Hollekreisch that took place that same Sabbath afternoon.

NOTES TO CHAPTER 4

R. Jacob Mulin, *Shut Maharil*, ed. Yitzchok Satz (Jerusalem, 1979), nos. 104–105.

1. For statistics concerning the medieval mortality rates, see Boswell, *Kindness of Strangers*, 13–17; Sarah Grieco, "Breastfeeding, Wet Nursing and Infant Mortality," in *Historical Perspectives on Breast Feeding*, eds. Sarah F. Matthews Grieco and Carlo A. Corsini (Florence, 1991), 15–62.

2. I will discuss children up to the age of roughly two years. In spite of the gendered nature of the Hebrew language, the word *tinoq* (child/infant), if not qualified in the source, may refer to either a male or a female child.

3. For example, in the writings of Bartholemaeus Anglicus (England), Raymond Llull (Spain), Phillippe de Nouvarre (Northern Italy), Konrad of Megenburg (Germany), and others. For a description of this genre, see Michael Goodich, *From Birth to Old Age*, (Lanham, 1989), 39–42, 83–104; A. George Rigg and Frank Anthony Carl Mantello, *Medieval Latin* (Washington, D.C., 1996), 416–21.

4. For example: Alexandre-Bidon and Closson, *L'enfant à l'ombre des cathédrales*; more recently, Riché and Alexandre-Bidon, *L'enfance au Moyen Age*.

5. As opposed to the lack of such encyclopedias in Ashkenaz, we possess such texts from Italy and Spain. See, for example, R. Menaḥem Ibn Zeraḥ, *Zeida laDerekh* (Warsaw, 1880), Part 1, Rule 3, chs. 13–14; and in medical manuscripts from Italy, MS Cambridge Ms. Dd. 68/10 (fourteenth century), fol. 22a–23d. The difference between Ashkenaz and Spain or Italy in this instance reflects the more general difference described above concerning medical texts from these different locations. Supra, chap. 1, pp. 45–46.

6. Shaḥar, *Childhood*, 53–54; Berkvam, *Enfance et maternité*, 47–49; Schultz, *Knowledge of Childhood*, 73.

7. In addition, as they believed that personality traits could be transmitted to the nursing infants through the milk they suckled, medieval people were reticent to feed their children animal milk. See Grieco, "Breast-feeding," 21.

8. Shaḥar, *Childhood*, 53–55; Eadem, "Infants, Infant Care, and Attitudes toward Infancy," 283–91.

9. For example: Klapisch-Zuber, "Blood Parents and Milk Parents," 132–63.

10. Vanessa Maher, "Breast-feeding in Cross Cultural Perspective," in *The Anthropology of Breastfeeding* (Oxford and Washington, D.C., 1992), 1–35, 9–11; Ortner, *Making Gender*, 14, 27–31.

11. Hastrup, "Breast-Feeding Patterns," 91–108. This idea is also expressed succinctly in Klapisch-Zuber's "Including Women," 2:3: "The roles assigned to women are assigned not by virtue of women's innate characteristics (their ability to bear children or their relative physical weakness compared to men) but by virtue of a series of arguments that taken together, constitute an ideological system."

12. R. Menaḥem Ibn Zeraḥ, Zeida laDerekh, Part 1, Rule 3, ch. 14.

13. A summary of this topic can be found in Shaḥar, *Childhood*, 1–6. This direction in research was very popular in the seventies among psychoanalysts. For example, De Mause, "Evolution of Childhood," 1–79, esp. 26–39.

14. Herlihy and Klapisch-Zuber, *Tuscans and Their Families*, 136–48.

15. Shaḥar, *Childhood*, is an outstanding example of this approach. In addition, see Hanawalt, *The Ties That Bound*; Gottlieb, *Family in the Western World*; Berkvam, *Enfance et maternité*. Some early modern scholars disagree over these same issues, as summarized in Cunningham, *Children and Childhood*.

16. Ephraim E. Urbach, "Al Grimat Mavet biShegagah uMavet ba'Arisa," *Asufot* 1(1987): 319–32. Urbach (p. 322) discusses a responsum of R. Meir b. Barukh (Maharam). See chapter 5 for further discussion of this responsum.

17. Simḥa Goldin, "Beziehung der jüdischen Familie," 211–56; Kanarfogel, "Attitudes toward Childhood," 1–35. In the appendix he brings a list of sources that discuss breast-feeding; Ta-Shma, "Children in Medieval Germanic Jewry," 263–80; Samuel Kottek, "HaHanaka beMekorot haYahadut : Historia veHalakha," *Sefer Asia* 4(1983): 275–86.

18. See introduction, pp. 2–3.

19. Some of the halakhic issues concerning breast-feeding have been summarized by Yisrael Z. Gilat, "The Obligation of Nursing Children," *Diné Israel* 18(1995–96): 321–69 [in Hebrew].

20. BT Bekhorot 7b.

21. On the margins of this discussion of breast-feeding obligations, we find a certain discomfort with the practice of breast-feeding. The Tosefta discusses whether or not breast-feeding is comparable to "sucking from an abomination," Tosefta, Niddah 2:3. Although this point of view did not prevail, it does come up in some of the sources.

22. BT Berakhot 31b. This idea is expressed in other cultures as well. See the examples brought by Grieco, "Breast-feeding," 24.

23. Ketubbot 5:4, 9.

24. BT Ta'anit 27a; Mishna Niddah 1:4. Like old women past menopause, pregnant women, and sterile women, a nursing mother was not obligated by the same laws as all other women.

25. Tosefta, Niddah 2:2; Mishna, Sotah 4:3.

26. While the halakhic formulas discuss the remarriage of widows and divorcées, this discussion includes not only women who are nursing their own children, but also hired wet nurses who are nursing the children of others. Two different cases are discussed in the Talmud, BT Ketubbot 60b, in which the same figure, R. Naḥman, ruled in two different ways. In one case he forbade a wet nurse to remarry during the period of her contract, while in the other case, he allowed a wet nurse who was employed by the head of the exile to remarry despite her commitment to nurse a child, arguing that she knew that if she broke her contract, her high-ranking employer would have her killed.

27. Ibid., PT Sotah 4:3. The PT also ruled that a mother whose child died within the nursing period could not remarry until the end of the twenty-four months. The PT does not give a reason for this ruling, but Urbach surmised, on the basis of the list of ḥilluqim (differences in customs) between Palestinian Jews and Easterners (Babylonians), that the motive for the different rulings is the fear that the woman might kill her child. See Urbach, "Mavet biShegaga," 320. See: HaḤiluqim sebein Anshei Mizraḥ uBnei Ereẓ Israel, ed. Mordekhai Margaliyot (Jerusalem, 1938), 75–76, where this fear is mentioned; another reason for this difference might have to do with sleeping habits. In Palestine, children slept in their parents' bed and overlying was more common, whereas in Babylon, children slept in cribs, Urbach, ibid.

28. BT Ketubbot 59b.

29. Oẓar haGeonim, Ketubbot, nos. 441–45. For another case: Halakhot Psukot min ha-Geonim, ed. Joel Müller (Krakau, 1893), no. 115 [in Hebrew].

30. She'eltot Rav Aḥai Gaon, ed. Samuel K. Mirsky (Jerusalem, 1959), 1: Gen., no. 13.

31. BT Ketubbot 60a. There is only one instance in which a difference between boys and girls is noted. One Gaonic response states that if the infant was female and her mother remarried after eighteen months, her marriage did not need to be annulled. See Lewin, Oẓar haGe'onim, Ketubbot, no. 222.

32. Tosefta, Niddah 2:6; BT Yevamot 34b.

33. Tosefta, Niddah 2:4.

34. Avodah Zara, 2:1.

35. This belief was part of Galenic medicine. See Thomasset, "The Nature of Women," 54; Laurent, Naître au moyen âge, 83.

36. BT Niddah 9a: "According to the view of R. Meir, menstrual blood decomposes and turns into milk, while according to the view of R. Jose, R. Judah and R. Simeon, the woman's limbs are disjointed and her natural vigor does not return before the lapse of twenty-four months."

37. David Herlihy, "Medieval Children," in Women, Family and Society in Medieval Europe. Collected Essays 1978–1991 (Providence, 1995), 113.

38. Idem, Medieval Households, 26–28.

39. Keith R. Bradley, "Wet Nursing at Rome: A Study in Social Relations," in The Family in Ancient Rome, ed. Beryl Rawson (London and Sydney, 1986), 201–29.

40. Brundage, Law, Sex and Christian Society, 182.

41. Avner Giladi, Infants, Parents and Wet-Nurses: Medieval Islamic Views on Breast-Feeding and Their Social Implications (Leiden, Boston, and Köln, 1999), 13–40, esp. 19–21; 91–94. At the root of this approach are questions related to understandings of purity and impurity. These issues were also the basis for the discussion of whether an infant who nurses from his/her mother is like one who sucks an "abomination" in Jewish texts (supra, n. 21), as well as in Christianity (Marilyn Yalom, History of the Breast (New York, 1997), 37–48).

42. For a similar metaphor in Christian literature, see Laurent, Nâitre au moyen âge, 101.

43. Maḥzor Vitry, no. 428.

44. Tosafot, Ketubbot 60a, s.v. "Rabbi Yehoshua." The time framework mentioned here is based on R. Joshua's statement in the Tosefta that some children nurse for up to four years. The repetition of these ages in the texts seems to indicate that this was not unusual.

45. Menaḥem Ibn Zeraḥ, *Sefer Ẓedah laDerekh*, part 1, rule 3, chapter 14.

46. R. Judah b. Nathan, *Perush Masekhet Yevamot leRabbenu Yehuda ben Nathan*, ed. Efraim Kupfer (Jerusalem, 1977), 42b, s.v., "*Memasmasa*" as well as Rashi's comment ad locum.

47. R. Solomon b. Isaac, *Responsa Rashi*, no. 217.

48. An additional method used to determine the duration of breast-feeding by demographers is the spacing of children. Unfortunately, the surviving documentation for medieval Jewish communities does not enable us to reach an unequivocal conclusion. See introduction, pp. 18–19.

49. This practice is one of the reasons it is so difficult to distinguish between nannies and wet nurses in medieval Latin sources, as the word *nutrix* serves for both functions: Grieco, "Breast-Feeding," 36–38; Valerie Fildes, *Wet Nursing: A History from Antiquity to the Present* (New York, 1988), 44.

50. Klapisch-Zuber, "Blood Parents," 144–45.

51. Grieco, "Breast-Feeding," 45–47; DeMaitre, "Idea of Childhood," 474.

52. R. Menaḥem Ibn Zeraḥ, supra n. 6; R. Moses of Couçy, *Semag*, negative commandment no. 81: "And she nurses him/her until s/he is twenty-four months old, and it is the same for male and for female."

53. For Christian society, see: Shahar, *Childhood*, 60–65; McLaughlin, "Survivors and Surrogates," 115–16; Shahar, "Infants, Infant Care," 288–91, 296–98. For Jewish sources, see Ketubbot 5:8; R. Moses b. Maimon, *Mishne Torah*, Hilkhot Ishut, ch. 21, nos. 5–6, who states that if a woman has two servants she need not nurse her children. Some texts reveal an interesting twist on this principle. It was customary that if a woman came from a family where women did not nurse their children, even if the man she married was not wealthy, she should not have to nurse her own children. Rashi, Ketubbot 61a, s.v. "*DeLav orḥa*."

54. Klapisch-Zuber, supra, n. 9.

55. We have no sources that provide a full description of these relationships from medieval Ashkenaz. A fascinating demonstration of the consequences of these social circumstances in early modern Italy can be found in Kathy Beller, *Jews before the Modenese Inquisition: 1600–1645*, Ph.D. Diss., Haifa University, (Haifa, 2002). I thank the author for sharing her findings with me.

56. Christiane Klapisch-Zuber discusses legal contracts in Christian society between the infant's family and the wet nurse's husband. See "Blood Parents," 143–53, 159. I do not know of any extant contracts from medieval Ashkenaz. Kenneth Stow discusses one such contract from sixteenth-century Rome (*Jews in Rome* (Leiden, New York, and Köln, 1995), 1: case 952).

57. R. Eliezer b. Nathan, *Sefer Even haEzer. Sefer Ra'avan* (Jerusalem, 1984), no. 294.

58. BT Bava Kama, 116b; Bava Meẓi'a 10a.

59. This source appeared in Moshe Weinberger, "Teshuvot Ḥakhmei Ashkenaz," in *Sefer haZikaron leRabbi Yaacov Beẓalel Zolty*, ed. Joseph Boxbaum (Jerusalem, 1987), 250. My thanks to Dr. Rami Reiner who referred me to this source.

60. Although the source does not explicitly state that the wet nurse was Jewish, I would suggest that, as the question is directed to a religious authority, this must be the case.

61. R. Asher b. Yeḥiel, *Shut haRosh*, rule 17, no. 7.

62. See rule 53, no. 2. This similarity applies to Christian Europe as a whole (with the exception of Iceland). Shahar, *Childhood*, 60–63.

63. Klapisch-Zuber demonstrated that in mid-fourteenth-century Florence, the average period that an infant stayed with a wet nurse was ten months. See "Blood Parents," 145.

64. Mordekhai, *Ketubbot*, no. 289; *Yevamot*, no. 3.

65. This emerges from Ra'avan's discussion of the issue, supra n. 57.

66. For example: R. Meir b. Barukh, *Shut Maharam* (Prague edition), no. 863; *Sefer Or Zaru'a*, 1: no. 740.

67. For Christian Society, see Klapisch-Zuber, "Blood Parents," 145–47. For Jewish cases, see above, pp. 129–30.

68. R. Solomon ben Aderet, *She'elot uTeshuvot*, 1: no. 723.

69. R. Moses of Couçy, *Semag*, negative commandment no. 81.
70. Natalie Zemon Davis, *The Gift in Sixteenth-Century France* (Madison, 2000), 51–53.
71. This is based on Esther 9:22.
72. At the beginning of this chapter, I pointed out the problems faced by scholars of Christianity in distinguishing between nannies and wet nurses; both these functions are designated by the Latin *nutrix*. The Hebrew, however, distinguishes between maids who took care of the infants and wet nurses, see chapter 5, p. 158.
73. R. Solomon b. Isaac, *Responsa Rashi*, no. 131 and parallels: *Mahzor Vitry*, no. 245; *Sepher haPardes, attributed to Rashi*, ed. Haym Judah Ehrenreich (Budapest, 1924), 255; R. Zidkiyah b. Abraham, *Shibbolei haLeket*, 158, no. 202. (In this source, the practice is forbidden by R. Kalonimus haZaken. Kalonimus was a contemporary of Rashi's, and Rashi might have studied with him); *Siddur Rashi*, 168; R. Abraham b. Nathan of Lunel, *Sefer haManhig* (Jerusalem, 1978), Massekhet Megillah, no. 26; MS Oxford Bodl., Opp. Add. 34 (641), fol. 135a, margins Laws of Purim. In all these sources, the custom of giving gifts to the Christian servants is referred to as improper and as something that should be prohibited.
74. R. Samson b. Zadok, *Sefer Tashbez*, no. 172 and in manuscripts: MS Parma 571, fol. 159a–b, no. 173; MS Paris héb. 327, fol. 86d, from 1386.
75. MS Montifiore 134, fol. 95a. For details of R. Menahem b. Jacob, see Urbach, *The Tosaphists*, p. 406.
76. Since no personal information about the wet nurses who were employed by Jews has reached us, we can draw no firm conclusions as to who they were. While it is probable that a woman who worked for a Jewish family made more money than a wet nurse who worked in a foundling house, as working in a Jewish home was against church laws, it was certainly not a desirable job. Beller, in her thesis, *Jews before the Modenese Inquisition: 1600–1645*, describes two cases of wet nurses brought before the Inquisition in Modena, one who worked for a wealthy family and the other who worked for a poorer family. Her description of the two women, and especially of the woman who worked for the poorer Jewish family, presents them as on the margins of Christian society.
77. For example: R. Menahem Ibn Zerah, *Zedah laDerekh*, part 1, rule 3, chap. 14: "The food the Blessed Name has prepared for the boy is milk, and anyone who wants to save him from illness will ensure that his food will not be anything but milk, but this is natural food. One should always choose a wet nurse between the ages of twenty and thirty of good complexion, without blemishes and of even temper, not thin or fat. And she should beware of intercourse that stimulates menstrual blood, so that she will have sweet white milk without a foul smell, not too thin and not too thick, but rather of medium quality. She should be of good qualities and not angry or cross, since these traits harm the milk. And the food that encourages good milk is sweet and fatty: the meat of lambs and young goats and moist fish and almond paste and other such things. And when the mother herself can nurse her son, this is best, because this is the food he was nourished with in the womb when the menstrual blood turned into milk. She should not nurse him too much so that he not lose the milk in his stomach, nor should she nurse him too little, for then his body will heat up. Rather, moderately, according to his strength. And when he is first born, his mother should not nurse him until eight days have passed by and her milk has evened out. . . . The wet nurse must make the baby happy and she should sing to him to make him cheerful and put him to sleep; for sleep is very good for him, and he should sleep in a dark place. And while he is awake, he should become accustomed to seeing the sun and the stars and to hearing all kinds of tunes, because every organ that is trained is strengthened. And they should teach him to talk, because infants imitate those who talk to them. Compare Goodich, *Birth to Old Age*, 80. Other Jewish sources also encourage maternal breast-feeding. For example: A Hebrew manuscript from fourteenth-century Italy details the care the mother and child should receive after birth. This manuscript provides detailed instructions for both maternal breast-feeding and employing a wet nurse. See Cambridge Ms. Dd. 68/10 fol. 22–24, *"MiTikun Shemirat haValad"*; supra n. 5.

78. See: Shaḥar, *Childhood*, 55–60; Atkinson, *Oldest Vocation*, 60–61.
79. This belief appears already in the Talmud, BT Ketubbot 61a, and in medieval sources: *Sefer Or Zaru'a*, 1: no. 630. For Christian society, see: Alexandre-Bidon and Closson, *L'enfant à l'ombre des cathedrales*, 121.
80. *Midrash Shemot Rabbah*, chapters I–XIV, ed. Avigdor Shinan (Jerusalem, 1984), 1:25. Compare: BT Sotah 12b.
81. See Schultz, *Knowledge of Childhood*, 73, and the sources reviewed there; Orme, *Medieval Children*, 11.
82. Berkvam, *Enfance et maternité*, 51; Alexandre-Bidon and Closson, *L'enfant à l'ombre des cathedrales*, 112–13.
83. This story is cited in Fildes, *Wet Nursing*, 43.
84. Many women nursed their own children along with a wet nurse in order to provide themselves with flexibility. Some noblewomen had up to four wet nurses. See ibid., 44.
85. McLaughlin suggests that until the eleventh century most children were nursed at home ("Survivors and Surrogates," 116). See also Shaḥar, *Childhood*, 60–69; Grieco, "Breast-Feeding," 34–35, n. 3.
86. For example: R. Asher b. Yeḥiel, *Shut haRosh*, no. 17; *Teshuvot Maimoniyot leSefer Nashim*, no. 24. The comments made about these women make it clear that these women were not always married. The Hagahot Maimoniyot, for example, comments about a specific wet nurse: "and some say she has a husband." From this comment we may learn that many of the wet nurses did not have husbands.
87. *Sefer Or Zaru'a*, 1: no. 657. The responsum was sent to R. Ḥayim haCohen b. Ḥananel, a student of R. Tam (Rami Reiner, *Rabbenu Tam: Rabbotav haZarfatim veTalmidav Benei Ashkenaz*, M.A. Thesis, Hebrew University (Jerusalem, 1997), 63 [in Hebrew]). This woman became pregnant while employed as a wet nurse. According to her testimony, her employer was the father of her next child. This source points to a practice that the Christian sources feared — sexual relations between the infant's father and the wet nurse. On this topic in a later period, see Horowitz, "Between Masters and Maidservants in the Jewish Society of Europe in Late Medieval and Early Modern Times," in *Sexuality and the Family in History: Collected Essays*, eds. Israel Bartal and Isaiah Gafni (Jerusalem, 1999), 193–212 [in Hebrew].
88. For an early example, see Amnon Linder, *The Jews in the Legal Sources of the Early Middle Ages* (Detroit and Jerusalem, 1997), 558, doc. 100: Rouen 1074: "De Judaeis canonicalis auctoritas, et Beati Gregorii decretum servetur, scilicet ne Christiana mancipia habeant, nec nutrices."
89. These sources were collected by Simonsohn and Grayzel: Simonsohn, *The Apostolic See*, 1: doc. 56 (before 1179), 79 (1205), 82 (1205), 134 (1233), 137 (1233), 171 (1244), 221 (1265–68), 232 (1267); Solomon Grayzel, *The Church and the Jews*, 1: doc. 14 (1205), 18 (1205), 69 (1233), 104 (1244), Third Lateran Council (296–97) (1215), Council of Montpellier (298–99) (1195), Council of Paris (306–307) (1213), Council of Narbonne (316–17) (1227), Regulations of Lord William of Bley (320–23) (1229), Synod of Worcester (330–31) (1240). Simonsohn argues that this prohibition was issued frequently after the third Lateran council (1215). Grayzel argued that this prohibition was new. However, as Amnon Linder has shown, we find this warning in the eleventh century as well (supra, n. 88).
90. For example, Aronius, *Regesten zur Geschichte der Juden*, no. 81, 168.
91. Mansi, *Sacrorum Conciliorum*, 22, col. 231: "Judaei sive Sarceni nec sub alendorum puerorum obtentu, nec pro servitio, nec alia causa, Christiana mancipia in domibus suis permittantur habere. Excommunicentur autem, qui cum eis praesumpserint habitare."
92. Mansi, ibid., col. 357; Simonsohn, *Apostolic See*, doc. 56: "Quod etiam obstetricibus et nutricibus eorum prohibere curetis, ne infantes Iudaeorum in eorundem domibus nutrire praesumant, quoniam Iudaeorum mores et nostri in nullo concordant et ipsi de facili ob continuam conversationem et assiduem familiaritatem, instigante humani generis inimico ad suam superstitionem et perfidiam simplicium animos inclinarent."

93. The practice of employing Christian women in Jewish homes is outlined fully in Jacob Katz, *Shabbes Goy*, where he discusses the specific halakhic issues raised by their employment on the Sabbath and holidays, rather than the general phenomenon. He notes (12, n. 4) that most of the cases in which the employment of Christian servants is mentioned have to do with these specific, problematic halakhic circumstances. By contrast, the employment of Christian wet nurses is mentioned in everyday contexts, and very few of the sources discussing the wet nurses mention Sabbath or holidays as an issue.

94. Grayzel, *Church and the Jews*, 1: doc. 25.

95. The Hebrew here states that the wet nurses argued between them and then indicates in the next sentence that their master was responsible for these arguments.

96. *SHP*, no. 159. See also Parma manuscript of Sefer Hasidim no. 159, which differs slightly from the printed edition.

97. *SHP*, no. 1439.

98. *Sefer Or Zaru'a*, 2: no. 48, no. 279; R. Hayim b. Isaac, *Piskei Halakha shel R. Hayim Or Zaru'a (Drashot Maharah)*, ed. Isaac Samson Lange (Jerusalem, 1973), 155; R. Moses b. Barukh, *Teshuvot, Minhagim uPesakim*, 1: no. 95, 2: no. 131 and parallels; MS Cambridge Or. 548, no. 106, fol. 30b–31a.

99. *SHP*, no. 1139.

100. For example, R. Yehiel of Paris ruled: "And feeding a minor from the lard which is called *bolieu* that is made from the *helev* of non-Jews, even if this is done by the hand of a Jewess, is permitted since the infant is like a sick person whose life is endangered," R. Yehiel b. Judah of Paris, *Piskei R. Yehiel miParis veHoraot meRabbanei Zarfat*, ed. Eliyahu Dov Pines (Jerusalem, 1977), no. 137. For an example concerning the laws of Sabbath, see: R. Moses of Couçy, *Semag*, Issur ve-Heter, rule 59, nos. 28–29: "And if the baby does not have what to eat he can tell a Canaanite to cook him pap on the Sabbath. And if the infant does not want to be fed by anyone but his mother, R. Samson of Couçy (d. 1221) replied that his mother is permitted to feed him, even from a broth of milk that was milked and cooked on the Sabbath by the Canaanite, since he is like a sick person whose life is in danger, as he does not want to eat from anyone else."

101. R. Moses Parnas, *Sefer haParnas*, no. 162 and in a slightly different version in manuscript MS Oxford Bodl., Mich. 455 (146), fol. 15b, no. 125; *SHP*, no. 1073.

102. Shoham, *Social Attitudes*, 96 n. 287; MS Paris Héb. 1122 fol. 5b; MS Oxford Bodl., Opp. 31 (271) fols. 88a–89b where the use of lard for a cream to ease the symptoms of a skin disease (*Shhin*) is mentioned; Barkai, *Les infortunes de Dinah*, 99–104. I thank Dr. Ephraim Shoham for referring me to these sources.

103. The word *min* means type (like a type of food) and is another name for heretics or, in many medieval texts, for Christianity. This passage plays with both these meanings.

104. *Sefer Or Zaru'a*, 4: no. 146.

105. R. Meir b. Barukh, *Teshuvot, Pesakim uMinhagim*, 2: no. 131.

106. Grayzel, *Church and the Jews*, 1:107, 115, 199, 211, 307, 317, 321–23, 329, 331. References to illicit relationships between Jews and their Christian wet nurses can also be found in other sources. For example: *SHP*, no. 19, which mentions a penance for someone who sinned with a Christian servant. See the comments of Goldin, "Beziehung der jüdischen Familie," 220–22.

107. For Innocent's accusation, see Grayzel, *Church and the Jews*, 1:114–15: "Faciunt enim Christianas filiorum suorum nutrices, cum in die ressurectionis Dominice illas recipere corpus et sanguinem Jesu Christi contingit, per triduum antequam eos lactent, lac effundere in latrinam." For Henrici de Segusio, see *Summa Aurea* (Venice, 1581), 1514–1515: "Nam sunt qui, quod nephandum est dicere, nutrices christianas habentes non permittunt lactare filios, com corpore Christi sumpserunt, nisi primo per triduum lac effuderint in latrinam: quasi intelligunt quod corpus Christi incorporetur et ad secessum descendat."

108. Rashi, Avodah Zara 26a, s.v. "*Menikah benah shel Yisrael bir'shutah.*"

109. R. Yehiel of Paris, *Vikuah R. Yehiel of Paris*, ed. Reuven Margaliqot (Jerusalem, 1928),

21. This is also the wording in MS Moscow Günzberg 1390 fol. 94b. The Latin version of the disputatiom does not include this passage, nor does the Hebrew version cited by Wagenseil in his *Tela Ignae Satanae*. For the different versions of the disputation, see Loeb, "La controverse de 1240," REJ (1880): 1:247–61; 2:248–70; 3:39–57, and especially 1:248 54.

110. Tosfot, Avodah Zara 26 a, s.v. *"Ovedet kokhavim menikah benah shel Yisrael."*

111. The phrase used to describe the supervision of the Jewish friends, *"Yoẓe venikhnas"* is a common phrase. See Rashi, Berakhot 34b, s.v. *"Ke'eved."*

112. R. Elḥanan b. Isaac, *Tos'foth*, ed. David Fränkel, (Husiatyn, 1901), 26a. R"i's other student, R. Samson of Sens also agrees with this opinion: Tosfot R. Samson b. Abraham of Sens, *Shitat Kadmonim al Massekhet Avodah Zora*, ed. Moses Judah Blau (New York, 1969), 26a.

113. R. Barukh was known in much of the literature as R. Barukh of Worms. Recently, Simḥa Emanuel has shown that he was from Paris ("Biographical Data on R. Baruch b. Isaac"). *Tarbiẓ* 69(2000): 423–40.

114. Urbach, *The Tosaphists*, 347–54.

115. R. Barukh b. Isaac, *Sefer haTerumah*, no. 152. This book was fairly popular during the Middle Ages, and these instructions can be found in many thirteenth-century manuscripts: MS Oxford Bodl., Opp. 73 (640), fol. 15, no. 145; MS Parma 813, fol. 187, no. 21. For a slightly different version, see MS Oxford Bodl., Opp. Add. 34 (641), fol. 14d, no. 149. It is interesting to note that R. Barukh's opinion opposes that of the other disciples of his mentor, R. Isaac of Damprierre, supra, n. 113.

116. R. Moses of Couçy, *Semag*, negative commandment no. 45.

117. R. Jacob b. Judah Ḥazan of London, *Eẓ Ḥayyim*, 2:331, *Hilkhot Avodah Zarah veGerim*. See also R. Abraham b. Ephraim, *Sefer Hamiẓvot*, MS Paris héb. 392, fol. 41b, no. 165.

118. This fear was certainly a valid one, as scholars have demonstrated over the years in discussions on adolescent converts. There is a major difference, however, between the influence a Christian family could exert over adolescents, and their possible influence on infants. For adolescent conversion, see Ivan Marcus, "Jews and Christians Imagining the Other in Medieval Europe," *Prooftexts* 15(1995): 222; and, more recently, William C. Jordan, "Adolescence and Conversion in the Middle Ages: A Research Agenda," in *Jews and Christians in Twelfth Century Europe*, ed. Michael A. Signer and John Van Engen (Notre Dame, 2001), 77–93; Alfred Haverkamp, "Baptised Jews in German Lands during the Twelfth Century," in *Jews and Christians in Twelfth Century Europe*, eds. Michael A. Signer and John Van Engen (Notre Dame, 2001), 255–310.

119. I attribute less importance to the fear that wet nurses would kill Jewish children than Goldin, "Jewish Children and Christian Missionizing," who sees this as a central consideration in child rearing. While I do not doubt that this fear existed, I do not think it was as menacing or as all-encompassing as Goldin suggests.

120. R. Barukh's ruling seems to accord well with what Urbach defined as his tendency to find solutions for halakhic issues dealing with Jewish-Christian daily relations. See Urbach, *The Tosaphists*, 350–51, especially since his opinion is different from that of some of his contemporaries, supra, n. 115.

121. For example: R. Eleazer b. Joel haLevi, (b. 1140), *Sefer Ra'aviah Avodah Zarah*, no. 1057.

122. R. Eleazar b. Judah, *Sefer Rokeaḥ*, (Fano, 1505), no. 472. This ruling can also be found in MS Paris héb. 363, fol. 179b. This manuscript was copied by Sabbetai b. Joseph, also known as Bon Fish, in 1452. This text is not included in the modern printed edition of *Sefer Rokeaḥ*, and its omission may be a case of modern editing of a halakhic text.

123. *Sefer Or Zaru'a*, 4: no. 145. Later German sources quote R. Barukh with few comments. For example: *Hagahot Maimoniyot* on Maimonides, *Hilkhot Ovdei Kokhavim*, 9:16; Mordekhai, *Avodah Zara*, no. 812.

124. Supra, n. 14.

125. Some scholars have suggested that the custom of employing a wet nurse was most prevalent in France where the business of wet nursing flourished in the Middle Ages. In these coun-

tries, wet nurses made more money than elsewhere, and it was more common to find children sent out to the homes of wet nurses, rather than cared for in their own homes (Fildes, *Wet Nursing*, 36–39). This difference might explain the distinction between the practices in Germany and those in northern France, and, perhaps, the German-Jewish texts' stronger reservations regarding sending children to the homes of Christian wet nurses.

126. Such an example appears in *Sefer Or Zaru'a*, 1: no. 657. In this case, it is clear that the woman was very poor when she sought employment.

127. Christian theological objections to other wet-nursing arrangements grounded in the superiority of Christianity to Judaism, or the fear of conversion of the wet nurses to Judaism, would not have applied to this practice. Only one source mentions this option, and it is from outside the geographical area under discussion. A thirteenth-century document from Valdolid, Spain, forbids Jewish and Muslim women to nurse Christian children, and Christian women to nurse Jewish and Muslim children. See Heath Dillard, *Daughters of the Reconquest: Women in Castillian Town Society 1100–1300* (Cambridge, 1984), 207.

128. Only R. Eliezer b. Nathan discusses the reasons a Jewish woman should not accept employment in a Christian home. He explains that if she were single, committing herself to be a wet nurse would restrict her ability to marry during the period of her employment, and if she were a married woman, working in a Christian home would cause her husband to be averse to her (*Sefer Ra'avan*, no. 294).

129. Aside from this ruling, Mordekhai, *Avodah Zara*, no. 813, some of the sources propose an alternate solution: The woman can express the milk and then throw it away. For example: R. Moses of Zurich, *Semak of Zurich*, no. 101; R. Meir b. Barukh, *Shut Maharam* (Prague edition), no. 41.

130. Rubin, *Gentile Tales*, 33.

131. This possibility is also linked with an insinuation against the Jews that appears in a *bulla* of Innocent III from 1208, that mentions that Jews sell the milk that their children do not drink to Christians: "Similar to this is what the Jewish women do with the milk which is publicly sold for the nourishment of children." It is not at all clear that this was breast milk, nor is it clear exactly what the Jewish women do (Grayzel, *Church and the Jews*, doc. 24, pp. 126–27). The entire document discusses practices of the Jews—such as selling non-kosher meat to Christians—that are derogatory to Christians, since they receive substances the Jews themselves refuse to consume. It seems, however, that it was common practice to express breast milk for infants and feed them with bottles. This practice was not allowed on the Sabbath. See: R. Yehiel of Paris, *Piskei R. Yehiel*, no. 9.

132. Maher, *Anthropology of Breast Feeding*, 18; Jane Khatib-Chahidi, "Milk Kinship in Shi'ite Islamic Iran," in *The Anthropology of Breast Feeding*, ed. Vanessa Maher (Oxford, 1992), 109–12.

133. Eric R. Wolf, "Kinship, Friendship and Patron-Client Relationships in Complex Societies," in *The Social Anthropology of Complex Societies*, ed. Michael Banton (Edinburgh, 1966), 1–18; Jane Schneider, "Introduction: The Analytic Strategies of Eric R. Wolf," *Articulating Hidden Histories: Exploring the Influence of Eric R. Wolf*, eds. Jane Schneider and Rayna Rapp (Berkeley, Los Angeles, and London, 1995), 7–9.

134. Chapter 1, pp. 49–52.

135. The main concern was that the nursing infant would die because s/he would refuse to nurse from someone other than his/her mother, or that a suitable wet nurse might not be found. Since this second pregnancy was within the family unit, there was no fear that the father or mother might be careless with their infant's life.

136. Jean-Paul Habicht et al., "The Contraceptive Role of Breast-Feeding," *Population Studies* 39(1989): 213–32; Ulla-Britt Lithell, "Breast-Feeding Habits and Their Relation to Infant Mortality and Marital Fertility," *Journal of Family History* 6(1981): 182–94.

137. One solution for this problem—coitus interruptus, was forbidden in Judaism as in Christianity. This suggestion and others are discussed in BT Yevamot 34b. As this method is discussed several times and repeatedly forbidden in medieval responsa, one can assume that like medieval Christians many Jews were aware of this method and practiced it.

138. For the Christian position, see Brundage, *Law, Sex and Christian Society*, 199, 242, 508. For the ancient Jewish discussion, see Tosefta, Niddah 2:6. The permission given to nursing women (as well as young girls and pregnant women) to use some form of contraception was not without objection. Others claimed that the issue was to be left to the mercy of the heavens and that no preventive measures should be taken.

139. Chapter 1, pp. 24–28.

140. R. Jacob b. Meir, *Sefer haYashar leRabbenu Tam, Ḥeleq haShe'elot vehaTeshuvot*, ed. Shraga Fish Rosenthal (Berlin, 1898), no. 166.

141. Note that in this source the mother is doing the hiring!

142. *SHP*, no. 1188.

143. BT Yevamot 12b and the comments made by the Tosaphot ad locum, s.v. "*Shalosh nashim meshamshot bemokh*." For two different discussions of this topic, see Cohen, "Be Fertile and Increase," 142; Judith Hauptman, *Rereading the Rabbis: A Woman's Voice* (Boulder, 1998), 130–41.

144. I would suggest adding this example to the list of shared ideas pertaining to fertility discussed in chapter 1.

145. The fact that contraception was women's business poses a challenge to historians who wish to study its history, as few written sources remain. Nevertheless, a number of studies have focused on this topic: Angus McLaren, *A History of Contraception* (Oxford, 1990), 101–40; John T. Noonan, *Contraception—A History of Its Treatment by the Catholic Theologians and Canonists* (Cambridge, Mass. and London, 1986), 170–257.

146. See the suggestion made by Soloveitchik, "Review Essay," 233–34.

147. Examples of exactly such behavior are well known in the history of *Niddah* (menstrual purity). For example, Cohen, "Purity, Piety and Polemic," 82–100.

148. R. Jacob b. Meir, *Sefer haYashar*, She'elot uTeshuvot, no. 166.

149. For example: R. Asher b. Yeḥiel, *Shut haRosh*, no. 53, 2, who determines that children should not be given in custody to those who are their potential heirs.

150. Recent scholars have estimated that divorce rates were high, especially after the Black Death. See Israel J. Yuval, "An Appeal against the Proliferation of Divorce in Fifteenth-Century Germany," *Zion* 48(1983): 177–216; and more recently: Grossman, *Pious and Rebellious*, 398–402. We do not know, however, how many women were widowed at a young age; nor do we have divorce statistics for the period before the Black Death.

151. In many questions, it is difficult to discern who is doing the asking, in part because of manuscript considerations.

152. About R. Samson see: Gross, *Gallia Judaica*, 477–78; Urbach, *The Tosaphists*, 118–20; Reiner, *Rabbenu Tam*, 57–60. For his rulings, see: R. Solomon b. Isaac, *Responsa Rashi*, no. 217, n. 13; *Teshuvot Ḥakhmei Provence*, ed. Abraham Schreiber (Sofer) (Jerusalem, 1967), no. 54.

153. R. Solomon B. Isaac, *Responsa Rashi*, no. 217, n. 13; R. Jacob b. Meir, *Sefer haYashar*, no. 11 and parallels: Tosafot, Yevamot 42a, s.v. "*stam*"; Tosafot, Ketubbot 60b, s.v. "*vehilkhata*"; Mordekhai, *Yevamot*, no. 3.

154. R. Solomon, b. Isaac, *Responsa Rashi*, no. 217; R. Jacob b. Meir, *Sefer haYashar*, She'elot uTeshuvot, no. 748.

155. This was the accepted opinion, that of the house of Shammai.

156. See Reiner, *Rabbenu Tam*, 57–60, and R. Jacob b. Meir, *Sefer haYashar*, She'elot uTeshuvot, no. 11. R. Tam bases his ruling on a Gaonic precedent set by R. Aḥai Gaon. This same ruling appears in *Sefer haNiyar*, ed. Gerson Appel (Jerusalem, 1994), 283.

157. Sotah 4:3.

158. BT Yevamot 42b.

159. R. Jacob b. Meir, *Sefer haYashar*, She'elot uTeshuvot, no. 11.

160. Supra, n. 158.

161. The appearance of women before rabbinical courts is a topic that requires further scrutiny.

For our purposes, I will note that R. Eliezer b. Nathan states that in his time, women frequented the courts: *Sefer Ra'avan*, no. 87.

162. Supra, n. 150.

163. For example: R. Meir b. Barukh, *Shut Maharam* (Prague), no. 655, nos. 863–64; R. Meir b. Barukh, *She'elot uTeshuvot* (Crimona), no. 161; R. Asher b. Yeḥiel, *Shut HaRosh*, no. 52; *Sefer Or Zaru'a*, 1: no. 740; Mordekhai, *Ketubbot*, no. 289; *Teshuvot Maimoniyot*, no. 24, and note 164.

164. For example: R. Jacob Hazan, *Eẓ Ḥayim*, Laws of Gittin, no. 9, 195, quotes a book called *Sefer haḤanokhi*, citing R. Samson's opinion and stating that R. Tam did not agree with him. *Sefer haḤanokhi* was written in the thirteenth century and has survived only in fragments quoted in other books. See: Simḥa Emanuel, *The Lost Halakhic Books of the Tosaphists*, Ph.D. Diss., Hebrew University (Jerusalem, 1993), 81, n. 3.

165. Tosafot, Yevamot 36b, s.v. *"VeLo ketanei"*: "And R. Joseph of Orleans ruled that one who marries a nursing woman does not need a divorce; rather, he should simply separate from her." This same ruling appears in Mordekhai, *Ketubbot*, no. 289, regarding a specific case in which a Jewish wet nurse had been hired for the infant and had sworn under grave oath that she would not leave her post before the end of her contract. For a description of how R. Tam's teachings spread in France, see Reiner, *Rabbenu Tam*, 68, and a summary of this topic on p. 113.

166. This was most probably a Jewish wet nurse. See also the discussion above, pp. 129–30.

167. For fairly detailed accounts, see: *Sefer Or Zaru'a*, 1: no. 640; MS Cincinnati 154, no. 5; R. Meir b. Barukh, *Shut Maharam* (Prague), nos. 863–64; R. Meir b. Barukh, *She'elot uTeshuvot* (Lvov), no. 362; MS Cambridge Or. 548, fol. 13, no. 74.

168. Israel M. Ta-Shma, "On the History of Polish Jewry in the Twelfth to Thirteenth Centuries." *Zion* 53(1988): 353–55 [in Hebrew]. Ta-Shma came to this conclusion based on the fact that parts of the manuscripts were torn out, as, for example, in the Cincinnati manuscript. See also Urbach, *The Tosaphists*, 488–91.

169. Ta-Shma cites this ruling, "History of Polish Jewry," 353. This opinion appears in a number of manuscripts: MS Paris héb. 392, fol. 23a; MS Paris héb. 393, fol. 15a; MS Vatican ebr. 176, fol. 50b–51a; MS Moscow Günzburg 1, fol. 22a; MS Parma 813, fol. 42b–43a.

170. For example: R. Meir b. Barukh, *Shut Maharam* (Prague), no. 864.

171. For example, R. Asher b. Yeḥiel, *Shut haRosh*, no. 53.

172. *Teshuvot Hakhmei Provence*, no. 53.

173. *Sefer Or Zaru'a*, 1: no. 740.

174. This fear is mentioned in other sources as well. For example, R. Asher b. Yeḥiel, supra, n. 171.

175. Ta-Shma, "History of Polish Jewry," 353, n. 22; idem, "Children in Medieval Germanic Jewry," 265.

176. Supra, n. 87.

177. In Islam, the situation was very different. See supra, n. 41. It should be noted, however, that while there were severe restrictions for divorcees in Islam, widows were allowed to remarry. A comparison of these matters certainly merits further investigation.

Notes to Chapter 5

Joseph Dan, *Iyyunim beSifrut Ḥasidei Ashkenaz* (Ramat Gan, 1975), 153, excerpted from MS Oxford Bodl., Opp. 540 (1567), fol. 3a.

1. For example: William F. MacLehose, "Nurturing Danger: High Medieval Medicine and the Problem(s) of the Child," in *Medieval Mothering*, eds. John Carmi Parsons and Bonnie Wheeler (New York and London, 1996), 3–24.

2. For example: Dhouda, *Manuel pour mon fils*: Introduction, texte critique, notes par Pierre Riché, traduit par Bernard de Vergille et Claude Mondesert S. J. (*Sources chrétiennes*, 225) (Paris,

1975); *The Goodman of Paris (Le ménagier de Paris)*: A Treatise on Moral and Domestic Economy (c. 1393), trans. Eileen Power (London, 1928).

3. The basis for the different commentaries is BT Kiddushin 30b–31a. The commandment is also explained in great detail in the Books of Commandments (*Sifrei mizvot*) that were popular during the Middle Ages in France: R. Moses of Couçy, *Semag*, Positive commandment, nos. 112–13; R. Joseph b. Isaac of Corbeil, *Semak*, nos. 9 and 50; *Book of Commandments of R. Abraham b. Ephraim* (student of R. Tuviah of Vienne), MS Parma 813, fol. 71a–b; Book of Commandments by an anonymous student of R. Yehiel of Paris, MS Montifiore 136, fol. 26a, no. 125; *Sefer Tosafot haShalem*, Jethro 20:12; R. Joseph Bekhor Shor, *Perushei R. Joseph Bekhor Shor al haTorah*, Kedoshim 19:2, "You shall be holy, for I, the Lord your God, am holy"; *Moshav Zekenim*, Jethro 20:12, "Honor your father."

4. This point is made clear in discussions of children's responsibility to feed and support their parents: BT Kiddushin 30b–31a. Some Christian commentators discuss the same issues. For example: Petrus Pictavensis, *Sentientiarum libri quinque*, PL, 211, 1108–109; Innocent III, *Libellus de elemosyna*, PL, 217, 757. Shulamith Shahar, *Growing Old*, trans. Yael Lotan (London and New York, 1997), 88–97, examines the obligations of children toward their parents as well. This was of interest to both Jews and Christians, as it was part of daily problems and difficulties. In medieval Jewish sources, see *SHP*, no. 126, 929–64, and, especially, 1319–38. In Responsa literature—R. Meir b. Barukh, *Shut Maharam* (Prague edition), no. 16. See also Michael A. Signer, "Honor the Hoary Head: The Aged in Medieval European Jewish Community," in *Aging and the Aged in Medieval Europe*, ed. Michael A. Sheehan (Toronto, 1990), 39–48.

5. *Perushei Joseph Bekhor Shor*, Jethro 20:12. The idea that the person who respects and honors his/her parents appropriately will know how to properly honor God appears in medieval Christian sources as well. See n. 9.

6. BT Kiddushin 31a.

7. MS Vatican ebr. 123, fol. 64b.

8. Besides the three-part relationship of God-father-mother, we cannot ignore the status of teachers/rabbis. The distinction between father and teacher is beyond the limits of our discussion, but has much to do with the further education of boys. For our purposes, it is important to note that the mother is always lowest in the hierarchy. In the Christian context this issue is discussed particularly in light of Jesus' words to his disciples: "He who loves his father and mother more than me is not worthy of me" (Matt. 10:37–38). Many medieval Christian commentators discussed this hierarchy. For example: Anselmus Lauduensis *Expositio in Mattaeum*, PL, 162, 1367–68; St. Bruno Signiensis, *Expositio in Exodum*, PL, 164, 280; 1386; Hugo de St. Victoris, *De sacramentis*, PL, 176, 355; Barbara Newman, *From Virile Woman*, 76–107. After the Reformation, the superiority of the father over the mother was emphasized further in this context. See Marianne Carbonnier-Burkard, "Les variations protestantes," *L'histoire des pères et de la paternité*, eds. Jacques Delemeau et Danîel Roche (Paris, 1990), 169; Ozment, *When Fathers Ruled*, 150–53.

9. BT Kiddushin 30a–31a; *Moshav Zekenim*, Leviticus 19:3.

10. R. Moses of Couçy, *Semag*, Positive commandment, no. 112. The reasoning given here is slightly different from that of the Talmud (BT Kiddushin 31a), where one is supposed to fear the father because he teaches his children Torah.

11. *Moshav Zekenim*, Lev. 19:3.

12. *Midrash aseret hadibrot, Beit haMidrash*, ed. Aaron Yellinek (repr. Jerusalem, 1967), 1:78. On the Midrash, see Joseph Dan, *HaSippur ha'Ivri beYemei haBenayim* (Jerusalem, 1974), 79–85. This idea is echoed in many commentaries from the Middle Ages. For example, MS Oxford Bodl., Mich. 558, fol. 5b.

13. For example, in an early modern book of prayers for the dead, the mother is thanked for bearing and caring for her children when they were small: *Sefer Ma'aneh Lashon. Seder Tefillat Ta'anit al Bet Almin* (Amsterdam, 1678), nos. 6, 7, 9.

14. Shahar, *Women in the Middle Ages*, 98–106; Vecchio, "Good Wife," 121–27.

15. Cadden, *Meanings of Sex Difference*, 117–30; Thomasset, "Nature of Woman," 58–60.
16. Shaḥar, *Women in the Middle Ages*, 98.
17. For example, B. Lanfrancus, *In D. Pauli Epist. Comment., Epist. I Ad Thess., PL,* 150, 334 "non nutrix filios alienos, sed nutrix fovens filios suos" (d. 1089); Herveus Burgidolensis, *Comment. in Epistolas Pauli., in Epist. I ad Thess., PL,* 181, 1361–62 (d. 1149); Petrus Lombardus, *Collectanea in Epist. D. Pauli, in Ep. I ad Thess., PL,* 192, 291–93 (d. 1160).
18. Helinandus, Sermones, XIX in Ass. BVM, *PL,* 212, 638: "Nos illi debemus honorem, quia est mater Domini nostri. Qui enim non honorat matrem, sine dubio inhonorat filium. Iterum Scriptura dicit: *Honora patrem tuum et matrem* (Ex. XX). Quid ergo dicemus fratres? Nonne ipsa est mater nostra. Per illam enim nati sumus, per illam nutrimur, crescimus per illam. Per illam nati sumus, non mundo, sed Deo; per illam nutrimur, non lacte carnis; . . . Per illam crescimus, non magnitude corporus, sed in virtute animae." Helinandus was a Cistercian monk (died 1219). Compare: S. Anselmus Lucensis Episcopi, *Meditatio super salve regina, PL,* 149, 586D; Petrus Cellensis, *Sermones,* In assumptione Beate Mariae Virginis, VIII, *PL,* 202, 868 (12th cent.); Helinandus, *Sermones,* XXI: In Nativitate B. Mariae Virginis I, *PL,* 212, 652. This same image appears in a commentary on Song of Songs 4:2 "Your teeth are like a flock of ewes climbing up from the washing pool." Bede explains: "Dentes sunt ecclesiae, quia panem verbi Dei parvulis illius ad quem mandendum ipsi non sufficiunt parant. Solent quippe piae nutrices particulas panis dentibus conficere et inter lactandum," Venerabilis Beda, *In Cantica Canticorum Allegorica Expositio, PL,* 91, 1130.
19. R. Simon b. Isaac b. Abun and his piyutim are discussed in Grossman, *Sages of Ashkenaz,* 86–102; Leopold Zunz, *Die Literaturgeschichte der synagogalen Poesie* (Berlin, 1865), 112–13.
20. The piyut was published by Avraham M. Haberman, *Liturgical poems of R. Shimon bar Yiẓḥaq* (Berlin and Jerusalem, 1938), 99–100.
21. Naomi, for example, is referred to as an *omenet* (Ruth 4:16), as is Mefiboshet's nurse (2 Sam. 4:4). Moses refers to himself as an *omen*, using the imagery of pregnancy and birth (Num. 11:12). By contrast, his mother, Yokheved, is called a *meneqet*, as is the nurse of Joash (2 Kings 11:2). No such distinction exists in Latin or English. From a feminist point of view, this term is fascinating as it provides a parallel to a mother for a figure who mothers. This is the thesis of many scholars following Nancy Chodorow, *The Reproduction of Mothering: Psychoanalysis and the Sociology of Gender* (Berkeley, Los Angeles, and London, 1978).
22. Rashi, Deut. 32:20, s.v. "*Emun.*"
23. See chapter 1, p. 29.
24. *SHB,* no. 589.
25. Supra, unnumbered note.
26. For example: R. Moses of Couçy, *Semag,* negative commandment no. 81.
27. Ibid., *Isur veheter,* no. 59, 28–29.
28. Both eating and washing are prohibited on Yom Kippur. The legal language uses the feminine in these cases. BT Yoma 77b; Rashi, ad locum, s.v. "*Isha mediḥa yada bemayim; Maḥzor Vitry,* no. 345; R. Jacob b. Meir, *Sefer haYashar, She'elot uTeshuvot,* nos. 52, 2.
29. MS Oxford Bodl., Opp. 77 (844), responses of R. Meir b. Barukh of Rothenburg from 1375, fol. 142, no. 95.
30. Tosafot, Shabbat 111b, s.v. "*Hai mesucraita.*"
31. For example, Bellette, the sister of R. Isaac b. Menahem, and Miriam, the wife of R. Tam, were known to instruct the women of their communities on the observance of precepts pertaining to women. Bellette is mentioned in a number of sources, *Maḥzor Vitry,* 610; R. Eleazer b. Yoel Halevi, *Sefer Ra'aviah,* 1: no. 185, 210; MS Montifiore 134, *Sefer Asufot,* fol. 48c; *Sefer Or Zaru'a,* 1: no. 363. Miriam is mentioned in *Hagahot Maymoniyot, K'dushat Hashem.* Hannah, the sister of R. Tam, is referred to in MS Montifiore 134, *Sefer Asufot,* 77a. All these women are mentioned in the context of laws of ritual purity, food preparation, candle lighting, or making *ẓiẓit,* another ritual task fulfilled by women.

32. R. Meir b. Barukh, *Shut Maharam* (Prague), no. 314 and parallels.

33. In general, the synagogue was a place that children frequented, especially after they reached the age of education, but at a younger age as well. See n. 36.

34. *SHP*, no. 432.

35. *Sefer HaOrah attributed to Rashi*, ed. Solomon Buber (Lemberg, 1905), 2: no. 133; for a slightly different wording of the story, see R. Solomon b. Isaac, *Responsa Rashi*, no. 344.

36. For example: *Midrash Yezirat haValad*, 1: 244; *SHP*, no. 432.

37. *SHP*, no. 484.

38. *SHP*, no. 432 discusses the possibility of the father not attending the synagogue because he was busy caring for his son.

39. Shahar, *Childhood*, 169, nn. 181–83; Berkvam, *Enfance et maternité*, 12.

40. For example: Berthold of Regensburg, a thirteenth-century Franciscan monk, stated that women's devotion to their children was comparable to God's devotion to humanity. Schultz, *Knowledge of Childhood*, 110. On Berthold, see Volker Mertens, "Berthold v. Regensburg," *LdM*, 1:2035–36.

41. Grayzel, *Church and Jews*, 1:180–83: "Ad quod illa respondit, quod cum puer adhuc infans existat, antea partum onerosus, dolorosus in partu, post partum laboriosus matrimonium quam patrimonium nuncupetur, dictus puer apud matrem quam apud patrem."

42. From here the passage is repeated in *SHP*, no. 962.

43. Until this point, I am quoting from *SHP*, no. 301. The end of this passage is from a parallel source, no. 962.

44. *SHP*, no. 301.

45. Shahar, *Childhood*, 169–74; Alain Molinier, "Nourrir, éduquer et transmettre," *L'histoire des pères et de la paternité*, eds. Jacques Delemeau et Daniêl Roche (Paris 1990), 100.

46. *SHP*, no. 302.

47. *SHP*, no. 15.

48. Supra, p. 17.

49. Shahar, *Childhood*, 169–74; Hufton, *The Prospects before Her: A History of Women in Western Europe, 1500–1800* (New York, 1995), 1:177–220.

50. Shahar, *Childhood*, 112–17.

51. R. Judah b. Samuel Hasid, *Perushei haTorah leRabbi Yehuda heHasid*, 1 Kings 3:16, 59.

52. JPS translates the word *tov* as beautiful, but, in this case, the commentator wishes to avoid exactly this translation.

53. The Hebrew word here is *banim*, literally sons. It is unclear, however, if the commentator sought to distinguish between genders in this case. More likely, he employed the male form to refer to male and female children alike.

54. *Sefer Tosafot haShalem*, Exod. 2:2, no. 7.

55. R. Jacob Mulin, *Shut Maharil*, no. 104–105.

56. For a summary of this research, see Hanawalt, "Medievalists and the Study of Childhood."

57. BT Mo'ed Katan 27b.

58. The story first appears in the Maccabees: 2 Macc. 2; 4 Macc. 15–16.

59. This story is attributed to Sefer Hasidim by the Tosafist commentary on BT Kiddushin 80b, s.v. "*K'hahi ma aseh*," which is centered around the verse in Lam. 3:39, "Of what shall a living man complain." I have not found this story in any print or manuscript version of the book. My thanks to Dr. Rami Reiner who discussed this passage with me.

60. *SHP*, no. 293.

61. Haberman, *Gezerot Ashkenaz veZarfat*, 166–67.

62. *SHP*, nos. 132, 322, 327, 541, 1019, 1184, 1526. Others mention this idea as well: Rashi, Ta'anit 8a, s.v. "*MeHulda vebor*"; R. Moses of Zurich, *Semak of Zurich*, no. 356 and no. 402.

63. *Sefer haGematriyot leRabbi Judah heHasid*, fol. 22b.

64. While this passage discusses the possible dire consequences of the sins of mothers and fa-

thers for the lives of children, the source emphasizes the father's responsibility and sorrow, a point I will discuss later.

65. SHP deviates here from the original meaning of the verse. The verse discusses the House of Jacob, who was told by the Lord, who redeemed Abraham, that it will be shamed no more. The commentator here has Jacob redeeming Abraham.

66. SHP, nos. 1526, 1916. For other examples: *Moshav Zekenim*, Gen. 29:31, s.v. "*Ki senu'a Leah.*"

67. SHB, no. 364.

68. SHP, no. 103. See also SHP, no. 102.

69. The Hebrew reads *baḥur gadol*.

70. SHP, no. 327.

71. SHP, no. 345.

72. Quoted in Shaḥar, *Childhood*, 152–52.

73. Supra, n. 70.

74. This distinction is discussed in medieval sources in *Sefer Or Zaru'a*, 2: no. 422; R. Solomon b. Isaac, *Responsa Rashi*, no. 188.

75. *Massekhet S'maḥot*, 3:2–3; BT Mo'ed Katan, 24b.

76. For example, they discuss whether or not a child should be eulogized, and distinguish between children younger and older than age three or five or seven (depending on the opinion). These sources are repeated in the medieval literature with few additions or comments. For example: R. Eliezer b. Nathan, *Even haEzer. Sefer Ra'avan*, Mo'ed Katan 184c–d; R. Moses of Zurich, *Semak of Zurich*, no. 402, Mordekhai, *Mo'ed Katan*, no. 912. We do not know if there were distinctions made in markings on childrens' graves, depending on the age of the child, as none of the medieval tombstones note the age of the child at death. The same is true of Christian gravestones. See Janet Nelson, "Parents, Children and the Church," 91–92.

77. *Sefer haGematriyot leRabbi Judah heḤasid*, fol. 22b.

78. This distinction between younger and older children can be found in the medieval Christian sources as well. See Schultz, *Knowledge of Childhood*, 52–62; Gottlieb, *Family in the Western World*, 155–58.

79. Introduction, p. 2.

80. Goldin, "Die Beziehung der jüdischen Familie," 211–56; Kanarfogel, "Attitudes Toward Childhood," 1–35. For a more moderate approach, see Ta-Shma, "Children in Medieval Germanic Jewry," 263–80.

81. SHP, no. 173.

82. The wife's rights varied from place to place. Scholars have pointed especially to differences between northern and southern Europe: Shaḥar, *Women in the Middle Ages*, 90–93; Leyser, *Medieval Women*, 168–86; James Brundage, "The Merry Widow's Serious Sister: Remarriage in Classical Canon Law," in *Matrons and Marginal Women in Medieval Society*, eds. Robert R. Edwards and Vickie Ziegler (Suffolk, 1995), 33; idem, "Widows As Disadvantaged Persons in Medieval Canon Law," in *Upon My Husband's Death: Widows in the Literature and Histories of Medieval Europe*, ed. Louise Mirrer (Ann Arbor, 1992), 194–205.

83. Klapisch-Zuber, "The Cruel Mother," 117–31, esp. 119–24; Brundage, "Widows As Disadvantaged Persons," 197–201; Elaine Clark, "Mothers at Risk of Poverty in the Medieval English Countryside," in *Poor Women and Children in the European Past*, eds. John Henderson and Richard Wall (London and New York, 1994), 140–42; Brundage, "Merry Widow's Serious Sister," 33–34, 45–48.

84. Leyser, *Medieval Women*, 168–69.

85. Several articles on this topic have been published by Cheryl Tallan, but a broader study is still a desideratum. Cheryl Tallan, "The Economic Productivity of Medieval Jewish Widows," WCJS 11 B1 (Jerusalem, 1994): 151–58; "Opportunities for Medieval Northern European Jewish Widows in the Public and Domestic Spheres," *Upon My Husband's Death*, ed. Louise Mirrer

(Ann Arbor, 1992), 195–206; "The Position of the Medieval Jewish Widow As a Function of Family Structure," *WCJS* 10 B2 (Jerusalem, 1990): 91–98.

86. Examples for this are many. See R. Eleazar b. Joel, *Sefer Ra'aviah*, 4: no. 914.

87. According to Jewish law, a woman was supposed to wait three months so as to be sure that she was not pregnant. However, even women of whom there was no doubt that they were not pregnant were required to wait three months. See, for example, *Sefer Or Zaru'a*, 1:628.

88. *SHP*, no. 1028.

89. For a survey of the studies on the topic, see Shahar, *Childhood*, 121–44. Of special importance is Boswell, *The Kindness of Strangers*, 428–34.

90. Brenda Bolton, "Received in His Name: Rome's Busy Baby Box," in *The Church and Childhood*, ed. Diana Wood (*Studies in Church History*, 31) (Oxford, 1994), 153–68; Toubert, "The Carolingian Moment," 386.

91. As Boswell and others have argued, this medieval practice was very different from abandonment practices in ancient times, in which fathers, even among the nobility, often decided to expose their children, and especially their daughters. Boswell, *Kindness of Strangers*, 183–227; Herlihy, *Medieval Households*, 25–26.

92. BT Yevamot 37a, 85a; BT Kiddushin 75a.

93. R. Jacob Ḥazan of London, *Sefer Eẓ Ḥayim*, 2:313–14. Compare Maimonides, *Issurei Bi'ah*, ch. 15, no. 30, 31.

94. Rashbam, Exod. 2:6, s.v. "*Vatir'ehu et hayeled.*"

95. R. Judah heḤasid, *Perushei haTorah*, Exod. 2:6.

96. MS Parma 86, fol. 29a (p. 55 in the manuscript), no. 103.

97. Boswell, *Kindness of Strangers*, 350–56 argued that while cases of abandonment existed in talmudic times, there were no such cases in the Middle Ages.

98. In the case above, it was clear that the infant was Jewish, but the question does not provide enough details to explain how this was made clear.

99. Shahar, *Childhood*, 121–39.

100. *SHP*, no. 171.

101. Shahar, *Childhood*, 207–209; 237–38.

102. Shahar, *Childhood*, 146–49.

103. Shahar, *Childhood*, 128–29.

104. *SHP*, no. 1917.

105. *SHP*, no. 1918. Compare Muntner, *Sefer Assaf, Korot* 4: no. 243.

106. Caesarius Heisterbacensis, *Dialogus miraculorum*, ed. Josephus Strange (Köln, 1851), Distinctio II, 24: "Ex quibus unus cum multa indugnatione parvulum (parvulam) pede apprehendens, allisit ad parietem."

107. In recent years, a tremendous amount of research on single mothers and illegitimate birth in the past has been conducted: Peter Landau, "Das Weihehindernis der Illegitimität in der Geschichte des kanonischen Rechts," in *Illegitimität im Spätmittelalter*, ed. Ludwig Schmugge (München, 1994), 15–21; Schultz, *Knowledge of Childhood*, 124; Yves Brissaud, "L'infanticide à la fin du Moyen Age, ses motivations psychologiques et sa répression," *Revue historique de droit français et étranger* 50(1972): 229–56; Marianne Carbonnier-Burkard, "Perenniser et concevoir," 90–94; Michael Mitterauer, *Ledige Mutter. Zur Geschichte unehelicher Geburten in Europa* (Munich, 1983), 13–21.

108. For example: *Sefer Or Zaru'a*, 1:652. Compare Bulst, "Illegitimate Kinder," 33–34.

109. For example: *Teshuvot Maimoniyot*, no. 8; R. Meir b. Barukh, *Shut Maharam* (Prague), no. 98; R. Solomon b. Aderet, *She'elot uTeshuvot*, 1: nos. 832–33; *SHP*, no. 126.

110. *SHP*, no. 1301.

111. Urbach, "*Mavet biShegaga,*" 319.

112. Barbara Kellum, "Infanticide in England in the Later Middle Ages," *History of Childhood Quarterly* 1(1973–74): 369–71 and more recently, Phillip Gavitt, "Infant Death in Late Medieval

Florence: The Smothering Hypothesis Reconsidered," in *Medieval Family Roles: A Book of Essays*, ed. Cathy Jorgensen Itnyre (New York and London, 1996), 137–53.

113. One should note that while we are familiar with penances in Christianity from the Early Middle Ages, there are few penances in Jewish culture in ancient times. Penances were popular among Ḥasidei Ashkenaz, and some scholars have suggested that the adoption of penitential practices by Jews was due to their immersion in Christian culture. See Yitzhak Baer, "The Religious-Social Tendency of 'Sepher Ḥassidim,'" 1–50; Fishman, "The Penitential System of Ḥasidei Ashkenaz," 201–30. These penitential practices were quickly and widely accepted.

114. MS Oxford Bodl., Opp. Add. 34, fol. 57b in the margins. My thanks to Professor Ivan Marcus who referred me to this manuscript.

115. MS Darmstadt, Cod. Or. 25, fol. 116d and with minor variations: MS Parma 86, fol. 29b, no. 104. The same penance is also attributed to R. Ḥayim Paltiel, MS Oxford Bodl., Mich. 84, fol. 27b: "My dear Samuel. I am deeply saddened by the incident, and you should know that the Ge'onim ruled that a woman who finds a child dead next to her [in bed], this is an accident that borders on a deliberate deed. Nevertheless, I cannot be stringent with the woman with regard to fasting. For some women miscarry as a result of excessive fasting. And her penance will be within a 365–day period, Mondays and Thursdays, or forty consecutive days, or three consecutive days and nights. But this is impossible for a pregnant woman. And it is good if she calculate how many Mondays and Thursdays are in a 365–day year, excluding Ḥanuka and the month of Nisan and Ḥol haMo'ed when one may not fast. And she should fast one day a week until she completes [her fasting period], and give as much charity as she can, and shalom to all, Ḥayim Paltiel." In the same manuscript on fol. 28 in the margins, we find: "And my teacher told me what his teacher R. Judah Katz said about women who find small children dead in their beds; he said that one should be strict with them, and that [the deaths of the children] are considered deliberate deeds and not accidental transgressions. And so I found in the responsa of Maharam." I thank Dr. Simḥa Emanuel who generously shared his vast knowledge of these manuscripts with me.

116. For example, R. Jacob Mulin, *Shut Maharil*, no. 45; Eisik Tirna, *Sefer haMinhagim*, ed. Shlomo J. Spitzer (Jerusalem, 1979), 89, n. 97.

117. The response, as it appears in the early modern literature, combines the different medieval responses. See Urbach, "*Mavet biShegaga*," 322, who quotes the later responsa but states that he could not find the medieval ones. For the early modern response, see Jacob Elbaum, *Repentance and Self-Flagellation in the Writings of the Sages of Germany and Poland 1348–1648* (Jerusalem, 1992), 48–49, n. 6, 230. The distinction between cradle and not-cradle cultures and the corresponding responsibility of parents for these deaths is found in Mishna Makkot, 2:1; Tosefta Makkot 2:4; PT Makkot chap. 2, no. 4. The Babylonian Talmud does not discuss the issue. For a discussion of these sources, see Urbach, "*Mavet biShegaga*," 319–20.

118. This attitude is demonstrated clearly in the sixteenth-century response. Urbach, "*Mavet biShegaga*," 321–22, quotes from R. Benjamin b. Abraham Selnik's responsa: "About the woman who laid her child down in the cradle and knows nothing more. [She knows not] how her child got [to her bed] from the cradle; she has no memory of when she laid the child lying dead in her arms. No one knows who hit him and when, and the servant says that when she gave the infant to his mother and that she put the breast in his mouth, and that the mother took the child from her. And, furthermore, the servant says that when she gave the child to his mother she got angry at the servant and cursed her. But the mother says she is unaware of all of this." Benjamin Aaron b. Abraham Selnik, *Mas'at Binyamin* (Krakow, 1633), no. 26.

119. McNeill and Gamer, *Medieval Handbooks of Penance*, 254, 275, 293, 302.

120. Alexandre-Bidon et Closson, *L'enfant à l'ombre des cathédrales*, 25.

121. Peter Abelard, *Ethica*, ed. and trans. David E. Luscombe (Oxford, 1971), 17, nos. 79–80.

122. Boswell suggested that oblation was also a form of abandonment: *Kindness of Strangers*, 225–28. On mothers who abandoned their children and joined monastic orders, see: Atkinson, *Oldest Vocation*, 167–91; Newman, *From Virile Woman*, 78–96.

123. Anneke Mulder-Bakker, *Sanctity and Motherhood: Essays on Holy Mothers in the Middle Ages* (New York, 1995), "Introduction," 7–8. These figures are popular from the eleventh century onward.

124. The story of Anna, mother of Mary, was also used in this context. According to the Protoevangelion of Jacob, a text widely accepted in the West during the Middle Ages, the Virgin Mary was also brought to the temple at a young age as an oblate. Newman, *From Virile Woman*, 78–96.

125. Newman, *From Virile Woman*, 84–99; Kleus Arnold, *Kind und Gesellschaft* (Paderborn, 1980), 38.

126. Newman, *From Virile Woman*, 76–89. For Griselda's story, see Geoffrey Chaucer, *Canterbury Tales*, ed. Walter W. Skeat (Oxford, 1940), 4: The Clerk's Tale, 1. 1081–85: "She bothe hir yonge children un-to hir calleth, And in hir armes pitously wepings, Embraceth hem and tendrely kissinge, Ful lyk a mooder, with her salte teres, She batheth both hir visage and hir heres." This story has been studied frequently in recent years. For other interpretations and historical analyses, see Atkinson, *The Oldest Vocation*, 144–93, esp. 144–49; and Klapisch-Zuber, "The Griselda Complex," 213–21.

127. Newman, *From Virile Woman*, 105–06.

128. Much has been written about the chronicles in recent years. See Marcus, "From Politics to Martyrdom: Shifting Paradigms in the Hebrew Narratives of the 1096 Crusade Riots," *Prooftexts* 2 (1982):40–52; Robert Chazan, *European Jewry and the First Crusade* (Berkeley, 1981); Jeremy Cohen, "'The Persecutions of 1096'—From Martyrdom to Martyrology: The Sociocultural Context of the Hebrew Crusade Chronicles," *Zion* 59 (1994):169–208 [in Hebrew]; Israel J. Yuval, "Vengeance and Damnation, Blood and Defamation: From Jewish Martyrdom to Blood Libel Accusations," *Zion* 58 (1993):33–90 [in Hebrew].

129. The theme of the Sacrifice of Isaac and the First Crusade has been explored at length: See Spiegel, "Me'aggadot haAkeda," in *Alexander Marx Jubilee Volume*, ed. Saul Lieberman (New York, 1959), Hebrew Section, 471–547; Marcus, "From Politics to Martyrdom," 40–52.

130. A hint of this can be found in the tradition of the four *tekufot* (seasons) of the year in which blood and water intermingle. This tradition posits that the spirit of Jephthe's daughter and that of Isaac hovers over the waters in the wells during the first four dangerous days at the beginning of each season. See *Mahzor Vitry*, no. 580 in the addenda, 14. I thank Professor Israel Yuval for pointing this passage out to me.

131. This is the narrative in *Sefer Yossipon*, ed. David Flusser (Jerusalem, 1978), 15:60–67, p. 74 as well as in the Crusade chronicles.

132. *Sefer Yossipon*, Flusser edition, 15:60–67, p. 74, and compare with *Sefer Yossipon*, Houminer edition (Jerusalem, 1955), 19:76.

133. 2 Macc. 7:20–23.

134. 4 Macc. 16:5–11.

135. This idea is expressed in many of the sources quoted by Mc Laughlin, "Survivors and Surrogates," 123–39.

136. The Jewish response to 1096 has never been examined in light of what it reflects about relations between parents and children.

137. For claims that the suicides during the Crusades were proof of the divergent attitudes of Jews and Christians toward their children: Goldin, "Jewish Children and Christian Missionizing," 98–99.

138. "But if a child was ushered into the other religion—how should this matter? . . . For he cannot distinguish between right and left," Mordekhai, *Mo'ed Katan*, no. 886; Mordekhai, *Sanhedrin*, no. 716.

139. For example: Haberman, *Gezerot Ashkenaz veZarfat*, 75; 56; 95; David Malkiel has recently suggested that many families were divided over the question of slaughtering their children: "Vestiges of Conflict in the Hebrew Crusade Chronicles," *Journal of Jewish Studies* 52(2001): 323–40.

140. Haberman, *Gezerot Ashkenaz veZarfat*, 37. This story has been discussed extensively in research in recent years: Chazan, *European Jewry*, 103–105; Cohen, "Persecutions," 185–95; Yuval, "Vengeance and Damnation," 68. My reading of this event differs slightly from that of Yuval's.

141. Haberman, *Gezerot Ashkenaz veZarfat*, 35, and in translation: Chazan, *European Jewry*, 238. I have changed the last two words of the second sentence from "in their pseudo-faith" as Chazan translated these with: "to their erroneous faith."

142. Haberman, *Gezerot Ashkenaz veZarfat*, 34.

143. Cohen, "*Persecutions*," 195–205, esp. 199–200, compares Rachel to the Virgin Mary in her aspect of *mater dolorosa*, a comparison that is very apt for my purposes here. He then proceeds to expand this comparison to include *synagoga* and *ecclesia*. For my purposes, the more immediate comparison and contrast between Hosea and Psalms should suffice.

144. Haberman, *Gezerot Ashkenaz veZarfat*, 96.

145. For example, ibid., 79, in which two women kill a newborn to prevent his falling into the hands of the Crusaders.

146. For the Christian response to these deeds, see: Albertis Aachenis, *Recueil des historiens des croisades*, Historiens occidentaux 2 (Paris, 1879), 293: "Matres pueris lactentibus, quod dictu nefas est, guttura ferro secabant, alios transforabant, volentes potius sic propriis manibus perire, quam incirconcisorum armis exstingui"; Yuval, "Vengeance and Damnation," 75–79; Minty, "*Kiddush haShem*," 214–47. I reject the suggestion of Magdalene Schultz that Christian anger was the result of their own feelings of inferiority because Christians believed Jews loved their children more than they did: "The Blood Libel: A Motif in the History of Childhood," *Journal of Psychohistory* 14(1986): 1–23, esp. 7–10.

147. It is interesting to note that the actions of Jewish women are mentioned mainly in the internal Jewish discourse and receive no comment in most of the Christian writings documenting this period. Albert of Aachens, quoted above, is an exception to this rule. See, for example, the cases discussed by Yuval, "Vengeance and Damnation," 76; Minty, "*Kiddush haShem*," 214–26.

Notes to Conclusion

1. For a comparison between the education of boys and girls, see Baumgarten, "Religious Education of Children in Medieval Jewish Society" (forthcoming).

2. See Appendix to chapter 2.

3. Haym Soloveitchik, "Religious Law and Change: The Medieval Ashkenazic Example," *AJS Review* 12(1986): 205–22. The author points to the self-image of the community during the eleventh and twelfth centuries, but does not inquire as to how this self-conception changed over time. See also: Israel J. Yuval, "Heilige Städte, Heilige Gemeinden. Mainz als des Jerusalem Deutschlands," in *Judische Gemeinden und Organisationsform*, eds. Robert Jütte und Abraham P. Kustermann (Wien, 1996), 91–101.

4. Marcus, "From Politics to Martyrdom," 40–52.

5. Susan Einbinder, "Jewish Women Martyrs: Changing Models of Representation," *Exempleria* 12(2000): 105–27.

6. Lett, *L'enfant des miracles*, 107–14; Taglia, "The Cultural Construction of Childhood," 255–88, esp. 258–65; Bolton, "Mulieres Sanctae," 77–95; Bynum, *Holy Feast and Holy Fast*, 21–23.

GLOSSARY

'Arvit—Evening prayers.
Ba'al brit (f. *ba'alat brit*, pl. *ba'alei brit, ba'alot brit*)—Figure chosen by parents to hold infant at circumcision ceremony.
Challah—Bread, the "obligation of challah" requires that the baker break off a piece of dough and burn it.
Cohen—Person of priestly (Aaronic) descent.
Get—Divorce writ.
Halakhah—Legal practices and observances of Judaism.
Ḥazan—Cantor.
Isha Ḥakhama—Lit. wise woman, midwife.
Kahal—Congregation.
Ketubbah—Marriage agreement that protects woman's monetary rights.
Kiddush haShem—Sanctifying the name of God.
Kindbett (Kindbetterin)/Maḥzor—Book of ritual prayers.
Meyaledet—Midwife.
Mikve—Ritual bath.
Mila—Circumcision.
Minḥa—Afternoon prayers.
Miẓvot Ḥannah—Three precepts that are considered women's commandments—challah, niddah, and lighting Sabbath candles.
Mohel (pl. *mohalim, mohalot*)—Circumciser.
Niddah—Impurity of menstruation.
Onah—Conjugal obligations of a husband toward his wife.
Piyut (pl. *piyutim*)—Liturgicpoem.
Rosh haShana—New Year.
Sandek—Synonym of ba'al brit.
Sefer Ḥasidim—Book of moral advice and instruction written primarily by R. Judah the Pious in early thirteenth-century Germany.
Sefer Miẓvot (pl. *Sifrei Miẓvot*)—Halakhic books of a popular genre in the thirteenth century that enumerate each commandment.
Shaḥarit—Morning prayers.
Shekhina—Presence of God in the world, term often used in mystical texts.
Shema—Prayer said twice a day, one of the first prayers children were taught.
Shushvin (pl. *shushvinim*)—Two shushvinim were chosen, one by the groom's side and one by the bride's side to represent each family before and during the wedding.
Streya—Witches.
Takkanah (pl. *takkanot*)—Regulations governing the internal life of communities.
Tefillin—Phylacteries.
Tekhine—Prayer.
Wimpel—A cloth diaper taken from the circumcision ceremony and made into a Torah binder.
Ẓiẓit—Ritual garment with fringes.

BIBLIOGRAPHY

Many Hebrew books contain English title pages. In order to enable non-Hebrew-speaking readers access to these titles, I have provided these titles whenever they were available. In these cases, I have not used the rules of transliteration adopted for this book. Rather, I have followed the spelling used by their authors.

Manuscripts

Cambridge, University Library
Add. 3127: Customs.
Dd. 68/10: Medical treatise.
Or: 548: Responsa of R. Meir b. Barukh.
Or. 786: *Midrash Shoher Tov*; Issur veHeter miBeit Midrasho shel Rashi.

Cincinnati Hebrew Union College
154: *Sefer Or Zaru'a*.

Darmstadt, Stadtarchiv
Cod. Or. 25: Responsa of R. Meir b. Barukh.

London, Jews College, Montifiore Collection
134: *Sefer Asufot*.
136: Customs of the student of R. Yehiel of Paris.

Moscow, Russian State Library, Günzburg Collection
1: *Sefer Mizvot of R. Abraham b. Ephraim*.
481: Sections of *Mahzor Vitry*.
1390: Disputation of R. Yehiel of Paris.

New York, Jewish Theological Seminary
Mic. 8092: *Mahzor Vitry*.

Oxford, Bodleian Library (numbers in Neubauer Catalog are listed in brackets)
Heb. d. 11 (2797): Creation of the fetus.
Hunt. 404, (794): Customs.
Mich. 9 (1531): Amulets.
Mich. 84 (784): Responsa of R. Meir b. Barukh; sections from *Sefer Hasidim*.
Mich. 365 (1208): Commentaries on *Piyutim*.
Mich. 455 (146): *Sefer ha Parnas*.
Mich. 558 (2256): Customs.
Opp. 31 (271): Medical treatise.

Opp. 59 (1100): *Maḥzor Vitry*.
Opp. 73 (640): *Sefer haTerumah*.
Opp. 77 (844): Responsa of R. Meir b. Barukh.
Opp. 170 (1205): Commentaries on *Piyutim*.
Opp. 317 (692): *Responsa*.
Opp. 642 (1106): *Customs*.
Opp. 687 (2138): *Book of Assaf haRofe*.
Opp. Add. 14 (1101): *Maḥzor Vitry*; legal rulings.
Opp. Add. 34 (641): Responsa; *Sefer Ḥasidim*; *Sefer haTerumah*.

Paris, Bibliothèque nationale

héb. 326: Legal rulings.
héb. 327: *Sefer Tashbez*.
héb. 363: *Sefer Rokeah*.
héb. 392: *Sefer Mizvot of R. Abraham b. Ephraim*.
héb. 393: *Sefer Mizvot of R. Abraham b. Ephraim*.
héb. 643: *Sefer Tashbez*; *Sefer Mizvot Katan*.
héb. 1120: Medical treatise.
héb. 1122: Medical treatise.
héb. 1408: legal rulings.

Parma, Biblioteca Paltaina

403: Siddur, *Maḥzor Vitry*.
563: Creation of the fetus.
571: *Sefer Tashbez*.
813: *Sefer haTerumah*, *Sefer Mizvot of Rabbi Abraham b. Ephraim*.
86: Responsa of R. Meir b. Barukh.
Pal. 2342: Cures and amulets.
Pal. 2757: Responsa of R. Meir b. Barukh.
Pal. 2897: *Sefer haTerumah*.

Vatican

ebr. 44: Creation of the fetus.
ebr. 123: Commentary on the Pentateuch.
ebr. 176: *Sefer Mizvot of R. Abraham b. Ephraim*.

Verona, Seminar

Heb. 34: Sections of *Maḥzor Vitry*.

Primary Sources

Aaron b. Jacob haCohen of Lunelle. *Sefer Orḥot Ḥayyim*, ed. Moses Schlesinger, 3 vols. (Berlin, 1912).
Abelardus, Petrus. *Ethica*, ed. and trans. David E. Luscombe (Oxford, 1971).
———. *The Letters of Abelard and Héloise*, trans. Betty Radice (Hammondsworth, 1974).

Abraham b. Nathan of Lunelle. *Sefer haManhig*. (Rulings and Customs), Introduction and Explanations by Yitzhak Raphael, 2 vols. (Jerusalem, 1978).
Albertus Aachensis. *Recueil des historiens des croisades (Historiens occidentaus* 2) (Paris, 1879).
Anselmus Lauduensis. *Expositio in Matthaeum, PL* 162: 1227–498.
Anselmus Lucensis. *Sermones, PL* 149: 475–85.
Asher b. Yeḥiel. *Shut haRosh*, ed. Shlomo Yudelov (Jerusalem, 1994).
Bartholomaeus Anglicus. *De genuinis rerum coelestium terrestrium et inferarum* (Frankfurt, 1601).
Barukh b. Isaac. *Sefer haTerumah* (Warsaw, 1897).
Beda Venerabilis. *Expositionis in Cantica Canticorum, PL* 91: 1065 1234.
Beit haMidrash, ed. Aaron Jellinek, 6 parts in 2 vols. (repr. Jerusalem, 1967).
Benjamin Aaron b. Abraham Selnik. *Mas'at Binyamin* (Krakow, 1633).
Bruno Episcopis Signiensis. *Expositio in Exodum, PL* 164: 233–376.
Burchardus Wormatiensis Episcopi. *Decretorum, PL* 140: 537–1096.
Caesarius Heisterbacensis. *Dialogus miraculorum*, ed. Josephus Strange (Köln, 1851).
Chaucer, Geoffrey. *Canterbury Tales*, ed. Walter W. Skeat (Oxford, 1940) (4th ed.).
Dhouda. *Manuel pour mon fils*, introduction, texte critique, notes par Pierre Riché, traduit par Bernard de Vergille et Claude Mondesert S.J., (*Sources chrétiennes*, 225) (Paris, 1975).
Eisik Tirna. *Sefer haMinhagim of Rabbi Eisik Tirna*, ed. Shlomo J. Spitzer (Jerusalem, 1979).
Eleazar b. Joel. *Sefer Ra'aviah*, ed. Victor Aptowizer, 4 vols. (Jerusalem, 1964[2]).
Eleazar b. Judah. *Perush haRokeah al haTorah* (A Commentary on the Bible of Rabbi Eleazar of Worms), ed. Chaim Kanyevsky, 5 vols. (Bnei Brak, 1986).
———. *Perushei Siddur HaTefila LaRokeach*, ed. Moshe Hershler and Judah Alter Hershler, 2 vols. (Jerusalem, 1992).
———. *Sefer Rokeaḥ* (Fano, 1505).
———. *Sefer haRokeaḥ haGadol* (Jerusalem, 1960).
Elḥanan b. Isaac of Dampierre. *Tosfot al Massakhet Avodah Zara* (Tos'foth zum Trac. Aboda Sara), ed. David Fränkel (Husiatyn, 1901).
Eliezer b. Nathan. *Sefer Even haEzer: Sefer Ra'avan* (Jerusalem, 1984).
Gershom b. Judah. *Teshuvot Rabbenu Gershom Me'or haGolah*, ed. Shlomo Eidelberg (New York, 1956).
Glückel bas Judah, *Memoirs*, trans. Marvin Lowenthal (New York, 1977).
The Goodman of Paris (Le ménagier de Paris): A Treatise on Moral and Domestic Economy (c. 1393), trans. Eileen Power (London, 1928).
HaḤiluqim shebein Anshei Mizraḥ uBnei Ereẓ Israel, ed. Mordekhai Margaliyot (Jerusalem, 1938).
Halakhot Pesukot min haGeonim (Kurze Geonäische Entscheidungen), ed. Joel Müller (Krakow, 1893).
Ḥayim b. Isaac. *Piskei Halakha shel R. Ḥayim Or Zaru'a (Drashot Maharaḥ)*, ed. Isaac Samson Lange (Jerusalem, 1973).
———. *Sefer She'elot uTeshuvot Maharaḥ Or Zaru'a*, ed. Isaac Alexander Rosenberg (Leipzig, 1860).
Helinandus frigidis montis monachis. *Sermones, PL* 212: 481–720.
Henricus de Segusio. *Summa Aurea* (Venice, 1581).

Hermann von der Hardt, *Juris Judaeorum canonici prodromus, De circumcisione* (Helmstadt, 1700).
Hermannus Boniensis. *Das Viaticum narrationem des Hermannus Boniensis*, ed. Alfons Hilka (Berlin, 1935).
Herveus Burgidolensis. *Commentaria in Isaiam*, PL 181: 18–590.
Hildegardis Bigensis. *Causae et curae*, ed. Paul Kaiser (Leipzig, 1903).
―――. *Liber subtilitateum diversarum naturam creaturarum*, ed. Charles Daremberg and F. A. Reuss, PL 197: 1177–1350.
―――. *Scivias*, ed. Adelgundis Führkötter O.S.B. collaborante Angela Carlevaris O.S.B., (*CCCM* 43) (Turnholti, 1978).
Hugo de St. Victoire. *Des sacramentis fidei Christianae*, PL 176: 173–612.
Innocentius III. *Libellus de elemosyna*, PL 217: 747–60.
Isaac b. Joseph of Corbeil. *Sefer'Amudei Golah haNikra Semak* (reprint Jerusalem, 1979).
Isaac b. Moses. *Sefer Or Zaru'a*, 4 parts, 2 vols. (Zhitomir, 1862).
Isaac b. Nathan, *Perush Rivan leMassekhet Yevamot*, ed. Efraim Kupfer (Jerusalem, 1977).
Jacob and Gershom the Circumcisers. *Sefer Zikhron Brit*, ed. Jacob Glassberg (Berlin, 1892).
Jacob b. Judah Ḥazar of London. *Eẓ Ḥayyim*, ed. Israel Brodie, 3 vols. (Jerusalem, 1962–64).
Jacob b. Meir. *Sefer haYashar leRabbenu Tam. Ḥeleq haḤidushim*, ed. Shimon Shlomo Schlesinger (Jerusalem, 1959).
―――. *Sefer haYashar leRabbenu Tam: Ḥeleq haShe'elot vehaTeshuvot*, ed. Shraga Fish Rosenthal (Berlin, 1898).
Jacob b. Moses Mulin. *Sefer Maharil: Minhagim* (The Book of Maharil: Customs by Rabbi Yaacov Mulin), ed. Shlomoh J. Spitzer (Jerusalem, 1989).
―――. *Shut Maharil* (Responsa of Rabbi Yaacov Molin-Maharil), ed. Yitzchok Satz (Jerusalem, 1979).
―――. *Shut Maharil haḤadashot* (New Responsa of Rabbi Yaacov Molin-Maharil), ed. Yitzchok Satz (Jerusalem, 1977).
Jacob Barukh b. Judah Landa. *Sefer haAgur haShalem*, ed. Moses Hershler (Jerusalem, 1960).
Jacob Weil. *She'elot uTeshuvot Mahari Weil*, ed. Yitzchok Satz (Jerusalem, 1988).
Jacobus de Voragine. *Legenda Aurea*, ed. Theodor Graesse (Dresden and Leipzig, 1845).
Johann Dominicus Mansi. *Sacrorum conciliorum nova et amplissima collectio*, 22 (Graz, 1961).
Joseph b. Moses. *Sefer Leket Yosher*, ed. Jacob Freimann (Berlin, 1904).
Joseph Bekhor Shor. *Perushei R. Joseph Bekhor Shor al haTorah*, ed. Yehoshafat Nevo (Jerusalem, 1994).
Joseph Juspa Hahn Neurlingen. *Sefer Yosef Omeẓ* (Frankfurt, 1928).
Joseph Juspa Kashman, *Noheg kaZon Yosef* (Tel Aviv, 1969).
Jousep (Juspa) Schammes. *Minhagim deKehilat Kodesh Wormeisa* (Wormser Minhagbuch), eds. Benjamin Salomon Hamburger and Erich Zimmer, 2 vols. (Jerusalem, 1988).
Judah Löw Kirchheim. *Minhagot Wormeisa* (The Customs of Worms Jewry), ed. Isaac Mordechai Peles (Jerusalem, 1987).

Judah b. Nathan. *Perush Masekhet Yevamot leRabbenu Yehuda ben Nathan*, ed. Efraim Kupfer (Jerusalem, 1977).
Judah b. Samuel. *Perushei haTorah leRabbi Yehuda heḤasid*, ed. Isaac Samson Lange (Jerusalem, 1975).
———. *Sefer Gematriot of R. Judah the Pious*, introduction by Daniel Abrams and Israel M. Ta-Shma (Los Angeles, 1998).
———. *Sefer Ḥasidim* (Das Buch der Frommen), ed. Judah Wistinetzki (Frankfurt, 1924²).
———. *Sefer Ḥasidim according to MS Parma H3280*, introduction by Ivan G. Marcus (Jerusalem, 1985).
———. *Sefer Ḥasidim*, ed. Reuven Margaliyot (Jerusalem, 1957) (based on Bologna edition).
Konrad von Megenberg. *Das Buch der Natur*, ed. Franz Pfiffer (Hildesheim, 1962).
Leon Modena. *Historia de riti hebraici* (Venice, 1678).
Maḥzor leYamim Nora'im, ed. Daniel Goldschmidt, 2 vols. (Jerusalem, 1970).
Maḥzor Pesach, ed. Jonah Frankel (Jerusalem, 1993).
Maḥzor Vitry, ed. Simon haLevi Horowitz (Nürnberg, 1892).
Massekhet Smakhot, ed. Michael Higger (New York, 1934).
Meir b. Barukh of Rothenburg. *Sefer Hilkhot Smakhot haShalem*, ed. Akiba Dov and Jacob Aaron Landa (Jerusalem, 1976).
———. *Sefer Minhagim deBei Maharam b. Barukh meRotenburg* (Sefer Minhagim of the School of Rabbi Meir ben Baruch of Rothenburg), ed. Israel Elfenbein (New York, 1938).
———. *Sefer Sha'arei Teshuvot Maharam b. Barukh*, Berlin ed., ed. Moses Arye Blakh (Berlin, 1891).
———. *Sefer She'elot uTeshuvot*, Crimona ed. (repr. Jerusalem, 1986).
———. *Sefer Shut Maharam b. Barukh*, Prague ed., ed. Moses Arye Blakh (Budapest, 1895).
———. *She'elot uTeshuvot*, ed. R. N. Rabinowitz (Lvov, 1860).
———. *Teshuvot Pesakim uMinhagim* (Responsa, Rulings, and Customs), ed. Isaac Ze'ev Cahana, 3 vols. (Jerusalem, 1957–62).
Menaḥem Ibn Zeraḥ. *Zeida laDerekh* (Warsaw, 1880).
Menaḥem b. Shlomo. *Midrash Sekhel Tov*, ed. Shlomo Buber (Berlin, 1900).
Midrash Eikha Rabbah, ed. Shlomo Buber (Vilna, 1899).
Midrash Rabbah, ed. Moses Arye Mirkin, 11 vols. (Tel Aviv, 1968²).
Midrash Shemot Rabbah. Chapters I–XIV, ed. Avigdor Shinan (Jerusalem, 1984).
Midrash Shemuel, ed. Shlomo Buber (Krakow, 1993).
Midrash Tanḥuma, ed. Ḥanokh Zundel (Jerusalem, 1969).
Midrash Tanḥuma, ed. Shlomo Buber, 2 vols. (repr. New York, 1946).
Midrash Tehillim haMekhune Shoḥer Tov, ed. Shlomo Buber (Vilna, 1891; repr. New York, 1947).
Midrash Wayyikra Rabbah, ed. Mordecai Margulies, 2 vols. (New York-Jerusalem, 1893³).
Moses b. Isaac Mintz. *She'elot uTeshuvot Rabbenu Moshe Mintz* (*Maharam Mintz*), ed. Jonathan Shraga Domb, 2 vols. (Jerusalem, 1991).
Moses b. Jacob of Couçy. *Sefer Miẓvot haGadol*, 2 vols. (Venice, 1547, repr. Jerusalem, 1961).

Moses Henochs Altschul-Jeruschalmi. *Brantspiegel*, ed. Sigrid Riedel (Frankfurt, 1992).
Moses of Zurich. *Sefer haSemak miZurich*, ed. Isaac Jacob Har-Shoshanim-Rosenberg, 3 vols. (Jerusalem, 1973).
Moses Parnas. *Sefer haParnas* (Vilna, 1897).
Moshav Zekenim al haTorah, ed. Shlomo David Sasson (London, 1959).
Nathan b. Yehiel. Sefer Arukh haShalem, ed. Alexander Kohut, 8 vols. (Vienna, 1926).
Nissim b. Jacob of Kirouan, *Hibbur haYafe min haYeshhu'a*, trans. and introduction by Hayim Z. Hirshberg (Jerusalem, 1954).
Ozar HaGaonim (Thesaurus of the Gaonic Responsa and Commentaries), ed. Benjamin M. Lewin, 13 vols. (Haifa-Jerusalem, 1930–43).
Ozar Midrashim: A Library of Two Hundred Minor Midrashim, ed. Judah David Eisenstein, 2 vols. (New York, 1915).
Petrus Cellensis. *Sermones, PL* 202: 637–928.
Petrus Lombardus. *Collectaneorum in epist: S. Pauli, PL* 192: 9–518.
Petrus Pictavensis. *Sententiarum libri quinque, PL* 211:783–1287.
Pirke deRabbi Eliezer, ed. Hayim M. Horowitz (Jerusalem, 1973).
Samson b. Abraham of Sens, *Shitat Kadmonim al Massekhet Avodah Zara*, ed. Moses Judah Blau (New York, 1969).
Samson b. Zadok, *Sefer haTashbez* (Warsaw, 1901).
Seder Rav Amram Gaon, ed. Daniel Goldschmidt (Jerusalem, 1972).
Sefer Assaf haRofe, ed. Züssman Muntner, *Korot* 3–5 (1966–71).
Sefer haNiyar, ed. Gerson Appel (Jerusalem, 1994).
Sefer Jossipon, ed. David Flusser, 2 vols. (Jerusalem, 1978).
Sefer Jossipon, ed. Hayim Houminer (Jerusalem, 1957).
Sefer Ma'aneh Lashon: Seder Tefillat Ta'anit al Bet Almin (Amsterdam, 1678).
Sefer Sha'arei Zedek: Teshuvot min haGeonim (Jerusalem, 1966).
Sefer Tosafot haShalem (Commentary on the Bible), ed. Jacob Gellis, 10 vols. (Jerusalem, 1982–95).
Sepher haPardes (Liturgical and Ritual Work, attributed to Rashi), ed. Haym Judah Ehrenreich (Budapest, 1924).
She'eltot Rav Ahai Gaon, ed. Samuel K. Mirsky, 5 vols. (Jerusalem, 1959).
Siddur R. Saadja Gaon, eds. Israel Davidson, Simha Assaf, and Issascar Joel (Jerusalem, 1941).
Siddur R. Shlomo b. R. Nathan haSigilmasi, ed. Shmuel Haggai (Jerusalem, 1995).
Siddur R. Solomon b. Samson of Worms, ed. Moshe Hershler (Jerusalem, 1971).
Simon b. Isaac. *Piyutei R. Shimon beRabbi Yizhaq* (Liturgical Poems of R. Shimon bar Yishaq), ed. Avraham Meir Haberman (Berlin-Jerusalem, 1938).
Solomon b. Aderet. *She'elot uTeshuvot* (Bnei Brak, 1958).
Solomon b. Isaac (Rashi). *HaOrah* (Ritualwerk), ed. Salomon Buber (Lemberg, 1905).
———. *Responsa Rashi*, ed. Israel Elfenbein (New York, 1943).
———. *Siddur Rashi* (Ritualwerk, R. Salomo ben Isaak zugeschreiben), ed. Jacob Freimann and Shlomo Buber (Berlin, 1911).
———. *Tosfot al Massekhet Mo'ed Katan* (Commentarius in Tractatum Mo'ed Qatan), ed. Efraim Kupfer (Jerusalem, 1961).
Soranus. *Gynaecology*, ed. Owsei Temkin (Baltimore, 1956).
Teshuvot uPsakim (Responsa et Decisiones), ed. Efraim Kupfer (Jerusalem, 1973).

Teshuvot Geonei Mizrah uMa'arav (Responsen der Lehrer des Ostens und Westens), ed. Joel Müller (Berlin, 1888).
Teshuvot Hakhmei Provence (Responsae of the Sages of Provence), ed. Abraham Schreiber (Sofer) (Jerusalem, 1967).
Vincent de Beauvais. *Speculum historiale* (Graz, 1964–65).
Wolfram von Eschenbach. *Willelhalm*, ed. Albert Letzmann (Tübingen, 1961).
Yehiel b. Judah of Paris. *Piskei R. Yehiel miParis veHoraot meRabbanei Zarfat*, ed. Eliyahu Dov Pines (Jerusalem, 1977).
———. *Vikuah R. Yehiel miParis meBa'alei haTosafot*, ed. Reuven Margaliyot (Jerusalem, 1928).
Yehiel b. Yekutiel haRofeh. *Sefer Tanya Rabbati* (Vilna, 1899).
Zidkiya b. Abraham. *Sefer Shibolei haLeqet haShalem*, ed. Shlomo Buber (Vilna, 1886).

SECONDARY SOURCES

Abrahams, Israel. *Jewish Life in the Middle Ages* (London, 1932).
Agus, Irving A. "The Development of the Money Clause in the Ashkenazic Ketubah," *JQR* 30 (1939/1940): 221–56.
———. *The Heroic Age of Franco-German Jewry* (New York, 1969).
———. *Urban Civilization in Pre-Crusade Europe: A Study of Organized Town-Life in Northwestern Europe during the Tenth and Eleventh Centuries based on the Responsa Literature* (New York, 1965).
Alexandre-Bidon, Danièle, and Monique Closson. *L'enfant à l'ombre des cathédrales* (Lyon and Paris, 1985).
Algazi, Gadi. "Abelard, Héloise and Astralabe." In *Women, Children and the Elderly: Essays in Honour of Shulamith Shahar*, eds. Miriam Eliav-Feldon and Yitzhak Hen (Jerusalem, 2001), 85–98 [in Hebrew].
Angenendt, Arnold. "Taufe und Politik im frühen Mittelalter," *Frühmittelalterliche Studien* 7 (1973): 143–68.
Ariès, Phillippe. *Centuries of Childhood: A Social History of Family Life*, trans. Robert Baldick (New York, 1962).
Arnold, Klaus. *Kind und Gesellschaft im Mittelalter und Renaissance* (Paderborn, 1980).
Aronius, Julius. *Regesten zur Geschichte der Juden im fränkischen und deutschen Reiche bis zum Jahre 1273* (Berlin, 1902, repr. Hildesheim and New York, 1970).
Ashley, Kathleen, and Pamela Sheingorn (eds.). *Interpreting Cultural Symbols, Saint Anne in Late Medieval Society* (Athens, GA., 1990).
Assaf, Simha: *Mekorot le-Toldot haHinukh*, 4 vols. (Tel Aviv, 1924).
Assis, Yom Tov. *The Golden Age of Aragonese Jewry: Community and Society in the Crown of Aragon 1213–1327* (London and Portland, Ore., 1997).
———. "'The 'Ordinance of Rabbenu Gershom' and Polygamous Marriages in Spain," *Zion* 46 (1981): 251–77 [in Hebrew].
Atkinson, Clarissa. *The Oldest Vocation: Christian Motherhood in the Middle Ages* (Ithaca, N.Y., and London, 1991).
Azmon, Yael (ed.). *A View into the Lives of Women in Jewish Societies* (Jerusalem, 1995) [in Hebrew].

Baader, Gerhard. "Die Hebammenkatechismus des Muscio — ein Zeugnis frühmittelalterlichen Geburtshilfe." In *Frauen in Spätantike und Frühmittelalter*, ed. Werner Affeldt (Sigmaringen, 1990), 126–35.
Badinter, Elisabeth. *L'amour en plus: L'histoire de l'amour maternel (XVIIe–XXe siècle)* (Paris, 1980).
Baer, Yitzhak F. "The Religious-Social Tendency of 'Sepher Hassidim,' " *Zion* 3 (1938): 1–50 [in Hebrew].
Baldwin, John. *The Language of Sex: Five Voices from Northern France around 1200*, (Chicago and London, 1994).
Banks, Amanda Carson. *Birthchairs, Midwives and Medicine* (Jackson, MS, 1999).
Bar-On, Ya'ara. *The Crowded Delivery Room: Gender and Public Opinion in Early Modern Gynecology* (Haifa, 2000) [in Hebrew].
Barkai, Ron. *A History of Jewish Gynaecological Texts in the Middle Ages* (Leiden, Boston, and Köln, 1998).
———. "Greek Medical Traditions and Their Impact on Conceptions of Women in the Gynaecological Writings in the Middle Ages." In *A View into the Lives of Women in Jewish Societies*, ed. Yael Azmon (Jerusalem, 1995) 115–42 [in Hebrew].
———. *Les infortunes de Dinah: Le livre de la generation, la gynécologie juive au moyen âge* (Paris, 1991).
———. "A Medieval Hebrew Treatise on Obstetrics," *Medical History* 33 (1988): 96–119.
Baron, Salo W. *A Social and Religious History of the Jews*, 18 vols. (Philadelphia, 1952–83).
Bartal, Israel, and Isaiah Gafni (eds.). *Sexuality and the Family in History: Collected Essays* (Jerusalem, 1999) [in Hebrew].
Barth, Lewis M. (ed.). *Berit Mila in the Reform Context* (New York, 1990).
Baskin, Judith R. "From Separation to Displacement: The Problem of Women in Sefer Hasidim," *AJS Review* 19 (1994): 1–18.
——— (ed.). *Jewish Women in Historical Perspective* (Detroit, 1998²).
———. "Silent Partners: Women As Wives in Rabbinic Literature." In *Active Voices: Women in Jewish Culture*, ed. Maurie Sacks (Urbana and Chicago, 1995), 19–37.
———. "Some Parallels in the Education of Medieval Jewish and Christian Women," *Jewish History* 5 (1991): 41–52.
Baumgarten, Elisheva. "Thus Sayeth the Wise Midwives: Midwives and Midwifery in Thirteenth-Century Germany," *Zion* 65 (2000): 45–74 [in Hebrew].
Beissel, Stephan. *Geschichte der Verehrung Marias im 16 und 17 Jahrhundert: Ein Beitrag zur Religionswissenschaft und Kunstgeschichte* (Freiburg, 1909).
Bell, Catherine. *Ritual Theory, Ritual Practice* (New York, 1992).
Beller, Katherine. *Jews before the Modenese Inquisition: 1600–1645*, Ph.D. diss., Haifa University (Haifa, 2002).
Bennett, Judith M. "Medievalism and Feminism." In *Studying Medieval Women: Sex, Gender and Feminism*, ed. Nancy Partner (Cambridge, Mass., 1993), 7–29.
———. "Medieval Women, Modern Women: Across the Great Divide." In *Culture and History 1350–1600: Essays on English Communities, Identities and Writings*, ed. David Aers (Detroit, 1992), 147–75.
Berger, David. *The Jewish Christian Debate in the High Middle Ages, A Critical Edition of The Nizzahon Vetus, with an Introduction, Translation and Commentary* (Philadelphia, 1979).

Berkvam, Doris Desclais. *Enfance et maternité dans la littérature française des XIIe et XIIIe siècles* (Paris, 1981).
Berliner, Adolf. *Aus dem inneren Leben der deutschen Juden im Mittelalter nach gedruckten und ungedruckten Quellen. Zugleich ein Beitrag für deutsche Kulturgeschichte* (Berlin, 1871).
Blumenkranz, Bernhard. *Les auteurs chrétiens latins du moyen âge sur les juifs et le judäisme* (Études juives, 4) (Paris, 1963).
Bock, Gisela. "Challenging Dichotomies: Perspectives on Women's History." In *Writing Women's History: International Perspectives*, eds. Karen Offen, Ruth Rouch Pierson, and Jane Randall (Bloomington and Indianapolis, 1991), 1–24.
Bolton, Brenda. "Mulieres Sanctae." In *Sanctity and Secularity: The Church and the World*, ed. Derek Baker (Studies in Church History, 10) (Oxford, 1973), 77–95.
———. "Received in His Name: Rome's Busy Baby Box." In *The Church and Childhood*, ed. Diana Wood (Studies in Church History, 31) (Oxford, 1994), 153–68.
Bonfil, Robert (Roberto). *Jewish Life in Renaissance Italy*, trans. Anthony Oldcorn (Berkeley, Los Angeles, and London, 1994).
———. *Rabbis and Jewish Communities in Renaissance Italy*, trans. Jonathan Chipman (London and Washington, 1993).
———. *Tra due mondi. Cultura ebraica e cultura cristiana nel Medioevo* (Napoli, 1996).
Borchers, Susanne. *Jüdisches Frauenleben im Mittelalter. Die Texte des Sefer Chasidim* (Frankfurt, Berlin, Bern, New York, Paris, and Vienna, 1998).
Bossy, John. "Blood and Baptism: Kinship, Community and Christianity in Western Europe from the Fourteenth to the Seventeenth Centuries." In *Sanctity and Secularity: The Church and the World*, ed. Derek Baker (Studies in Church History, 10) (Oxford, 1973), 129–43.
———. "Godparenthood: The Fortunes of a Social Institution in Early Modern Christianity." In *Religion and Society in Early Modern Europe 1500–1800*, ed. Kaspar von Greyerz (London, Boston, and Sydney, 1984), 194–201.
Boswell, John. *The Kindness of Strangers: The Abandonment of Children in Western Europe from Late Antiquity to the Renaissance* (New York, 1989).
Bouhot, Jean-Paul. "Explications du rituel baptismal à l'époque carolingienne," *Revue des études Augustiennes* 24 (1978): 278–301.
Bourdieu, Pierre. *Esquisse d'une théorie de la pratique: précédé de trois études d'ethnologie kabyle* (Genève-Paris, 1972).
———. "Rites As Acts of Institution." In *Honor and Grace in Anthropology*, eds. John G. Peristiany and Julian Pitt-Rivers (Cambridge, 1992), 81–88.
Bradley, Keith R. "Wet Nursing at Rome: A Study in Social Relations." In *The Family in Ancient Rome*, ed. Beryl Rawson (London and Sydney, 1986), 201–29.
Brandenberg, Tony. "Saint Anne: A Holy Grandmother and Her Children." In *Sanctity and Motherhood: Essays on Holy Mothers in the Middle Ages*, ed. Anneke B. Mulder-Bakker (New York and London, 1995), 31–65.
Bresc Henri, "Europe: Town and Country." In *History of the Family*, eds. André Burguière, Christiane Klapisch-Zuber et al. (Cambridge, Mass., 1996), 430–66.
Breuer, Mordechai. "The 'Black Death' and Antisemitism." In *Antisemitism Through the Ages: A Collection of Essays*, ed. Shmuel Almog (Jerusalem, 1980), 139–52 [in Hebrew].

Brill, Jacques. *Lilith ou la mère obscure* (Paris, 1981).
Brissaud, Yves. "L'Infanticide à la fin du Moyen Age, ses motivations psychologiques et sa répression," *Revue historique de droit français et étranger* 50 (1972): 229–56.
Brody, Robert. "The Enigma of *Seder Rav* 'Amram." In *Knesset Ezra: Literature and Life in the Synagogue: Studies Presented to Ezra Fleischer*, ed. Shulamith Elizur et al. (Jerusalem, 1994), 21–34 [in Hebrew].
Brooke, Christopher. *The Medieval Idea of Marriage* (Oxford, 1989).
Bröwe, Peter S. J. *Beiträge zur Sexualethik des Mittelalters* (Breslau, 1932).
Brühl, Carlrichard. *Deutschland-Frankreich: Die Geburt zweier Völker*, (Köln and Vienna, 1990).
Brundage, James. *Law, Sex and Christian Society in Medieval Europe* (Chicago, 1988).
———. "The Merry Widow's Serious Sister: Remarriage in Classical Canon Law." In *Matrons and Marginal Women in Medieval Society*, eds. Robert R. Edwards and Vickie Ziegler (Suffolk, 1995), 33–48.
———. "Widows As Disadvantaged Persons in Medieval Canon Law." In *Upon My Husband's Death: Widows in the Literature and Histories of Medieval Europe*, ed. Louise Mirrer (Ann Arbor, 1992), 194–205.
Bullough, Vern. "Medieval Medical and Scientific Views of Women," *Viator* 4 (1973): 485–501.
Bulst, Neithard. "Illegitime Kinder—viele oder wenige? Quantitative Aspekte der Illegitimität im spätmittelalterlichen Europa." In *Illegitimität im Spätmittelalter*, ed. Ludwig Schmugge (Munich, 1994), 21–40.
Bynum, Caroline W. *Fragmentation and Redemption: Essays on Gender and the Human Body in Medieval Religion* (New York, 1991).
———. *Holy Feast and Holy Fast: The Religious Significance of Food to Medieval Women* (Berkeley, 1987).
Cadden, Joan. *Meanings of Sex Difference in the Middle Ages: Medicine, Science and Culture* (Cambridge, 1991).
Callaway, Helen. "The Most Essentially Female Function of All: Giving Birth." In *Defining Females: The Nature of Women in Society*, ed. Shirley Ardener (Oxford and Providence, 1993), 146–67.
Carbonnier-Burkard, Marianne. "Les variations protestantes." In *L'histoire des pères et de la paternité*, eds. Jacques Delemeau et Danîel Roche (Paris, 1990), 155–78.
Carlebach, Elisheva. "Early Modern Ashkenaz in the Writings of Jacob Katz." In *Pride of Jacob: Essays on Jacob Katz and His Work*, ed. Jay M. Harris (Cambridge, Mass., 2002), 65–83.
Casey, James. *History of the Family* (New York, 1989).
Caspers, Charles. "Leviticus 12, Mary and Wax: Purification and Churching in Late Medieval Christianity." In *Purity and Holiness: The Heritage of Leviticus*, eds. M. J. H. M. Poorthus and Joshua Schwartz (Leiden, Boston, and Köln, 2000), 295–309.
Chazan, Robert. *European Jewry and the First Crusade* (Berkeley, 1987).
Chodorow, Nancy. *The Reproduction of Mothering: Psychoanalysis and the Sociology of Gender* (Berkeley, Los Angeles, and London, 1978).
Clark, Elaine. "Mothers at Risk of Poverty in the Medieval English Countryside." In *Poor Women and Children in the European Past*, eds. John Henderson and Richard Wall (London and New York, 1994), 139–59.
Cohen, Esther, and Elliott Horowitz. "In Search of the Sacred: Jews, Christians and

Rituals of Marriage in the Later Middle Ages," *Journal of Medieval and Renaissance Studies* 20 (1990): 225–50.

Cohen, Jeremy. *"Be Fertile and Increase. Fill the Earth and Master It": The Ancient and Medieval Career of a Biblical Text* (Ithaca and London, 1989).

———. "Between Martyrdom and Apostasy: Doubt and Self-Definition in Twelfth-Century Ashkenaz," *Journal of Medieval and Early Modern Studies* 29 (1999), 431–71.

———. "Conjugal Sex inRaABaD," *Jewish History* 6 (1992): 65–78.

———. "'The Persecutions of 1096'—From Martyrdom to Martyrology: The Sociocultural Context of the Hebrew Crusade Chronicles," *Zion* 59 (1994): 169–208 [in Hebrew].

Cohen, Richard I. *Jewish Icons: Art and Society in Modern Europe* (Berkeley and London, 1998).

Cohen, Shaye J. D. "Purity, Piety and Polemic: Medieval Rabbinic Denunciation of 'Incorrect' Purification Practices." In *Women and Water: Menstruation in Jewish Life and Law*, ed. Rahel R. Wasserfall (Hanover, N.H. and London, 1999), 82–100.

———. "Why Aren't Jewish Women Circumcised?" *Gender and History* 9 (1997): 560–78.

Cohen, Steven M., and Paula Hyman (eds.). *The Jewish Family: Myths and Reality* (New York, 1986).

Cohn, Norman. *Europe's Inner Demons: The Demonization of Christians in Medieval Christendom* (London, 1993).

Coster, William. "Purity, Profanity and Puritanism: The Churching of Women, 1500–1700." In *Women in the Church*, eds. W. J. Sheilds and Diana Wood (*Studies in Church History*, 27) (Oxford, 1990), 377–87.

Cramer, Peter. *Baptism and Change in the Early Middle Ages, c. 200–c. 1150* (Cambridge, 1993).

Cressy, David. *Birth, Marriage and Death: Ritual, Religion and the Life-Cycle in Tudor and Stuart England* (New York, 1997).

———. "Purification, Thanksgiving and the Churching of Women in Post-Reformation England," *Past and Present* 141 (1993): 106–46.

Cunningham, Hugh. *Children and Childhood in Western Society since 1500* (London and New York, 1995).

Dan, Joseph. *HaSippur ha'Ivri beYemei haBenayim* (Jerusalem, 1974).

———. *Iyyunim beSifrut Ḥasidei Ashkenaz* (Ramat Gan, 1975).

———. "Sippurim Demonologim miKitvei R. Judah heḤasid." In *The Religious and Social Ideas of the Jewish Pietists in Medieval Germany*, ed. Ivan G. Marcus (Jerusalem, 1987), 165–82.

Darmsteter, Arsène, and David S. Blondheim. *Le glosses françaises dans les commentaires talmudiques de Raschi* (Paris, 1929).

Darnton, Robert. *The Great Cat Massacre and Other Episodes in French Cultural History* (New York, 1985).

Davidman, Lynn, and Shelley Tennenbaum (eds.). *Feminist Perspectives on Jewish Studies* (New Haven, 1994).

Davidson, Israel. *Thesaurus of Medieval Hebrew Poetry*, 4 vols. (New York, 1970) [in Hebrew].

Davis, Natalie Zemon. *The Gift in Sixteenth-Century France* (Madison, 2000).

———. *Society and Culture in Early Modern France* (Stanford, 1975).
Delumeau, Jean, and Danîel Roche (eds.). *Histoire des pères et de la paternité* (Paris, 1990).
DeMaitre, Luke. "The Idea of Childhood and Childcare in Medical Writings of the Middle Ages," *Journal of Psychohistory* 4 (1976/77): 461–90.
Demand, Nancy. *Birth, Death and Motherhood in Classical Greece* (Baltimore and London, 1994).
Despres, Denis L. "Immaculate Flesh and the Social Body: Mary and the Jews." *Jewish History* 12 (1998): 47–70.
Diemling Maria, `Christliche Ethnographien' über Juden und Judentum in der Frühen Neuzeit: Die Konvertiten Victor von Carben und Anthonius Margaritha und ihre Darstellung jüdischen Lebens und jüdischer Religion, Dissertation zur Erlangung des Doktorgrades der Philosophie eingericht an der Geisteswissenschaftlichen Fakultät der Universität Wien (Vienna, 1999).
Dienst, Heidi. "Zur Rolle der Frau in Magischen Vorstellungen." In *Frauen in Spätantike und Frühmittelalter. Lebensbedingungen—Lebensnormen–Lebensformen*, eds. Werner Affeldt et al. (Sigmaringen, 1990), 173–94.
Dillard, Heath. *Daughters of the Reconquest: Women in Castillian Town Society 1100–1300* (Cambridge, 1984).
Dinari, Yedidya Alter. *The Rabbis of Germany and Austria at the Close of the Middle Ages: Their Conceptions and Halacha-Writings* (Jerusalem, 1984) [in Hebrew].
Dockray-Miller, Mary. *Motherhood and Mothering in Anglo-Saxon England* (London, 2000).
Douglas, Mary. *Purity and Danger: An Analysis of the Concepts of Pollution and Taboo* (London, 1989).
Duby, Georges. *Medieval Marriage: Two Models from Twelfth-Century France*, trans. Elborg Foster (Baltimore and London, 1978).
Dupâquier, Jacques (ed.). *Marriage and Remarriage in the Populations of the Past* (London, 1981).
Eilberg-Schwartz, Howard. *The Savage in Judaism: An Anthropology of the Israelite Religion and Ancient Judaism* (Bloomington and Indianapolis, 1990).
Einbinder, Susan L. "Jewish Women Martyrs: Changing Models of Representation," *Exemplaria* 12 (2000): 105–27.
Erlbaum, Jacob. *Repentance and Self-Flagellation in the Writings of the Sages of Germany and Poland 1348–1648* (Jerusalem, 1992) [in Hebrew].
Elliott, Dyan. *Spiritual Marriage: Sexual Abstinence in Medieval Wedlock* (Princeton, 1993).
Elsakkers, Marianne. "In Pain You Shall Bear Children: Medieval Prayers for a Safe Delivery." In *Women and Miracle Stories: A Multidisciplinary Explanation*, ed. Anne Marie Korte (Leiden, Köln, and Boston, 2001), 179–210.
Emanuel, Simḥa. "Biographical Data on R. Baruch b. Isaac," *Tarbiẓ* 69 (2000): 423–40 [in Hebrew].
———. "LeInyano shel Maḥzor Vitry," *Alei Sefer* 12 (1986): 129–30.
———. *The Lost Halakhic Books of the Tosaphists*, Ph.D. diss., Hebrew University (Jerusalem, 1993) [in Hebrew].
Falk, Zeev. *Jewish Matrimonial Law in the Middle Ages* (Oxford, 1966).
———. *Marriage and Divorce: Reforms in the Family Law of German-French Jewry* (Jerusalem, 1961) [in Hebrew].

Feldman, William Moses. *The Jewish Child: Its History, Folklore, Biology and Sociology* (London, 1917).
Feuchtwanger-Sarig, Naomi. *Torah Binders from Denmark*, Ph.D. diss., Hebrew University (Jerusalem, 1999).
Fildes, Valerie. *Wet Nursing: A History from Antiquity to the Present* (New York, 1988).
Finkelstein, Louis. *Jewish Self-Government in the Middle Ages* (New York, 1964).
Fisher, John D. C. *Christian Initiation: Baptism in the Medieval West: A Research in the Disintegration of the Primitive Rite of Initiation (Alcuin Club Collection 47)* (London, 1965).
Fishman, Talya. "The Penitential System of Hasidei Ashkenaz and the Problem of Cultural Boundaries," *Journal of Jewish Thought and Philosophy* 8 (1999): 201–30.
——— . "A Kabbalistic Perspective on Gender Specific Commandments: On the Interplay of Symbols and Society," *AJS Review* 17 (1992): 199–245.
Flandrin, Jean Louis. *Familles: parenté, maison, sexualité dans l'ancienne société* (Paris, 1984).
Fonrobert, Charlotte Elisheva. *Menstrual Purity: Rabbinic and Christian Reconstructions of Biblical Gender* (Stanford, 2000).
Franz, Adolf. *Die kirchlichen Benediktionen im Mittelalter* (Freiburg, 1909).
Freimann, Abraham Ḥaim. *Seder Kiddushin veNissuin Aharei Ḥatimat haTalmud. Meḥkar Histori Dogmati beDinei Yisrael* (Jerusalem, 1945).
Gaudemet, Jean. *Le mariage en Occident: Les moeurs et le droit* (Paris, 1987).
Gavitt, Phillip. "Infant Death in Late Medieval Florence: The Smothering Hypothesis Reconsidered." In *Medieval Family Roles: A Book of Essays*, ed. Cathy Jorgensen Itnyre (New York and London, 1996), 137–53.
Gélis, Jacques. *L'arbre et le fruit: La naissance dans l'occident moderne XVI–XIX siècle* (Paris, 1984).
Germania Judaica, vol. 1, eds. Ismar Elbogen, Abraham Freimann and Haim Tykocinski (Tübingen, 1963).
Germania Judaica, vol. 2, ed. Zvi Avneri (Tübingen, 1968).
Gibson, Gail McMurray. "Blessing from Sun and Moon: Churching As Women's Theater." In *Bodies and Disciplines: Intersections of Literature and History in Fifteenth-Century England*, eds. Barbara A. Hanawalt and David Wallace (Minneapolis and London, 1996), 139–57.
——— . "Scene and Obscene: Seeing and Performing Late Medieval Childbirth," *Journal of Medieval and Early Modern Studies* 29 (1999): 7–24.
Giladi, Avner. *Infants, Parents and Wet Nurses: Medieval Islamic Views on Breast-Feeding and Their Social Implications* (Leiden, Boston, Köln, 1999).
Gilat, Yisrael Zvi. "The Obligation of Nursing Children," *Diné Israel* 18 (1995–96): 321–369 [in Hebrew].
Ginzberg, Louis. *Geonica: The Geonim and Their Halakic Writings*, 2 vols. (New York, 1909).
——— . *The Legends of the Jews*, 7 vols. (Philadelphia, 1947).
Goitein, Shlomo Dov. *A Mediterranean Society: The Jewish Communities of the Arab World As Portrayed in the Documents of the Cairo Geniza*, 6 vols. (Berkeley, Los Angeles, and London, 1967–93).
Goldberg, Harvey E. "Coming of Age of Jewish Studies, or Anthropology Is Counted in the Minyan," *Jewish Social Studies* (n.s.) 4 (1997): 29–63.

Goldin, Simḥa. "Die Beziehung der jüdischen Familie im Mittelalter zu Kind und Kindheit," *Jahrbuch der Kindheit* 6 (1989): 211–56.

———. "Jewish Children and Christian Missionizing." In *Sexuality and the Family in History: Collected Essays*, eds. Israel Bartal and Isaiah Gafni (Jerusalem, 1999), 97–118 [in Hebrew].

———. "The Synagogue in Medieval Jewish Community As an Integral Institution," *Journal of Ritual Studies* 9 (1995): 15–39.

———. *Uniqueness and Togetherness: The Enigma of the Survival of the Jews in the Middle Ages* (Tel Aviv, 1997) [in Hebrew].

Goodich, Michael E. *From Birth to Old Age* (Lanham, 1989).

Goody, Jack. "Against 'Ritual': Loosely Structured Thoughts on a Loosely Defined Topic." In *Secular Ritual*, eds. Sally F. Moore and Barbara G. Myerhoff (Assen, 1977): 25–35.

———. *Production and Reproduction: A Comparative Study of the Domestic Domain* (Cambridge, 1976).

Gottlieb, Beatrice. *The Family in the Western World from the Black Death to the Industrial Revolution* (New York, 1993).

Goshen-Gottstein, Moshe. "Likrat Ḥeker haShekiin shel Masorot haTirgumim haArami'im.: In *Studies in Rabbinic Literature, Bible and Jewish History, Ezra Zion Melammed Festschrift*. eds. Isaac D. Gilat, Hayim Y. Levine and Tzvi M. Rabinowitz (Ramat Gan, 1982), 43–47.

Grayzel, Solomon. *The Church and the Jews in the Thirteenth Century*, vol. 1 (New York, 1966).

Green, Monica H. "The Development of the Trotula," *Revue d'histoire des textes*, 16 (1996): 119–203.

———. "A Handlist of Latin and Vernacular Manuscripts of the So-called Trotula Texts" *Scriptorum*, 50 (1996): 137–75; 51 (1997): 81–103.

——— (ed.). *The Trotula: An English Translation of the Medieval Compendium of Women's Medicine* (Philadelphia, 2002).

———. "Women's Medical Practice and Health Care in Medieval Europe," *Signs* 14 (1989): 434–73.

Grieco, Sarah F. Matthews. "Breast-feeding, Wet Nursing and Infant Mortality in Europe (1400–1800)." In *Historical Perspectives on Breast-Feeding*, eds. Sarah F. Matthews Grieco and Carlo A. Corsini (Florence, 1991), 15–62.

Grimm, Jacob. *Deutsche Mythologie*, ed. Elard Hugo Meyer, 3 vols. (Tübingen, 1953).

Gross, Henri. *Gallia Judaica*, ed. Simon Schwarzfuchs (Amsterdam, 1969).

Grossman, Avraham. "Background to Family Ordinances—R. Gershom Me'or haGolah." In *Jewish History: Essays in Honor of Chimen Abramsky*, eds. Ada Rappaport-Albert and Steven J. Zipperstein (London, 1988), 3–24.

———. *The Early Sages of Ashkenaz: Their Lives, Leadership and Works (900–1096)* (Jerusalem, 2001³) [in Hebrew].

———. *The Early Sages of France: Their Lives, Leadership and Works* (Jerusalem, 2001³) [in Hebrew].

———. "The Origins and Essence of the Custom of 'Stopping the Service,'" *Milet* 1 (1983): 199–219 [in Hebrew].

———. *Pious and Rebellious: Jewish Women in Europe in the Middle Ages* (Jerusalem, 2001) [in Hebrew].

---. "The Status of Jewish Women in Germany (10th–12th Century)." In *Zur Geschichte der jüdischen Frau in Deutschland*, ed. Julius Carlebach (Berlin, 1993), 17–36.
Güdemann, Moshe. *Sefer haTorah veHeḤayim beArẓot Ashkenaz beYemei haBenayim*, 3 vols. (Warsaw, 1897).
Guggenheim, Florence. "Houlekraasch," *Israelitisches Wochenblatt Zürich* 24 (1958): 32.
Gutmann, Joseph. *The Jewish Life Cycle* (Leiden, 1987).
Haberman, Abraham M. *Sefer Gezerot Ashkenaz veZarfat* (Jerusalem, 1946).
Habicht, Jean-Paul, et al. "The Contraceptive Role of Breast Feeding," *Population Studies* 39 (1989): 213–32.
Hamburger, Benjamin Shlomo. *Shorshei Minhag Ashkenaz* (Bnei Brak, 1995).
Hanawalt, Barbara. *Growing Up in Medieval London* (New York and Oxford, 1993).
---. "Medievalists and the Study of Childhood," *Speculum* 77 (2002): 440–60.
---. *The Ties That Bound: Peasant Families in Medieval England* (New York, 1986).
Handwörterbuch des deutschen Aberglaubens, ed. Hanns Bächtold-Stäubli, 10 vols. (Berlin, 1927–41).
Hastrup, Kirsten. "A Question of Reason: Breast-Feeding Patterns in Seventeenth- and Eighteenth-Century Iceland." In *Anthropology of Breast-Feeding: Cross Cultural Perspectives on Breast-Feeding*, ed. Vanessa Maher (Oxford, Providence, Berg, and New York, 1992), 91–108.
---. "The Semantics of Biology: Virginity." In *Defining Females: The Nature of Women in Society*, ed. Shirley Ardener (Oxford and Providence, 1993), 34–50.
Hauptman, Judith. *Rereading the Rabbis: A Woman's Voice* (Boulder, 1998).
Haverkampf, Alfred. "Baptised Jews in German Lands during the Twelfth Century." In *Jews and Christians in Twelfth-Century Europe*, eds. Michael A. Signer and John Van Engen (Notre Dame, 2001), 255–310.
---. "'Concivilitas' von Christen und Juden in Aschkenas im Mittelalter." In *Jüdische Gemeinden und Organisationsformen von der Antike bis zur Gegenwart*, eds. Robert Jütte und Abraham P. Kustermann (Vienna, Köln, and Weiman, 1996), 103–36.
Herdt, Gilbert H. "Sambia Nosebleeding Rites and Male Proximity to Women." In *Cultural Psychology: Essays on Comparative Human Development*, eds. James W. Stigler, Richard A. Shweder, and Gilbert Herdt (Cambridge and New York, 1990), 366–400.
Herlihy, David. "Medieval Children." In *Women, Family and Society in Medieval Europe: Collected Essays 1978–1991* (Providence, 1995), 215–43.
---. *Medieval Households* (Cambridge, Mass. and London, 1985).
Herlihy, David, and Christiane Klapisch-Zuber. *Tuscans and Their Families: A Study of the Florentine Catasto of 1427* (New Haven, 1985).
Herweg, Rachel Monika. *Die jüdische Mutter. Das verborgene Matriarchat* (Darmstadt, 1994).
Hess, Ann Giardina. "Midwifery Practice among the Quakers in Southern Rural England in the Late Seventeenth Century." In *The Art of Midwifery: Early Modern Midwives in Europe*, ed. Hilary Marland (London and New York, 1993), 49–76.
Hidiroglou, Patricia. *Les rites de naissance dans le Judaïsme* (Paris, 1997).
Hirsch, Marianne. "Feminism and the Maternal Divide: A Diary." In *The Politics of Motherhood: Activist Voices from Left to Right*, eds. Alexis Jetter, Annelise Orleck, and Dianna Taylor (Hanover, N.H. and London, 1997), 352–68.

Hoffman, Lawrence A. *The Cannonization of the Synagogue Service* (Notre Dame and London, 1979).
———. *Covenant of Blood: Circumcision and Gender in Rabbinic Judaism* (Chicago and London, 1996).
Holmes, Urban T. *Daily Living in the Twelfth Century, Based on the Observations of Alexander Neckam in London and Paris* (Madison, 1952).
Horowitz, Elliot. "Between Masters and Maidservants in the Jewish Society of Europe in Late Medieval and Early Modern Times." In *Sexuality and the Family in History: Collected Essays*, eds. Israel Bartal and Isaiah Gafni (Jerusalem, 1999), 193–212 [in Hebrew].
———. "Coffee, Coffeehouses and Nocturnal Rituals," *AJS Review* 14 (1990): 17–46.
———. "'A Different Mode of Civility': Lancelot Addison on the Jews of Barbary." In *Christianity and Judaism*, ed. Diana Wood (*Studies in Church History*, 29) (Oxford, 1992), 309–25.
———. "The Eve of Circumcision: A Chapter in the History of Jewish Nightlife," *Journal of Social History* 13 (1989/90): 45–69.
Ḥoshen, Dalia. "Sexual Relations between Husband and Wife," *S'vara* 3 (1993): 39–45.
Howell, Martha. *The Marriage Exchange: Property, Social Place and Gender in Cities of the Low Countries, 1300–1550* (Chicago and London, 1998).
Hufton, Olwen. *The Prospects Before Her: A History of Women in Western Europe, 1500–1800*, 1 (New York, 1995).
Huneycutt, Lois L. "Public Lives, Private Ties: The Royal Mothers in England and Scotland, 1070–1204." In *Medieval Mothering*, eds. John Carmi Parsons and Bonnie Wheeler (New York, 1996), 295–312.
Hurwitz, Siegmund. *Lilith die erste Eva. Eine Studie über dunkle Aspekte des Weiblichen* (Zurich, 1980).
Jeremias, Joachim. *Die Kindertaufe in den ersten vier Jahrhunderten* (Göttingen, 1958²).
Johnson, Elizabeth A. "Marian Devotion in the Western Church." In *Christian Spirituality: High Middle Ages and Reformation*, ed. Jill Raitt (London and New York, 1987), 2: 392–414.
Johnson, Penelope. *Equal in Monastic Profession: Religious Women in Medieval France* (Chicago and London, 1991).
Jordan, William C. "A travers le regard des enfants," *Provence Historique* 37 (1987): 531–43.
———. "Adolescence and Conversion in the Middle Ages: A Research Agenda." In *Jews and Christians in Twelfth-Century Europe*, eds. Michael A. Signer and John Van Engen (Notre Dame, 2001), 77–93.
———. *The French Monarchy and the Jews: From Philip Augustus to the Last Capetians* (Philadelphia, 1989).
———. "Jews on Top: Women and the Availability of Consumption Loans in Northern France in the Mid–Thirteenth Century," *Journal of Jewish Studies* 29 (1978): 39–56.
———. "Marian Devotion and the Talmud Trial of 1240." In *Religionsgespräche im Mittelalter*, eds. Bernard Lewis and Friedrich Niewöhner (Wiesbaden, 1992), 61–76.
———. *Women and Credit in Pre-Industrial and Developing Societies* (Philadelphia, 1993).
Jorgenson Itnyre, Cathy (ed.). *Medieval Family Roles: A Book of Essays* (New York, 1996).

Jussen, Bernhard. *Patenschaft und Adoption im frühen Mittelalter: Künstliche Verwandtschaft als soziale Praxis* (Göttingen, 1991).

———. "Le parrainage à la fin du Moyen Age: Savior public, attentes théologiques et usages sociaux," *Annales E.S.C.* 47 (1992): 467–502.

———. *Spiritual Kinship As Social Practice: Godparenthood and Adoption in the Early Middle Ages*, trans. Pamela Selwyn (Newark and London, 2000).

Kanarfogel, Ephraim. "Attitudes Toward Childhood and Children in Medieval Jewish Society," *Approaches to Judaism in Medieval Times*, 2 (1985): 1–35.

———. *Jewish Education and Society in the High Middle Ages* (Detroit, 1992).

Karant-Nunn, Susan C. *The Reformation of Ritual* (London and New York, 1997).

Katz, Eli. "Zeman Netinat Shem leBen uleBat," *Zefunot* 6 (1990): 41–45.

Katz, Jacob. *Exclusiveness and Tolerance: Studies in Jewish-Gentile Relations in Medieval and Modern Times* (London, 1961).

———. "Marriage and Sexual Life among the Jews at the Close of the Middle Ages," *Zion* 10 (1945): 21–54 [in Hebrew].

———. *The "Shabbes Goy": A Study in Halakhic Flexibility*, trans. Yoel Lerner (Philadelphia, 1989).

———. *Tradition and Crisis: Jewish Society at the End of the Middle Ages*, trans. Bernard Dov Cooperman (New York, 1993).

Kellum, Barbara. "Infanticide in England in the Later Middle Ages," *History of Childhood Quarterly* 1 (1973–74): 367–88.

Khatib-Chahidi, Jane. "Milk Kinship in Shi'ite Islamic Iran." In *The Anthropology of Breast-Feeding: Cross Cultural Perspectives on Breast-Feeding*, ed. Vanessa Maher (Oxford, Berg, Providence, and New York, 1992), 109–32.

Kieckhefer, Richard. "Major Currents in Late Medieval Devotion." In *Christian Spirituality: High Middle Ages and Reformation*, ed. Jill Raitt, 2 (London and New York, 1987) 89–93.

Kirshenblatt-Gimblett, Barbara. "The Cut That Binds: The Western Ashkenazic Torah Binder As Nexus between Torah and Circumcision." In *Celebration: Studies in Festivity and Ritual*, ed. Victor Turner (Washington, D.C., 1982) 136–45.

Klapisch-Zuber, Christiane. *A History of Women in the West: Silences of the Middle Ages*, vol. 2 (London and Cambridge, Mass., 1992).

———. "Au péril des commères: L'Alliance spirituelle par les femmes à Florence." In *Femmes, marriages, lignages, XIIe–XIVe siècles, Melanges offerts à George Duby*, eds. Pierre Toubert et al. (Brussels, 1992), 215–32.

———. "Les femmes dans les rituels de l'alliance et de la naissance à Florence." In *Riti e rituali nelle società medievali*, eds. Jacques Chiffoleau, Laura Martiers, and Agostino Paravicini Bagliani (Spoleto, 1994), 3–22.

———. *Women, Family and Ritual in Renaissance Italy*, trans. Lydia Cochrane (Chicago, 1985).

Klein, Michelle. *A Time to Be Born: Customs and Folklore of Jewish Birth* (Philadelphia and New York, 1999).

Klirs, Tracy Guren (ed.). *The Merit of Our Mothers: A Bilingual Anthology of Jewish Women's Prayers* (Cincinnati, 1992).

Knibiehler, Yvonne, and Catherine Fouquet. *L'histoire des mères du Moyen Age à nos jours* (Paris, 1980).

———. *Les pères aussi ont une histoire* (Paris, 1987).

Kobler, Franz. *Her Children Call Her Blessed: A Portrait of the Jewish Mother* (New York, 1955).
Kottek, Samuel. "HaHanaka beMekorot haYahadut: Historia veHalakha," *Sefer Asia* 4 (1983): 275–86 [in Hebrew].
Krautheimer, Richard. *Batei Knesset beYemei haBenayim*, trans. Amos Goren (Jerusalem, 1994).
Kwasman, Theodore. "Die Mittelalterlichen jüdischen Grabsteine in Rothenburg o.d. Tauber." In *Zur Geschichte der mittelalterlichen jüdischen Gemeinde in Rothenburg ob der Tauber: Rabbi Meir ben Baruch von Rothenburg zum Gedenken an seinen 700 Todestag*, ed. Hilde Merz (Rothenburg ob der Tauber, 1993), 35–180.
Landau, Peter. "Das Weihehindernis der Illegitimität in der Geschichte des kanonischen Rechts." In *Illegitimität im Spätmittelalter*, ed. Ludwig Schmugge (Munich, 1994), 41–53.
Langmuir, Gavin I. *History, Religion and Antisemitismr* (Berkeley, 1990).
Lasker, Daniel. "Transubstantiation, Elijah's Chair, Plato and the Jewish-Christian Debate," *REJ* 143 (1984): 31–58.
Laurent, Sylvie. *Naître au moyen âge: De la conception à la naissance: La grossesse et l'accouchement XIIe–XVe siècle* (Paris, 1989).
Lee, Becky Rose. "*Women ben purifyid of her childeryn*": *The Purification of Women after Childbirth in Medieval England*, Ph.D. diss., University of Toronto (Toronto, 1998).
Lett, Didier. *L'enfant des miracles. Enfance et société au Moyen Age (XIIe–XIIIe siècle)* (Paris, 1997).
Levine-Melammed, Renée, ed. *"Lift Up Your Voice": Women's Voices and Feminist Interpretation in Jewish Studies* (Tel Aviv, 2001) [in Hebrew].
Leyser, Henrietta. *Medieval Women: A Social History of Women in England 450–1500* (London, 1995).
Linder, Amnon. *The Jews in the Legal Sources of the Early Middle Ages* (Detroit and Jerusalem, 1997).
Lipton, Sara. *Images of Intolerance: The Representation of Jews and Judaism in the Bible moralisée* (Berkeley, 1999).
Lithell, Ulla-Britt. "Breast-Feeding Habits and Their Relation to Infant Mortality and Marital Fertility," *Journal of Family History* 6 (1981): 182–94.
Loeb, Isidore. "La controverse de 1240 sur le Talmud," *REJ* 1 (1880): 247–61; 2 (1881): 248–70; 3 (1882): 39–57.
Löw, Leopold. *Die Lebensalter in der jüdischen Literatur, von Physiologischem, Rechts, Sitten und Religionsgeschichtlichem Standpunkte betrachtet* (Szegedin, Hungary, 1875; repr. Jerusalem, 1969).
———. *Der Synagogale Ritus* (Krotoschin, 1884).
Lukes, Stephen. "Political Ritual and Social Integration," *Sociology* 9 (1975): 289–308.
Lynch, Joseph H. *Godparenthood and Kinship in Early Medieval Europe* (Princeton, 1986).
———. "Spiritale Vinculum: The Vocabulary of Spiritual Kinship in Early Medieval Europe." In *Religion, Culture, and Society in the Early Middle Ages: Studies in Honor of Robert E. Sullivan*, eds. Thomas F. X. Noble and John J. Contreni (Kalamazoo, Mich., 1987), 181–204.
MacFarlane, Alan. *Marriage and Love in England: Modes of Reproduction 300–1840* (Oxford, 1986).

MacLehose, William F. "Nurturing Danger: High Medieval Medicine and the Problem(s) of the Child." In *Medieval Mothering*, eds. John Carmi Parsons and Bonnie Wheeler (New York and London, 1996), 3–24.

Macrides, Ruth. "The Byzantine Godfather," *Byzantine and Modern Greek Studies* 11 (1987): 139–62.

Maher, Vanessa. "Breast-Feeding in Cross-Cultural Perspective: Paradoxes and Proposals." In *The Anthropology of Breast-Feeding: Natural Law or Social Construct* (Oxford and Washington, D.C., 1992), 1–35.

Malkiel, David. "Vestiges of Conflict in the Hebrew Crusade Chronicles, *Journal of Jewish Studies* 52 (2001): 323–410.

Marcus, Ivan G. "From Politics to Martyrdom: Shifting Paradigms in the Hebrew Narratives of the 1096 Crusade Riots," *Prooftexts* 2 (1982): 40–52.

———. "Jews and Christians Imagining the Other in Medieval Europe," *Prooftexts* 15 (1995): 204–26.

———. "Mothers, Martyrs and Moneymakers: Some Jewish Women in Medieval Europe," *Conservative Judaism* 38 (1986): 34–45.

———, (ed.). *The Religious and Social Ideas of the Jewish Pietists in Medieval Germany: Collected Essays* (Jerusalem, 1986) [in Hebrew].

———. *Rituals of Childhood: Jewish Acculturation in Medieval Europe* (New Haven and London, 1996).

Mause, Lloyd De (ed.). *The History of Childhood* (New York, 1974).

McLaren, Angus. *A History of Contraception* (Oxford, 1990).

McLaughlin, Mary Martin. "Survivors and Surrogates: Children and Parents from the Ninth to the Thirteenth Centuries." In *The History of Childhood*, ed. Lloyd De Mause (New York, 1974), 101–82.

McNeill, John T., and Helena M. Gamer. *Medieval Handbooks of Penance: A Translation of the Principal Libri Poenitentiales* (New York, 1990).

Melchoir-Bonnet, Sabine. "La Désignation du père." In *L'Histoire des pères et de la paternité*, eds. Jean Dulemeau and Danîel Roche (Paris, 1990), 55–70.

Mentgen, Gerd. *Die Juden des Mittelrhein-Mosel-Gebietes im Hochmittelalter unter besonderer Berücksichtigung der Kreuzzugsverfolgungen* (Bonn, 1995).

Minty, Mary. "'Judengasse' into Christian Quarter: The Phenomenon of the Converted Synagogue in the Late Medieval and Early Modern Holy Roman Empire." In *Popular Religion in Germany and Central Europe 1400–1800*, eds. Bob Scribner and Trevor Johnson (Basingstoke, England, 1996), 58–86.

———. "Kiddush HaShem in German Christian Eyes in the Middle Ages," *Zion* 59 (1994): 214–47 [in Hebrew].

Mintz, Sidney W. "Culture: An Anthropological View," *The Yale Review* (1982): 506–508.

Mintz, Sidney W., and Eric R. Wolf. "An Analysis of Ritual Co-Parenthood," *Southwestern Journal of Anthropology* 6 (1950): 341–68.

Mitterauer, Michael. *Historische-Anthropologische Familienforschung. Fragestellungen und Zugangsweisen* (Vienna, 1990).

———. *Ledige Mutter. Zur Geschichte unehelicher Geburten in Europa* (Munich, 1983).

Molinier, Alain. "Nourrir, éduquer et transmettre." In *L'histoire des pères et de la paternité*, eds. Jacques Delemeau et Danîel Roche (Paris, 1990), 95–120.

Molle, Marie Magdalene van. "Les fonctions du parrainage des enfants en Occident: Leur apogée et leur degradation (du VIe au Xe siècle)," *Paroisse et Liturgie* 46 (1964): 121–46.

Mooney, Catherine M. "Claire of Assisi and Her Interpreters." In *Gendered Voices: Medieval Saints and Their Interpreters* (Philadelphia, 1999), 52–77.

Motz, Lotte. "The Winter Goddesses: Percht, Holda and Related Figures," *Folklore* 116 (1984): 151–66.

Muir, Edward. *Ritual in Early Modern Europe* (Cambridge and New York, 1997).

Mulder-Bakker, Anneke B. (ed.). *Sanctity and Motherhood: Essays on Holy Mothers in the Middle Ages* (New York, 1995).

Murray, Jacqueline. "On the Origins and the Role of 'Wise Women' in Causes for Annulment on the Grounds of Male Impotence," *Journal of Medieval History* 16 (1990): 235–50.

Nelson, Janet. "Parents, Children and the Church." In *The Church and Childhood*, ed. Diana Wood (*Studies in Church History*, 31) (Oxford, 1994), 81–115.

Newman, Barbara. *From Virile Woman to WomanChrist: Studies in Medieval Religion and Literature* (Philadelphia, 1995).

———. "Hildegard and Her Hagiographers: The Remaking of Female Sainthood." In *Gendered Voices: Medieval Saints and Their Interpreters*, ed. Catherine Mooney (Philadelphia, 1999), 16–34.

———. *Sister of Wisdom: St. Hildegard's Theology of the Feminine* (Berkeley and Los Angeles, 1998^2).

Nichols, John A., and Lillian Thomas Shanks (eds.). *Distant Echoes: Medieval Religious Women*, 1 (Kalamazoo Mich., 1984)

Nirenberg, David. *Communities of Violence: Persecution of Minorities in the Middle Ages* (Princeton, 1996).

Noonan, John T. *Contraception—A History of Its Treatment by the Catholic Theologians and Canonists* (Cambridge, Mass. and London, 1986).

Nutton, Vivian. "Medicine in Medieval Western Europe 1000–1500." In *The Western Medical Tradition 800 B.C. to A.D. 1800*, eds. Lawrence I. Conrad et al. (Cambridge, 1995), 139–205.

Orme, Nicholas. "The Culture of Childhood in Medieval England," *Past and Present* 148 (1995): 48–88.

———. *From Childhood to Chivalry: The Education of English Kings and Aristocracy, 1066–1530* (London, 1984).

———. *Medieval Children* (New Haven, 2001).

Ortner, Sherry B. "Is Female to Male As Nature Is to Culture?" In *Making Gender: The Politics and Erotics of Culture* (Boston, 1996), 21–42.

Ozment, Steven. *When Fathers Ruled: Family Life in Reformation Europe* (Cambridge, Mass., 1983).

Paige, Karen Erikson and Jeffrey M. *The Politics of Reproductive Ritual* (Berkeley, Los Angeles, and London, 1981).

Parsons, John Carmi, and Bonnie Wheeler (eds.). *Medieval Mothering* (New York and London, 1996).

Paterson, Linda. "L'enfant dans la littérature occitane avant 1230," *Cahiers de civilization mediévale Xe–XIIe siècle* 32 (1989): 233–45.

Patlegean, Evelyn. "Christianisation et parents rituelles: Le domaine de Byzance," *Annales E.S.C.* 33 (1978): 625–36.
Pelikan, Jaroslav. *The Growth of Medieval Theology, 600–1300, The Christian Tradition: A History of the Development of Doctrine*, vol. 3 (Chicago and London, 1978).
Perles, Joseph. "Die Berner Handschrift des kleinen Aruch," *Jubelschrift zum siebzigsten Geburtstage des Prof. Dr. H. Graetz* (Breslau, 1887), 1–38.
Peskowitz, Miriam, and Laura Levitt. *Judaism since Gender* (New York, 1997).
Peuckert, Will-Erich. *Deutscher Volksglaube des Spätmittelalters* (Stuttgart, 1942).
Pinthus, Alexander. *Die Judensiedlungen der deutsche Städte. Eine stadtbiologische Studie* (Berlin, 1931).
Pollack, Herman. *Jewish Folkways in Germanic Lands (1648–1806): Studies in Aspects of Daily Life* (Cambridge, Mass., 1971).
Pollock, Linda. *Forgotten Children: Parent-Child Relationships from 1500–1900* (Cambridge and New York, 1983).
Powicke, Frederick M., and Christopher R. Cheney (eds.). *Councils and Synods with Other Documents Relating to the English Church* (Oxford, 1964).
Rawclifffe, Carole. *Medicine and Society in Later Medieval England* (Gloucester, 1995).
Reiner, Elḥanan. "From Joshua to Jesus: The Transformation of a Biblical Story into a Local Myth; A Chapter in the Religious History of the Galilean Jews." In *Sharing the Sacred: Religious Contacts and Conflicts in the Holy Land, First to Fifteenth Centuries C.E.*, eds. Arieh Kofsky and Guy Stroumsa (Jerusalem, 1998), 223–71.
Reiner, Rami. *Rabbenu Tam: Rabbotav haZarfatim veTalmidav Benei Ashkenaz*, M.A. thesis, Hebrew University (Jerusalem, 1997).
Riché, Pierre, and Danièle Alexandre-Bidon. *L'enfance au Moyen Age* (Paris, 1994).
Rieder, Paula M. *Between the Pure and the Polluted: The Churching of Women in Medieval Northern France 1100–1500*, Ph.D. diss., University of Illinois (Urbana and Champagne, 2000).
―――. "The Implications of Exclusion: The Regulation of Churching in Medieval Northern France," *Essays in Medieval Studies* 15 (1998): 71–80.
Rigg, A. George, and Frank Anthony Carl Mantello (eds.). *Medieval Latin* (Washington, D.C., 1996).
Röckelein, Hedwig. "Marienverehrung und Judenfeindlichkeit in Mittelalter und früher Neuzeit." In *Maria in der Welt. Marienverehrung im Kontext der Sozialgeschichte 10.–18. Jahrhundert*, eds. Claudia Opitz, Hedwig Röckelein, Gisela Signori, and Guy P. Marchal (Zürich, 1993), 279–307.
―――. "Vom Umgang der Christen mit Synagogen und jüdischen Friedhöfen," *Aschkenas* 5 (1995): 11–45.
Roemer Nils, "Turning Defeat into Victory: *Wissenschaft des Judentums* and the Martyrs of 1096," *Jewish History*, 13 (1999), 65–80.
Rokéaḥ, Zefira Entin. "The State, the Church and the Jews in Medieval England." In *Antisemitism Through the Ages: A Collection of Essays*, ed. Shmuel Almog (Jerusalem, 1980), 99–126.
Roper, Lyndal. *Oedipus and the Devil: Witchcraft, Sexuality and Religion in Early Modern Europe* (London, 1994).
Roth, Ernst N. Z. "Al haHollekreisch," *Yeda Am* 7 [52] (1962): 86–8.

Rubin, Miri. *Gentile Tales: The Narrative Assault on Late Medieval Jews* (New Haven, 1999).
Rubin, Nissan. *The Beginning of Life: Rites of Birth, Circumcision and Redemption of the Firstborn in the Talmud and Midrash* (Tel Aviv, 1995) [in Hebrew].
———. "Review of L. A. Hoffman, 'Covenant of Blood: Circumcision and Gender in Rabbinic Judaism,'" *Zion* 63 (1998): 225–31 [in Hebrew].
Rublack, Ulrike. "Pregnancy, Childbirth and the Female Body in Early Modern Germany," *Past and Present* 150 (1996): 84–110.
Ruddick, Sara. "Rethinking 'Maternal' Politics." In *The Politics of Motherhood: Activist Voices from Left to Right*, eds. Alexis Jetter, Annelise Orleck, and Dianna Taylor (Hanover, N.H. and London, 1997), 369–81.
Sabean, David Warren. "Kinship and Prohibited Marriages in Baroque Germany: Divergent Strategies among Jewish and Christian Populations," *Leo Baeck Institute Year Book* 47 (2002): 91–103.
Salfeld, Sigmund. *Martyrologium des Nürnberger Memorbuches* (Berlin, 1898).
Salvat, Michel. "L'accouchement dans la littérature scientifique médiévale," *L'enfant au moyen âge, Littérature et Civilisation* 9 (1980): 87–106.
Satlow, Michael. *Jewish Marriage in Antiquity* (Princeton, 2001).
Satz, Isaac. "Hagahat haGaon R. Israel b. haGaon Shalom Shakhna miLublin beInyan Zurat haOtiyot," *Moriah* 11 [7–8] (1982): 4–10.
Saxer, Victor. *Les rites de l'initiation chrétienne du IIe au VIe siècle. Esquisse, historique et signification d'après leurs principaux témoins* (Spoleto, Italy, 1988).
Schechter, Solomon. "The Child in Jewish Literature," *Studies in Judaism*, ser. 1 (Philadelphia, 1896), 282–313.
Schenk, Richard. "Covenant Initiation: Thomas Aquinas and Robert Kilwardy on the Sacrament of Circumcision." In *Ordo Sapientis et Amoris. Hommage au Professeur Jean-Pierre Torrell*, ed. Carlos-Josaphat Pinto de Oliveira (Fribourg, Switzerland, 1993), 555–93.
Schneider, Jane. "Introduction: The Analytic Strategies of Eric R. Wolf." In *Articulating Hidden Histories: Exploring the Influence of Eric R. Wolf*, eds. Jane Schneider and Rayna Rapp (Berkeley, Los Angeles, and London, 1995), 7–32.
Schulenburg, Jane Tibbets. *Forgetful of Their Sex: Female Sanctity and Society, ca. 500–1100* (Chicago, 1998).
Schultz, James. *The Knowledge of Childhood in the German Middle Ages, 1100–1350* (Philadelphia, 1995).
Schultz, Magdalene. "The Blood Libel: A Motif in the History of Childhood," *Journal of Psychohistory* 14 (1986): 1–23.
Scott, Joan W. *Gender and the Politics of History* (New York, 1988).
Sedan, Dov. *Shay Olamot: Three Hundred and Ten Worlds: Twelve Folkloristic Studies*, ed. Dov Noy (Jerusalem, 1990) [in Hebrew].
Shaḥar, Shulamith. *Childhood in the Middle Ages* (London and New York, 1990).
———. *The Fourth Estate: A History of Women in the Middle Ages*, trans. Chaya Galai (London and New York, 1983).
———. *Growing Old in the Middle Ages: "Winter Clothes Us in Shadow and Pain,"* trans. Yael Lotan (London, 1997).
———. "Infants, Infant Care, and Attitudes toward Infancy in the Medieval Lives of Saints," *Journal of Psychohistory* 10 (1982/83): 283–91.

Shatzmiller, Joseph. "Doctors and Medical Practices in Germany around the Year 1200: The Evidence of *Sefer Asaph*," *PAAJR* 50 (1983): 149–64.

———. "Doctors and Medical Practices in Germany around the Year 1200: The Evidence of *Sefer Hasidim*," *Journal of Jewish Studies* 33 (1982): 583–93.

———. *Jews, Medicine and Medieval Society* (Berkeley, Los Angeles, and London, 1994).

———. *Recherches sur la communauté juive de Manosque au Moyen Age, 1241–1329* (Paris, 1973).

Sheehan, Michael M. "Illegitimacy in Late Medieval England." *Illegitimität im Spätmittelalter*, ed. Ludwig Schmugge (München, 1994), 115–21.

Shoham-Steiner, Ephraim. *Social Attitudes Towards Marginal Individuals in Medieval European Society*, Ph.D. diss., Hebrew University (Jerusalem, 2002) [in Hebrew].

Sieder, Reinhard, and Michael Mitterauer. "The Reconstruction of the Family Life Course: Theoretical Problems and Empirical Results." In *Family Forms in Historic Europe*, ed. Richard Wall in collaboration with Jean Robin and Peter Laslett (Cambridge, 1983), 309–46.

Signer, Michael A. "Honor the Hoary Head: The Aged in Medieval European Jewish Community." In *Aging and the Aged in Medieval Europe*, ed. Michael A. Sheehan (Toronto, 1990), 39–48.

Simek, Rudolf. *Dictionary of Northern Mythology*, trans. Angela Hall (Cambridge, 1996).

Simonsohn, Shlomo. *The Apostolic See and the Jews*, 8 vols. (Toronto, 1988–91).

Soloveitchik, Haym. "Piety, Pietism and German Pietism: 'Sefer Hasidim I' and the Influence of 'Hasidei Ashkenaz,'" *JQR* 92 (2002): 455–93.

———. "Religious Law and Change: The Medieval Ashkenazic Example," *AJS Review* 12 (1986): 205–22.

———. "Review Essay of *Olam KeMinhago Noheg*," *AJS Review* 23 (1998): 223–34.

Sperber, Daniel. *Minhagei Yisrael*, 7 vols. (Jerusalem, 1989–98).

Spiegel, Gabrielle M. "History, Historicism and the Social Logic of the Text in the Middle Ages," *Speculum* 65 (1990): 59–86.

Spiegel, Shalom. "Me'aggadot haAkeda." In *Alexander Marx Jubilee Volume*, ed. Saul Lieberman (New York, 1959), Hebrew Section, 471–547.

Spiegel, Yaacov S. "Woman As Ritual Circumciser—the Halakhah and Its Development," *Sidra* 5 (1989): 149–57 [in Hebrew].

Stern, Moritz. "Verzeichnis der Judenbürger zu Nürnberg, 1338," *Die Israelitische Bevölkerung der deutschen Städte* 3 (1893/4): 9–14.

Stern, Sacha. *Jewish Identity in Early Rabbinic Writings* (Leiden, 1995).

Stone, Lawrence. *The Family, Sex and Marriage in England 1500–1800* (New York, 1977).

Stow, Kenneth. "The Jewish Family in the Rhineland: Form and Function," *American Historical Review* 92 (1987): 1085–110.

———. *The Jews in Rome, 1536–1551*, 2 vols. (Leiden, New York, Köln, 1995–96).

Swanson, Jenny. "Childhood and Child Rearing in *ad status* Sermons by Later Thirteenth Century Friars," *Journal of Medieval History* 16 (1990): 309–30.

Ta-Shma, Israel. "Al Kama Inyanei Mahzor Vitry," *Alei Sefer* 11 (1984): 81–89.

———. "Children in Medieval Germanic Jewry: A Perspective on Ariès from Jewish Sources," *Studies in Medieval and Renaissance History*, 12 (1991), 263–80.

———. "The Earliest Literary Sources for the Bar Mitzva Ritual and Festivity," *Tarbiz* 68 (1999): 587–98 [in Hebrew].
———. *Early Franco-German Ritual and Custom* (Jerusalem, 1992) [in Hebrew].
———. "On the History of Polish Jewry in the Twelfth to Thirteenth Centuries," *Zion* 53 (1988): 347–69.
———. "Response to Simha Emmanuel," *Alei Sefer* 12 (1986): 132 [in Hebrew].
———. "Review of Ivan Marcus, *Rituals of Childhood*," *JQR*, 87 (1996/7), 236–37.
———. *Ritual, Custom and Reality in Franco-Germany, 1000–1350* (Jerusalem, 1996) [in Hebrew].
———. "Synagogal Sanctity—Symbolism and Reality." In *Knesset Ezra: Literature and Life in the Synagogue: Studies Presented to Ezra Fleischer*, ed. Shulamith Elizur et al. (Jerusalem, 1994), 351–64 [in Hebrew].
Taglia, Kathryn Ann. "The Cultural Construction of Childhood: Baptism, Communion and Confirmation." In *Women, Marriage and Family in Medieval Christendom: Essays in Memory of Michael M. Sheehan*, eds. Constance M. Rousseau and Joel T. Rosenthal (Kalamazoo, Mich., 1998), 255–88.
Tallan, Cheryl. "The Economic Productivity of Medieval Jewish Widows," *WCJS* 11 B1 (Jerusalem, 1994): 151–58.
———. "Opportunities for Medieval Northern-European Jewish Widows in the Public and Domestic Spheres." In *Upon my Husband's Death*, ed. Louise Mirrer (Ann Arbor, 1992), 195–206.
———. "The Position of the Medieval Jewish Widow As a Function of Family Structure," *WCJS* 10 B2 (Jerusalem, 1990): 91–98.
Tarayre, Michael. *La vierge et le miracle. Le 'Speculum historiale' de Vincent de Beauvais* (Paris, 1999).
Thomas, Keith. *Religion and the Decline of Magic: Studies in Popular Beliefs in Sixteenth- and Seventeenth-Century England* (London, 1971).
Thomasset, Claude. "Quelques principes de l'embryologie médiévale," *L'enfant au moyen âge, Litterature et Civilisation* 9 (1980): 107–21.
———. "The Nature of Woman." In *A History of Women in the West*, ed. Christiane Klapisch-Zuber (Cambridge Mass., 1992), 2: 43–69.
Tilly, Louise A. "Women's History and Family History: A Fruitful Collaboration or Missed Connection," *Journal of Family History* 12 (1987): 303–15.
Tilley, Louise A., and Miriam Cohen. "Does the Family Have a History? A Review of Theory and Practice in Family History," *Social Science History* 6 (1982): 131–79.
Toch, Michael. "The Formation of a Diaspora: The Settlement of Jews in the Medieval German Reich," *Aschkenas* 7 (1997): 55–78.
———. *Die Juden im mittelalterlichen Reich* (*Enzyklopädie deutscher Geschichte*, 44) (Munich, 1998).
Toubert, Pierre, "The Carolingian Moment." In *A History of the Family*, ed. André Burgiére et al., trans. Sarah Hanbury Tenison, et al. (Cambridge, Mass., 1996), 379–406.
Trachtenberg, Joshua. *The Devil and the Jews: The Medieval Conception of the Jew and Its Relation to Modern Antisemitism* (New Haven, 1943).
———. *Jewish Magic and Superstition: A Study in Folk Religion* (New York, 1939).
Tubach, Frederic C. *Index Exemplorum* (Helsinki, 1969).
Tuitto, Eleazar. "Shitato haParshanit shel Rashbam al Reka haMeziut haHistorit shel

Zemano." In *Studies in Rabbinic Literature, Bible and Jewish History*, ed. Yizhak D. Gilat, Chaim Levine, and Zvi Meir Rabinowitz, (Ramat Gan, 1982), 48–74 [in Hebrew].

Tur-Sinai, Naftali. "*Shushvin*." In *Sefer Assaf. Kovetz Ma'amarei Mehkar*, eds. M. D. Cassuto, Joseph Klausner, and Joshua Guttman (Jerusalem, 1954), 316–22 [in Hebrew].

Urbach, Ephraim Elimelech. "Al Grimat Mavet biShegagah uMavet ba'Arisa," *Asufot* 1 (1987): 319–32.

———. *The Tosaphists: Their History, Writings and Methods* (Jerusalem, 1980, 4th ed.) [in Hebrew].

Vecchio, Silvana. "The Good Wife." In *History of Women in the West*, ed. Christiane Klapisch-Zuber (London and Cambridge, Mass., 1992), 2: 105–35.

Vogel, Cyrille. *Medieval Liturgy: An Introduction to the Sources*, trans. and revised by William Storey and Niels Rasmussen (Washington, D.C., 1986).

Vooys, C.G.N. de, *Middelnederlandse Merialegenden* (Leiden, 1903).

Walle, Etienne van de. "Recent Approaches to Past Childhoods." In *The Family in History: Interdisciplinary Essays*, eds. Theodore K. Rabb and Robert I. Rothberg (New York, Hagerstown, San Francisco, and London, 1973), 171–78.

Warner, Marina. *Alone of All Her Sex: The Myth and the Cult of the Virgin Mary* (New York, 1976).

Waschnitius, Viktor. *Perht, Holda und Verwandte Gestalten (Sitzungsberichte der kaiserlichen Akademie der Wissenschaften in Wien. Philosophisch-Historische Klasse*, 174) (Vienna, 1913).

Weinberger, Moshe. "Teshuvot Hakhmei Ashkenaz." In *Sefer haZikaron leRabbi Yaacov Bezalel Zolty*, ed. Joseph Boxbaum (Jerusalem, 1987), 248–50.

Weinstein, Roni. "Impotence and the Preservation of the Family in the Jewish Community of Italy in the Early Modern Period." In *Sexuality and the Family in History*, eds. Israel Bartal and Isiah Gafni (Jerusalem, 1999), 159–176 [in Hebrew].

———. *Jewish Marriage in Italy during the Early Modern Era: A Chapter in Social History and History of Mentality*, Ph.D. diss., Hebrew University (Jerusalem, 1995) [in Hebrew].

Weisner, Merry E. "The Midwives of South Germany and the Public/Private Dichotomy," In *The Art of Midwifery. Early Modern Midwives in Europe*, ed. Hilary Marland (London and New York, 1993).

———. *Working Women in Renaissance Germany* (New Brunswick, N.J., 1986).

Weissler, Chava. "For the Human Soul Is the Lamp of the Lord": The Tkhine for 'Laying Wicks' by Sarah bas Tovim," *Polin: Studies in Polish Jewry* 10 (1997): 39–65.

———. "The Missing Half and the Other Half: A Feminist and Anthropological Response," *Jewish Social Studies* 2 (1996): 98–105; 108–15.

———. *Voices of the Matriarchs: Listening to the Prayers of Early Modern Jewish Women* (Boston, 1998).

Wenninger, Markus J. "Zur Topographie der Judenviertel in den mittelalterlichen deutschen Städten anhand österreichischer Beispiele." In *Juden in der Stadt*, eds. Fritz Mayrhofer and Ferdinand Opll (Linz, 1999), 81–117.

Westreich, Elimelech. "Polygamy and Compulsory Divorce of the Wife in the Decisions of the Rabbis of Ashkenaz in the Eleventh and Twelfth Centuries," *Bar Ilan Law Studies* 6 (1988): 118–64.

———. *Transitions in the Legal Status of the Wife in Jewish Law*, (Jerusalem, 2002) [in Hebrew].

Whiting, John W. M. "Adolescent Rituals and Identity Conflicts." In *Cultural Psychology*, eds. James W. Stigler, Richard A. Schweder, and Gilbert Herdt (Cambridge, 1990), 357–65.

Whyte, Martin King. *The Status of Women in Preindustrial Society* (Princeton, 1978).

Wilson, Adrian. "The Ceremony of Childbirth and Its Interpretation." In *Women As Mothers in Pre-Industrial England, Essays in Memory of Dorothy McLaren*, ed. Valerie Fildes (London and New York, 1990), 68–107.

Wolf, Eric R. "Kinship, Friendship and Patron-Client Relationships in Complex Societies." In *The Social Anthropology of Complex Societies*, ed. Michael Banton (Edinburgh, 1966), 1–18.

Woolf, Jeffrey Robert. "Medieval Models of Purity and Sanctity: Ashkenzic Women in the Synagogue." In *Purity and Holiness: The Heritage of Leviticus*, ed. M. J. H. M. Poorthuis and Joshua Schwartz (Leiden, Boston, and Köln, 2000), 263–80.

Yalom, Marilyn. *History of the Breast* (New York, 1997).

Young, Frank W. *Initiation Ceremonies: A Cross-Cultural Study of Status Dramatization* (Indianapolis and New York, 1965).

Yuval, Israel J. "An Appeal against the Proliferation of Divorce in Fifteenth-Century Germany," *Zion* 48 (1983): 177–216 [in Hebrew].

———. "HaHesderim haKaspiyim shel haNissuin beAshkenaz beYemei haBenayim." In *Religion and Economy Connections and Interactions: Collected Essays*, ed. Menahem Ben Sasson (Jerusalem, 1995), 191–207.

———. "Heilige Städte, Heilige Gemeinden. Mainz als des Jerusalem Deutschlands." In *Jüdische Gemeinden und Organisationsform*, eds. Robert Jütte und Abraham P. Kustermann (Vienna, 1996), 91–101.

———. *Scholars in Their Time: The Religious Leadership of German Jewry in the Late Middle Ages* (Jerusalem, 1988) [in Hebrew].

"Two Nations in Your Womb": Perceptions of Jews and Christians (Tel Aviv, 2000) [in Hebrew].

———. "Vengeance and Damnation, Blood and Defamation: From Jewish Martyrdom to Blood Libel Accusations," *Zion* 58 (1993): 33–90 [in Hebrew].

Zimmer, Eric. *Society and Its Customs: Studies in the History and Metamorphosis of Jewish Customs* (Jerusalem, 1996) [in Hebrew].

Ziwes, Franz-Josef. *Studien zur Geschichte der Juden im mittleren Rheingebiet während des hohen und späten Mittelalters* (Hanover, 1995).

Zunz, Leopold. *Die gottesdienstlichen Vorträge der Juden historisch entwickelt: ein Beitrag zur Alterthumskunde und biblischen Kritik, zur Literatur- und Religionsgeschichte* (Frankfurt, 1892).

———. *Die Literaturgeschichte der synagogalen Poesie* (Berlin, 1865).

———. *Der Ritus des synagogalen Gottesdienstes, geschichtlich entwickelt* (Berlin, 1919^2).

INDEX

Aḥai Gaon, 230n.156
Aaron, 27, 173
abandonment of children, 152, 165, 169, 172–74, 178, 180, 236n.97, 237n.122
Abelard, Peter, 1, 177
abortion, 175
Abraham b. David of Posquières (Ra'abad: *Sefer Ba'alei haNefesh*), 26–27
Abrahams, Israel, 10, 15
Adam, 93, 117
adolescence, 187
adultery, 148–49, 174–75
aetitites, 48
Alexander III (pope), 136
Alexandre-Bidon, Danièle, 2
Amram Gaon, 57
amulets and charms, 9, 31, 43, 48–49, 53, 98, 107, 109
Anna (mother of Mary), 238n.124
Ariès, Philippe, 2, 14–15, 121, 164–65, 169
Aristotle, 41
Asher b. Yeḥiel, 129–30
Ashkenazic culture, 4–7, 10–12, 18, 39, 49–50, 56, 64–65, 68–69, 80, 91–92, 96, 100, 105, 116, 124, 128–29, 133, 147–49, 155, 158, 169, 177, 184, 189, 215n.7
Atkinson, Clarissa, 2, 178
atonement, 104, 108, 110, 115, 165–66, 186
Austria, 6

ba'al brit (masc. sing.), 65–70, 80–81, 99; and alternative names, 80; changing roles of, 70–72, 73–76, 86; and choice of, 67–68, 85; and importance of role, 67, 70; and origin of role, 68–70
ba'alat brit (fem. sing.), 70–75, 85–88
ba'alei brit (plural), 65–67
Babylon, 223n.27
Babylonian Talmud, 123, 170
baptism, 52, 55–56, 58, 92, 97, 98, 100, 110, 116, 181, and circumcision, 59–60; in emergency, 58, 97–98; history of, 57–59; women's roles, 88–89
Barkai, Ron, 38–39
Baron, Salo, 10
Bartholomaeus Anglicus, 155, 119, 221n.3

Barukh b. Isaac (*Sefer haTeruma*), 141–42
Befania, 97
Beila (the midwife), 204n.125
Beit Hillel and Beit Shammai, 29, 123, 148
Beller, Kathy, 225n.76
Bellete, 233n.31
Benjamin b. Abraham Selnik, 237n.118
Berla (the midwife), 204n.125
Bernard of Clairvaux, 134
Berthold of Regensburg, 234n.40
bible moralisée, 59
birth, 7, 9, 13, 20, 22–24, 37–39, 42, 112, 115, 161, 178, 186, 200n.45, 233n.21; and death, 39–41, 202n.91; as metaphor, 39–40; as perilous, 39–41; rituals of, 92, 101–16, 185
birth control, 124, 127
birthing chamber, 49. See also *Kindbett*
Black Death, 5, 230n.150
blood, 125
Bohemia, 6
Bologna, 27
Bonfil, Robert, 9
Bossy, John, 81–82, 84
Boswell, John, 172, 174, 236 nn. 91 and 97, 237n.122
Bourdieu, Pierre, 61–62
Bourlon, 134
breast-feeding, 18, 20, 29, 154, 225n.77; anthropology of, 120, 144; as contraceptive method, 145; divorcée's obligation for, 123–24; duration of, 123, 124, 126–28, 170, 223n.31; and infant mortality, 119–20, 229n.135; maternal, 120, 121–22; 124, 133–34, 144, 164; in mishnaic and talmudic era, 122–25; widow's obligation for, 122–24. See also wet nurses
Burchard of Worms, 37, 97–98
burial practices, 168
business, 6, 8–9, 19
Bynum, Caroline, 25
Byzantine Empire, 58, 70, 106

Caesarius of Heisterbach, 175
candles, 101, 106–7, 115, 217n.46
canon law, 121, 176

cantilles, 99, 217n.40
Carolingian period, 5, 6, 57–58, 61, 81, 106
Catherine of Sienna, 134
Causae et curae, 46. *See also* Hildegard of Bingen
celibacy, 13, 25, 27
charms. *See* amulets and charms; demons
charity, 103, 131–33, 167
Chaucer, Geoffrey, 178
child brides, 19
childbirth. *See* birth
childcare, 9, 14–15, 20, 119, 144, 158, 177–78, 184, 188–89; 225n.77
children and childhood, 2–4, 13–15, ages of, 161; attitudes toward, 121, 164–65; and Jewish studies, 14–15, 121; obligations of, toward parents, 155–58; and religious observance, 186–87
christening cloth, 107
Church, 49–50, 106–9, 160
churching (*Kirchengang, Aussegnung*), 101, 105–10; liturgy, 108, 218n.59; and *Shabbat Yeẓiat haYoledet*, 110–15
circumcisers, 46, 51, 54, 62, 63–65, 80 185; female circumcisers, 65, 88
circumcision, 16, 53, 78–79, 92, 94, 98, 100–102, 110, 116, 173, 187; anthropological approaches, 55–56; and baptism, 55, 59, 64, 79–83; liturgy of, 56–57, 61; as male ritual, 87; mothers' and women's role in, 56, 77–78, 83, 207n.8; and naming, 63; participants in, 62–79; as religious obligation, 55
Closson, Monique, 2
clothing, 102, 118
Cohen (of Aaronic descent), 150, 173
Cohen, Esther, 9
Cohen, Jeremy, 25–27
Cohen, Miriam, 14
communion, 138
conception, 29–30, 32, 166
confession, 52
conjugal obligations, 26
contraception, 145–47, 200n.45, 229n.135, 230n.145. *See also* birth control
conversion, 51–52, 136–38, 139, 160–61, 181–82, 228n.118
co-parents, 58–59, 76, 80–83, 100
courts, 149, 230n.161
cradles, 93, 177, 223n.27, 237n.117
crib death, 121, 176–78

cripples, 159, 174
custody, 159, 171. *See also* guardianship

Davis, Natalie Zemon, 111
Day of Atonement. *See* Yom Kippur
death: at childbirth, 39–41, 53–54, 109; of children, 2, 102, 119, 121, 127, 139, 151, 165–69, 170–71, 181–82; and circumcision, 64
demography, 18, 120–21, 135, 224n.48
demons, 93, 98, 109–10, 113, 116, 215n.5, 220n.82. *See also* amulets and charms; *streya*; witchcraft
Dinah, 29, 203n.107
divorce, 37–38, 100, 147, 159, 169, 202n.78, 230n.150; divorcée, 123–24, 127, 148–53, 171, 185
Douglas, Mary, 86
dowry, 84–85

education, 1, 18, 123, 127, 138, 160–61, 198n.6; age for beginning, 160, 184; of boys, 16, 90, 184; as father's obligation, 162–63; of girls, 22, 184
Egypt, 39, 41
Eilberg-Schwartz, Howard, 56
Einbinder, Susan, 187
Elḥanan b. Isaac, 50, 140–41
Eleazar b. Judah, 142, 166.
Eleazer b. Joel haLevi (Ra'aviah: *Sefer Ra'aviah*), 31, 35–36
Eliezer b. Nathan (Ra'aban: *Even haEzer*), 33–34, 129, 229n.128, 231n.161
Elijah, 62; Elijah's chair, 57, 69
Emanuel, Simḥa, 141
embryology, 21, 28–29, 41–42, 157
England, 6, 91, 107–9
Ephraim of Regensburg, 132
Esau, 42
Eucharist, 57, 167
Eve, 40–41, 117
excommunication, 136

Falaise, 148
fasting, 77–78, 88, 123, 162, 168, 176–77, 204n.122, 237n.115; and women, 88
fathers and fatherhood, 3, 120, 125, 155–58; and circumcision, 63–64, 67; obligations toward, 138, 155–58; paternal love, 158–65
Feast of Purification, 106–8

feminism, 2, 3, 4, 22, 38
fertility, 21, 26, 30, 38–43, 97, 146, 218n.63, 230n.145; and witchcraft, 47–48. *See also* infertility
First Crusade, 160, 179–80, 183
Fishman, Talya, 27
Florence, 121
food, 48, 102, 117–18, 176; baked goods, 97; for wet nurses, 133, 138–39; nonkosher, 137–38, 227n.100, 229n.131, its preparation on Sabbath, 159
foundlings, 172–74
France, 59, 91, 100, 139, 150, 228n.125. *See also* northern France
Frankfurt, 113
Frau Holle, 97–100, 107; and Virgin Mary, 216n.26
Frau Rose, 97
Freyja, 97
Frieda, 150

Galenus, 28, 45, 223n.35
Garden of Eden, 64
Geonim, 35, 55–56, 57, 65, 77
gender, 110, 112, 116, 122, 156, 172; gender studies, 3–4, 11, 14, 18, 188, 195n.53
Germanic traditions, 97
Germany, 5–6, 17, 27, 45, 58, 65, 70, 98, 100, 105, 107, 109, 129–30, 135, 138, 142, 143, 152, 229n.125
Gershom b. Jacob haGozer (the circumciser), 46, 48, 51, 54
Gershom b. Judah (Light of the Exile), 33–34, 37, 201n.57
ghettos, 8, 194n.51
Gibson, Gail McMurray, 54, 107–8
gifts, 131–32
Glückel of Hamel, 104
godparents, 71–72. *See also* co-parents
Goitein, Shlomo Dov, 13, 198n.96
Goldin, Simḥa, 14, 228n.119
Gratian, 26
gravestones, 17, 44, 235n.76
Green, Monica, 201n.59, 204n.121
Gregory IX (pope), 160–61
Gregory the Great (pope), 108
Griselda, 178
Grossman, Avraham, 12, 197n.82, 202n.78, 210n.59
guardianship, 162–63
Güdemann, Moritz (Moshe), 10, 97

Hamburger Shlomo, 104, 216n.16, 217n.43, 218n.49
Hanawalt, Barbara, 2
Hannah, 203n.96, 215n.7
Hannah (sister of Jacob b. Meir), 233n.31
Hanuka, 176
Hasidei Ashkenaz, 17, 27, 42, 159, 160, 163, 168
Hayim haCohen b. Ḥananel, 226n.87
ḥazan, 102, 109
Héloise, 1
Henricus Segusius, 138
Herlihy, David, 120–21, 139
High Holidays, 166
Hildegard of Bingen, 46, 48
Hoffman, Lawrence, 55–56, 197n.80
Holda, 97. *See also* Frau Holle
holidays, 176
Hollekreisch, 92, 93–100, 110, 113, 115
Horowitz, Elliot, 9
Ḥoshen, Dalia, 26–27

Iceland, 120
impotence, 31, 32, 34–36, 202n.78
impurity: after birth, 78, 111–12, 115; and menstruation, 123, 223n.41
incest, 58, 81–82, 84, 126
infanticide, 123, 125, 152, 165, 169–70, 174–78, 236n.91
infants: born out of wedlock, 129; welfare of, 151–52, 164. *See also* childcare
infertility, 21, 23–24, 28, 30–32; as grounds for divorce, 32–38
Innocent III (pope), 138, 172
Isaac (the Patriarch), 23, 93; circumcision of, 72–73; sacrifice of, 178, 180
Isaac b. Avraham (Rizba), 35–36
Isaac b. David, 182
Isaac b. Moses, 50, 69, 77, 80, 133, 135, 137–38, 142, 150, 151. See also *Sefer Or Zaru'a*
Isaac of Dampierre (R'i haZaken), 50, 140, 159–60, 228n.112
Isaac of Rouen, 150
Islam, 7, 11, 12, 125, 136, 231n.177
Israel b. Shalom Shakhna, 96
Italy, 6, 13, 58, 68–69, 105, 133, 224n.55, 225n.77
Ivo of Chartres, 26

Jacob (the Patriarch), 24, 42, 93
Jacob Ḥazan of London, 142, 173, 231n.164

Jacob b. Gershom haGozer (the circumciser), 46, 63, 71, 72, 75, 77
Jacob b. Meir (Rabbenu Tam), 35, 88, 147, 148–54, 159–60, 170, 181–82, 206n.169, 211n.64, 226n.87, 233n.31
Jacob b. Moses Mulin (Maharil), 63, 67, 72, 75–76, 77, 113, 119, 164
Jacob Savra haCohen of Krakow, 150
Jacobus de Voragine (*Golden Legend*), 106
Jacob Weil, 215n.1
Jephte, 178, 180, 238n.128
Jerusalem, 106
Jesus Christ, 26, 49, 59, 106, 134, 211n.87
Jewish-Christian relations, 7–9, 11, 16, 27, 100, 120, 143–44, 160–61, 184, 188–89; and medicine, 49–52, 140–41; and polemics, 8, 24–28, 59–61, 113–16
Joel Ibn Falquera (*Sefer Zori haGuf*), 45
John, 59, 207n.10
Jordan River, 59
Joseph b. Moses (*Sefer Leket Yosher*), 76
Joseph Bekhor Shor of Orleans, 149, 155–56, 231n.165
Joseph Juspa Hahn Neurlingen (*Sefer Yosef Omez*), 96, 113
Joshua, 59
Judah, 42; and Tamar, 39
Judah b. Asher, 51
Judah b. Isaac, 160
Judah b. Nathan (Riban), 127
Judah b. Samuel the Pious (Hasid), 23, 47, 53, 154, 163–64, 168, 173. See also *Sefer Hasidim*
Judaizers, 109
Juspa Hahn Kashman, 113
Juspa Shammes of Worms, 101, 117–18
Jussen, Bernhard, 82, 84

kaddish, 102
Kalonimus haZaken, 225n.73
Kanarfogel, Ephraim, 14
Karant-Nunn, Susan, 111
Katz, Jacob, 10
ketubbah, 34–36, 164, 171
Kiddush haShem, 178, 179–83
Kindbett and *Kindbetterin*, 53, 76, 107, 186
Kirchengang, Aussegnung. See churching
Klalei haMila. See Jacob b. Gershom and Gershom b. Jacob
Klapich-Zuber, Christiane, 4, 58–59, 120–21, 139
Köln, 27

Konrad of Megenburg, 221n.3
Koran, 126
Krakow, 150, 170

labor, division of, 154, 157–58, 160, 185
language, 8, 42, 193n.35
Leah (the Matriarch), 24
leprosy, 203n.96
Lett, Didier, 2
Lichtmess, 106, 220n.101
Likutei haPardes, 41
Lilith, 49, 98–100, 110, 113, 117, 217n.36, 221n.103
Linder, Amnon, 226, nn. 88 and 89
liturgy, 56, 61, 93, 108, 207n.8
living conditions, 18–19, 177
London, 142, 173
Löw Leopold, 101, 207n.4, 217n.43
Lublin, 96
lullabies, 137
lying-in period, 53, 102–5, 107, 111–13, 219n.69

Mahzor Vitry, 62, 64–66, 70–72, 77, 93–94, 99, 100, 127, 209n.38
Maccabbean Era, 165
Maccabbees, books of, 65, 180
Maimonides, 26–27, 173
Mainz, 6, 182
Marcus, Ivan, 9, 16, 113, 186–87
marketplace, 19
marriage, 3, 7, 12, 25–26, 30, 38, 61, 81, 83–85, 123, 196n.60, 217n.48; and infertility, 30–31; and monetary payments, 84–85
martyrs, 165, 178–83
Mary, 28, 41, 48–49, 52, 97, 106–11, 114–15, 134, 157–58, 178, 219n.66, 220n.101, 238n.124, 239n.143; Marian devotion, 26, 106, 114–15
Massekhet Smahot, 168
Matriarchs, 49. See also Sarah, Rebecca, Rachel, Leah
medicine, 7, 9, 13, 32, 44, 50–52, 65, 125, 133, 137, 140–41, 155
Mefiboshet, 233n.21
Meir b. Barukh of Rothenburg (Maharam), 36, 38, 67–68, 71–72, 75–76, 86–88, 90–91, 132, 138, 173, 176–77, 187, 212n.89
Menahem Ibn Zerah (*Sefer Zeidah laDerekh*), 225n.77
Menahhem b. Jacob, 132
menstruation and menstrual purity, 40, 47,

88, 105, 113, 125, 219n.77, 223n.36, 225n.77. *See also* impurity and mikve
Messiah, 175
Metz, 182
mizvot Hannah, 40, 113, 233n.31
Midrash, 21, 87
Midrash Aseret haDibrot, 156
Midrash Lekah Tov, 31
Midrash Shoher Tov, 68
Midrash Tanhuma, 40, 41
Midrash Yezirat haValad, 41
midwives and midwifery, 16, 20, 31, 39, 41, 43–54, 58, 97, 107, 175, 185–86, 210n.51; and witchcraft, 47–48
mikve, 43, 47, 53, 63, 67, 105, 115, 210n.62. *See also* menstruation and impurity
Minna (the midwife), 204n.125
minority culture, 9–10, 13, 174, 189
Mintz, Sidney, 59, 80, 82
minyan, 91
Miriam (the midwife), 204n.125
Miriam (sister of Moses), 133–34, 203n.96
Miriam (wife of Jacob b. Meir), 233n.31
miscarriage, 21, 46, 48
Modena, 225n.76
modesty, 87
monastic life, 25, 27, 48, 88, 172, 178–79
money-lending, 8
Montpellier (Council of), 226n.89
Mordekhai, 131
Mordekhai b. Hillel, 144
Moses, 39, 133–134, 164, 173, 233n.21
Moses b. Jacob of Couçy (*Sefer Mizvot Gadol*), 141–42, 159, 227n.100
Moses haDoeg b. Nathan, 150
Moses Mintz, 93, 96, 100
mother and seven sons, 165, 180–81
mothers and motherhood, 1, 2–4, 14, 22–24, 34, 108, 111–12, 120, 154, 186; as nurturers, 161; and circumcision, 64, 115; honoring of, 155–58; and maternal cruelty, 178, 182; obligations of toward children, 122; and maternal love, 158–65, 171, 180, 182; single mothers, 173–74, 175, 236n.107
mourning, 65, 67, 166–68, 181, 235n.76. *See also* death

naming, 93–94, 97
Naomi, 233n.21
Narbonne, 226n.89
Nathan b. Yehiel (*Sefer haArukh*), 68
New Moons (Rosh Hodesh), 176

New Testament, 93, 108
Newman, Barbara, 178–79
Nicholas of Verdun, 73
Niddah. *See* menstruation and menstrual purity
Ninth of Av, 61
Nissim Gaon, 69
northern France, 5–6, 17, 27, 65, 70, 98, 138, 142–43, 152, 229n.125
Nürnberg, 44, 204n.125
nursing. *See* breast-feeding
nutrix, 158, 224n.49, 225n.72. *See also* wet nurse

oblation, 237n.122, 238n.124
Ogia (the midwife), 204n.125
omen, 158
Orme, Nicholas, 2, 91, 134
orphans, 162
oublies, 99, 217n.40

Paige, Karen, and Mark Paige, 85–86
Palestine, 223n.27
Palestinian Talmud, 123, 170
parents and parenthood, 154, 155–58; and parental love, 120–21, 161–65, 169
Paris, 27, 139, 141, 142, 226n.89
Parturient, 38–40, 48–50, 52, 54, 75, 77–78, 203n.96. *See also* Sabbath of the Parturient and birth
Paschal sacrifice, 63
paternity, recognition of, 63–64
Patriarchs, 63. *See also* Abraham, Isaac, and Jacob
patriarchy, 16, 22, 38, 85, 112–13, 186
penance, 163, 167–68, 176–78, 186, 237n.113
Pentateuch, 93, 215n.7
Perchta, 97
Perles, Joseph, 97
phantoms, 167
Pharaoh's daughter, 133–34, 173
Phillippe de Nouvarre, 155, 221n.3
Physica, 46. *See also* Hildegard of Bingen
pilgrimage, 174
Pinthus, Alexander, 19
Pirkei deRabbi Eliezer, 69
piyut, 17, 23, 158
Poland, 5, 105, 193n.29
polygamy, 33, 37, 202n.65
poverty, 131–32, 177
prayers, 78–79, 102, 117–18; and women, 44
pregnancy, 18, 28, 39, 41–43, 53, 125, 145–46, 173–76, 180, 233n.21, 236n.87

procreation, 13, 20, 22, 24–30, 33–38, 145–46, 156, 198n.2
Protestants, 51
Provence, 7, 13, 45, 65, 217n.37
Prum, 37
Puerto Rico, 59, 82
purification, 105, 106–8, 110, 115, 219n.66, 221n.103
Purim, 100, 131–32, 176

Quakers, 51

Rabbenu Tam. *See* Jacob b. Meir
Rachel (the Matriarch), 23, 203n.96
Rachel b. R. Isaac b. Asher, wife of R. Judah, 182
Rashi. *See* Solomon b. Isaac
Rebecca (the Matriarch), 23, 203n.96
Reformation, 109, 115
Regensburg, 132, 182
Regensburg Pentateuch, 72
Reginus of Prum, 37
remarriage, 29, 124–25, 147–52, 169–72, 185, 223n.27
Rhine Valley, 6, 37, 50
Riché, Pierre, 2
Rieder, Paula, 105–6, 108, 111–12, 219n.64
Rikhzena (the midwife), 44
ritual, 9, 13, 16, 19–20, 56, 61–62, 81–82, 85–86, 112, 186–87
Roman society, 125
Rome, 68
Rosh haShana, 23, 39–40
Rothenburg, 203n.125
Rouen, 150
Rubin, Nissan, 55–56

Sa'adiah Gaon, 57
Sabbath, 42, 61, 70, 93, 100, 109, 117–18, 143, 159, 160, 176, 194n.40, 227n.93
Sabbath of the Parturient (*Shabbat Yeziat haYoledet*), 92, 100–105, 110–18
sacrifice, 102–3
Sefer haHanokhi, 231n.164
saint's lives, 155
Salernus, 45
Samson, 211n.87
Samson b. Zadok (*Sefer Tashbez*), 71–75, 132
Samson of Couçy, 227n.100
Samson of Falaise, 148, 231n.164
Samson of Sens, 228n.112
Samuel, 178, 215n.7

Samuel b. Meir (Rashbam), 173
Samuel the Pious (Hasid), 163
sandek, 68–70, 80, 211n.72
Sanoi, Sansoi, and Samengloff, 117. *See also* Lilith
Sarah (the Matriarch), 23–24, 182, 203n.96
Schönfraw, (the midwife) 44
Schultz, James, 2
Sefer Hasidim, 14, 17, 24, 27, 29, 40, 42, 51, 70, 72, 84, 93–94, 136–37, 146, 158–63, 165–67, 170–72, 174–76, 234n.59. *See also* Judah b. Samuel
Sefer Huqqei haTorah, 215n.7
Sefer Assaf haRofe, 45–46, 50
Sefer haGematriyot leRabbi Yehuda heHasid, 168–69
Sefer haToladot, 48
Sefer Nizahon Vetus, 27–28, 59, 106
Sefer Or Zaru'a, 98, 135, 137, 142, 150. *See also* Isaac b. Moses
Sefer haRokeah, 142. *See also* Eleazar b. Judah
Sefer Tashbez, 71–72. *See also* Samson b. Zadok
Sefer Yossipon, 180
Seklin (the midwife), 44
Sergius, 106
servants, 8, 70, 102, 136, 220n.101, 227n.93
Shahar, Shulamith, 2, 163
Shabbat Yeziat haYoledet. *See* Sabbath of the Parturient
Shavu'a haBat and *Shavu'a haBen*, 99
shem hol, 94–95
Sherira Gaon, 69
shrouds, 118
shushvin, 83–84, 213 nn. 123 and 128
Sifrei Mizvot, 17, 232n.3
Simeon, 106
Simeon b. Yohai, 102
Simon b. Isaac b. Abun, 158
Simonsohn, Shlomo, 226n.89
Solomon, 163–64
Solomon b. Aderet (Rashba), 131, 170
Solomon b. Isaac (Rashi), 28, 34–35, 37, 41, 47, 63, 78, 92, 96, 131–32, 139–40, 148, 160, 206n.169, 214n.128, 225n.73
Solomon b. Samson, 182
Soreh bas Toyvim, 104
Spain, 7, 11, 12, 13, 39, 45, 48, 65, 120, 127, 130, 133, 193n.32, 202 nn. 65 and 82, 217n.37, 229n.127
Spiegel, Yaacov S., 65
Speyer, 6, 37, 193n.39

St. Felicitas, 178–79
St. Julita, 178
St. Margaret, 48
St. Symphorosa, 178
St. Thomas Aquinas, 26, 157
Stampa, 97
step-parents, 147, 171–72
Stow, Kenneth, 19
Strasbourg, 160
streya, 98, 216n.24. *See also* witchcraft
swaddling, 52
synagogue, 18–19, 35–36, 61–62, 70, 71, 76, 79, 100, 102, 104–5, 109, 113, 117, 160, 234n.33; women's presence in, 77–78, 86–88
Synod of Canterbury, 58

Taglia, Kathryn, 91
Tallan, Cheryl, 171
Ta-Shma, Israel, 14, 150–52
tax-lists, 44
teachers, 232n.8
tefillin, 88, 90–91, 186
tekhine, 104
Temple, 103–5, 106
Ten commandments, 155–58
testimony of women, 34, 54
thanksgiving, 104, 108, 110, 115
Third Lateran Council, 50, 226n.89
Thomas Aquinas. *See* St. Thomas Aquinas
Thomas Cantimpratanus, 167
Thomas, Keith, 110
Tiber River, 172
Tilly, Louise, 14
time-bound commandments (*mizvot ʿaseh shehazman graman*), 88–89
Torah, 99, 102, 109, 118, 163, 167
Tosafist, 127, 140, 157, 164, 195n.56
Trier, 37
Trotula, 32, 45
Turner, Victor, 111
Tuviah b. Eliezer (*Midrah Lekaḥ Tov*), 31
Tuviah of Vienne, 150
twins and multiple births, 42

Urbach, Ephraim E., 121, 177, 223n.27

Van Gennep, Arnold, 111
veil, 102, 110, 217n.48
Vienne, 150
vigils, 100
Vincent de Beauvais, 52

violence, 81–83
virginity, 83

Wachnacht, 92, 99–100, 110, 113, 115
Wagenseil, Johannes Christoph, 228n.109
Warner, Marina, 218n.63
Waschnitius, Viktor, 97
werewolves, 98. *See also* demons and *streya*
Westreich, Elimelekh, 33
wet nurses, 16, 20, 119, 121, 124–25, 128–33, 135–36, 155, 169, 223n.26, 225n.77, 226n.84; Christian, 8, 49–50, 120, 124–25, 131–44; contracts and employment of, 125, 127–31, 137, 150; Jewish, 124–25, 129–30, 133–35, 143–44, 151, 225n.76, 226n.86; Muslim, 126, 229n.127; and sexual exploitation, 226n.87, 227n.106
widows, 45, 48, 123–24, 127, 129, 148–53, 170–72, 193n.40
widowers, 151
William of Bley, 226n.89
Wilson, Adrian, 111, 220n.87
wimpel (windel), 102, 109, 117–18, 221 nn. 106 and 112
wine, 77
Winheim, 204n.125
Wissenschaft des Judentums, 7, 13
witchcraft, 30, 46–48, 98, 201n.55
Wolf, Eric, 59, 80, 82
Wolfram von Eschenbach, 55
women, 2–4, 12, 14–15, 110, 185–86; as candlemakers, 101, 217n.46; and conjugal obligations, 122–23, 126; as halakhic authorities, 160; and religious practices and obligations, 28, 88–89, 98, 186–88
Worcester, 226n.89
Worms, 6, 37, 98, 101, 132, 166, 182, 204n.125
Würzburg, 204n.125

Yeḥiel of Paris, 139–40, 227n.100
Yoḥani bat Retavi, 47–48
Yom Kippur (Day of Atonement), 61, 159, 206n.148, 233n.28
Yuda Levy Kirkhum (*Sefer Minhagot Wormeisa*), 102
Yuta (the midwife), 204n.125

zaddik, 165–66
Zarlieb (the midwife), 204n.125
zizit, 88, 186, 233 n.31
Zipporah, 65
Zipporah of Worms, 182